Building Partnerships in the Americas

Building Partnerships in the Americas

A Guide for

Global Health Workers

Edited by

Margo J. Krasnoff, MD

DARTMOUTH COLLEGE PRESS

Hanover, New Hampshire

DARTMOUTH COLLEGE PRESS

An imprint of University Press of New England

www.upne.com

© 2013 Trustees of Dartmouth College

Manufactured in the United States of America

Typeset in Scala and Clio by Integrated Publishing Solutions

University Press of New England is a member of the Green Press Initiative.
The paper used in this book meets their minimum requirement for recycled paper.

For permission to reproduce any of the material in this book, contact
Permissions, University Press of New England, One Court Street, Suite 250,
Lebanon NH 03766; or visit www.upne.com

Library of Congress Cataloging-in-Publication Data

Building partnerships in the Americas : a guide for global health workers / edited by
Margo J. Krasnoff.

  p. ; cm.

Includes bibliographical references and index.

ISBN 978-1-61168-444-5 (cloth : alk. paper) — ISBN 978-1-61168-420-9 (pbk. : alk.
paper) — ISBN 978-1-61168-409-4 (ebook)

I. Krasnoff, Margo J., editor of compilation.

[DNLM: 1. Medically Underserved Area—Central America. 2. Medically
Underserved Area—Mexico. 3. Medically Underserved Area—West Indies.
4. Voluntary Workers—Central America. 5. Voluntary Workers—Mexico.
6. Voluntary Workers—West Indies. 7. Medical Missions, Official—Central
America. 8. Medical Missions, Official—Mexico. 9. Medical Missions, Official—
West Indies. 10. Relief Work—Central America. 11. Relief Work—Mexico.
12. Relief Work—West Indies. 13. Voluntary Health Agencies—Central America.
14. Voluntary Health Agencies—Mexico. 15. Voluntary Health Agencies—West
Indies. 16. World Health—Central America. 17. World Health—Mexico.
18. World Health—West Indies. WA 395]

RA418.5.P6

362.1—dc23   2013004432

5 4 3 2 1

For my parents

Contents

Acknowledgments

I would like to thank the authors of these essays and their in-country collaborators for sharing insider perspectives and wisdom, and for their extraordinary commitment to the people they serve and their communities.

Additionally, I would like to thank Charlene Gates, Dr. Eric Manheimer, Connie O'Leary, and especially Bob Wanamaker for their help and support. Thanks also to Dr. Walter E. Little, PhD, Dr. Ronald E. Pust, and Maria Hamlin Zuniga, MPH, whose insightful comments greatly improved the manuscript. I would also like to thank Dr. Jack Turco, the Tucker Foundation of Dartmouth College, the Geisel School of Medicine at Dartmouth, and the staff of Bridges to Community for supporting my trips to Nicaragua. Special appreciation goes to Dr. Phyllis Deutsch, editor-in-chief of University Press of New England, for her guidance at every juncture.

Introduction

When the media and social networking bring global poverty, disease, and natural disasters into our living rooms, there is an instinctive human reaction to try to help. This book is a response to the question, "How can I, with the skills that I possess, best contribute to addressing this widespread suffering in a shared way?" Understanding the cultural context of the communities being served is essential for the long-term success of any healthcare program. The direction must come from the culture itself—a collaborative approach is crucial for effective healthcare delivery.

Global health problems are symptoms of underlying societal issues that reach far beyond disease, such as poverty, economics, and the social environment. In recent years the field of global health has attracted people with diverse talents, skills, and levels of experience. There are many opportunities for both short- and long-term volunteers to serve patients and to promote health equity in the context of the ethical practices put forth by humanitarian organizations.[1] Health practitioners and students (including those in medicine, surgery, nursing, dentistry, optometry, rehabilitation, and public health) should try to link their efforts to programs that promote sustainable development.[2] Other fields essential to the broad efforts to improve community health include (but are not limited to) agriculture, engineering, education, anthropology, social work, and other applied social sciences. Volunteers can range from high school and university students to professionals, as well as those who find themselves with more freedom and flexibility in their lives and want to "give back" to the world.

This book focuses on opportunities for global health service in Mexico, Guatemala, El Salvador, Honduras, Nicaragua, Haiti, and the Dominican Republic (DR). Two chapters on Nicaragua examine different parts of the country and diverse medical and dental interventions. Although Mexico is a more developed country than the others, the Mexico chapter focuses on Chiapas, a state with a large indigenous population that has commonalities but also has important differences from its neighbors in Central America. This book does not cover Costa Rica, which has a long democratic tradition and is the wealthiest country in Central America.[3] It has consistently dedicated significant resources to health and education, resulting in a population with a life expectancy almost equal to that of the United States.[4]

While Mexico is technically part of North America, it is often included in discussions of Latin America because of its history as part of the Spanish empire. The definition of Latin America is thus more of a concept than an exact geographic location. Often, all nations south of the Rio Grande are included, with some inconsistency about including the English-speaking islands of the Caribbean. Here, we will follow the tradition of abbreviating Latin America and the Caribbean as LAC.

This volume goes beyond standard handbooks of the region by providing the rich historical and healthcare context for each country discussed. The essays that comprise the chapters are based on the unique, insider perspectives of people who have been devoting their lives to improving the health and well-being of Latin Americans. Although the essays differ in style and emphasis, each one offers a look at how historical developments, geopolitical significance, and environmental factors have resulted in contemporary healthcare issues and challenges, especially for the poor. The essay authors describe current structural and socioeconomic factors that create or sustain inequalities in healthcare services specific to each country. They discuss cultural and ethical issues as well as medical topics including maternal and child health, interventions for noncommunicable diseases (NCDs) such as diabetes, and strategies for volunteer surgical missions. Infectious diseases such as HIV/AIDS, tuberculosis, and cholera are featured, as well as dengue fever and Chagas disease. The authors describe the local health infrastructure, and provide examples of the *social gradient* of health and the role of gender. As these essays show, the poorer the person the worse his or her health, with women and children at higher risk. Indigenous populations fare worst of all—the Maya in Guatemala and Chiapas, the Moskitos on the Caribbean Coast of Nicaragua, and marginalized populations such as the Haitians living in the DR.[5]

Although chapters can be read individually, we recommend that you peruse the entire volume. These countries are geographically close and share much history and culture. Your experience will be greatly enriched—and your understanding of the region deepened—by the historical, political, and cultural cross-hatchings that tie chapters together. The authors of the El Salvador chapter explain the principles of social medicine, a useful framework for understanding health disparities. Chapters on the Dominican Republic, Mexico, and El Salvador describe how Latin Americans living and working in the United States send funds home to help their families (*remittances*) that predominantly benefit poor households.[6] Cultural beliefs about health are salient across LAC, and among these, the hot-cold dichotomy is presented in the Mexico chapter. The importance of the command of Mayan languages and cultural sensitivities is emphasized especially in the Guatemala chapter, but these issues are central to effective healthcare across the region. Spirituality and religion are vital aspects of life in LAC, and the chapter on Honduras, as well as the second chapter on Nicaragua, describes the health-related functions of several faith-based organizations (FBOS).

This introduction is organized into three sections that correspond to the core skills for the global health volunteer: (1) strategies to develop linguistic and cultural competence, (2) background knowledge of the historical and po-litical landscape, and (3) consideration of the social determinants of health. The book concludes with a chapter in which the authors explain how they de-veloped their long-term commitments to the people of LAC and became com-petent in the people's respective cultural practices.

Linguistic and Cultural Competency

Cultural competency refers to the skills that allow one to interact effectively and openly with people from different cultures. Culturally and linguistically appropriate clinical care is crucial because a misdiagnosis based on a lack of understanding can be fatal for patients. Becoming more culturally competent lets us develop more effective partnerships with local organizations. Cultural competency is a developmental process that evolves over time and involves one's self-awareness, knowledge, communication skills, and attitudes. A key question all global health volunteers should ask themselves before embarking on any service activity is, "How can individual efforts align with the work of others who are already creating change in the community?" A common mis-conception is to conflate culture with poverty and, then, to ignore how cultural practices that are freed from the constraints of poverty can serve as powerful means to deliver better healthcare to more people. Wuqu' Kawoq, the NGO described in the chapter on Guatemala and Acción Médica Cristiana (AMC) in Nicaragua, are excellent examples of how it can work.

Strategic Alliances

The distinction between solidarity (*solidaridad*) and charity (*caridad*) was described by Jorge, an activist-teacher in a medical Spanish program in Quez-taltenango, Guatemala: Caridad implies an action taken by an individual for an individual—for example, offering money or food to a poor person. Soli-daridad implies that one accepts the complexity of the situation and strives to become part of a collective solution. According to Jorge, the first priority for health providers is to understand and respect the traditions and needs of the local community; our personal agendas are of secondary importance. Mean-ingful service entails not just what we do, but also our attitudes, our motives, and our willingness to work with the local community and take seriously the significant cultural and practical knowledge it brings to the table.

Cultivating a "global state of mind" about the world and our place in it has been advocated as a strategy for developing a personal ethic for global health.[7] Humility and empathy have been recognized as essential for the promotion of solidarity and mutual caring. Globalization affects everyone and challenges us to understand how foreign and domestic issues are linked in our complex world.

Solidarity has recently been reframed to mean, "It's not about us helping them. It's about joining forces to help all of us."[8]

The idea of *accompaniment* is one version of solidarity that gets a lot of support in this volume. Daniel Palazuelos, MD, MPH, a coauthor of the Mexico chapter, defines the term: "To 'accompany' a process is to find the balance between dedication and humility, knowing that while we may individually have something to offer, true and lasting solutions will demand that we share this vision with teams that we trust. Call it solidarity or friendship—either way, we need to do whatever it takes to do what we know needs to get done" (see Palazuelos in Contributors). The authors included in this volume describe their close professional collaborations with their colleagues, and have invited their partners to contribute their perspectives; these are highlighted as boxes in each chapter and illustrate the challenges of working with few resources.

Several essays in this volume advocate creating strategic alliances with local communities—whether with paid or unpaid workers—to ensure the best and longest-lasting results. Community health workers (CHWs)—*promotoras, doctorcitas, trabajadores comunitarios* in Latin countries and *accompagnateurs* in Haiti—are laypeople with basic medical training who educate and assist members of the community to improve their health. They come from the communities they serve, and they work on teams to provide services where needed. CHWs are an invaluable source of local knowledge and networks for global health workers. Partners in Health (PIH) has refined a model for over twenty years in Haiti, Mexico, Guatemala, and elsewhere, in which trained CHWs are paid to deliver medication to the sick in their homes and ensure that they receive the care needed. CHWs provide essential adherence support and psychological counseling to patients.[9]

Strategic alliances are fostered when organizations seek to work collaboratively with local partners. For example, Doctors for Global Health (DGH) works only in communities where it has been invited. Its work in El Salvador and Mexico is featured in this book. A theme that runs through these essays is that health-focused organizations have a role in promoting local values, as well as the awareness that "foreign" interventions can disrupt local authority and control.

In Central America, accompaniment goes beyond the health arena and is used as a tool by human rights organizations such as Witness for Peace. Volunteer accompaniers serve by being physically present in volatile communities to monitor elections, report on human rights, and alert the international community to any abuses. The authors of the El Salvador chapter describe the steps that DGH volunteers took to accompany the Salvadoran community in response to the 2009–2011 murders of four environmental activists in the neighboring town to the community where they work.

Engaging in Dialogue

The concept of *citizen diplomacy* gives a framework for individual volunteers to engage in mutually beneficial dialogue:

LISTEN . . . to others with compassion and an open mind

LEARN . . . about history, culture, and ways of life and thinking different from your own

RESPECT . . . people's rights to views and approaches other than your own

EXPLORE . . . other cultures and places with curiosity and openness

ACT . . . to understand, engage, and work with people from around the world

EMBRACE . . . a role as someone who can connect and make a positive difference in the global community.[10]

Language skills help make global health workers much more effective. The payoff is well worth the effort. With the exceptions of Haiti and the indigenous communities of Guatemala and Mexico, Spanish is spoken throughout the other countries discussed. Prior to participating in health-focused experiences, global health workers may want to spend some time in the host country improving their Spanish. Language immersion programs with a home-stay experience can also foster cultural familiarity. Because so many programs are available, it's helpful to have the language school provide references, so prior participants can be contacted for feedback on the quality of the educational experience.

As a global health volunteer, you will need cultural guidance to help cultivate a global state of mind. There is no substitute for speaking with a mentor or local host about recommended standards for appropriate professional conduct in the setting where you will be working. This will help you integrate into a project or organization and establish the necessary relationships to become an effective participant. As you prepare for your journey, it's beneficial to reflect on your motivations and what you hope to get out of the experience.[11] Ryan Alaniz, PhD, a coauthor of the chapter on Honduras, offers important advice: "We each come into the country with particular stereotypes about what we are going to find. It is important to be 'self-reflexive' or constantly question-ing ourselves about how our beliefs about the place and the people may be coloring our work and interactions. Self-reflexivity also enables us to address 'white privilege' or our own 'US privilege' that we may be taking for granted. The more we think about and question not only our motives but also our as-sumptions, the closer we grow to true empathy and solidarity."[12]

Historical Overview

History, politics, economics, language, and culture are all related to the ways that health is conceived and the medical conditions that practitioners face today. A vital aspect of global health work is to prepare yourself by learn-ing about the background of the place and the people you will be working with, as well as the evolving political and social environment. What follows is a brief summary of some of the key historical events and economic factors that are relevant to LAC today. The authors of the Guatemala chapter provide essential background on the broad region of Mesoamerica prior to and after the arrival of the Spanish.

The Conquest

The original inhabitants of the Americas were diverse peoples who lived in settled agricultural communities for several millennia before the arrival of the Europeans. The Spaniards called them *Indios* to distinguish the original Americans from the Europeans, but they were not a uniform tribe or society. Christopher Columbus landed in the Bahamas in 1492, and soon afterward explored the islands of Hispaniola (home of present-day Haiti and the Do-minican Republic) and Cuba. In 1493, on his second voyage, Columbus in-troduced sugar cane to Hispaniola, and it flourished there.[13] Seeking gold and silver, the conquistadors sent expeditions to Mexico and Central America, and conquered the Aztec and later Maya lands in the 1520s.

Within a century of the arrival of the Europeans, approximately 90 percent of the indigenous people were decimated: a loss of 50 million Indians, with only 5 million survivors.[14] The Spanish conquistadors infected the Indians with diseases to which they had no immunity—including smallpox, typhus, and measles. The Spanish settlers relied on the Indians for food, imposing conditions that were so harsh that many Indians died of overwork and depri-vation, and others committed suicide.[15] In response to the loss of the Indians living in the Caribbean, the Spanish crown met its need for labor by allowing the systematic importation of slaves from Africa. Over the next fifty years, more than 130,000 slaves arrived in the Spanish colonies to work the sugar and coffee plantations.[16]

The island of Hispaniola was initially colonized by Spain, which ceded the territory of Haiti to France by treaty in 1697. The two colonies had vastly different numbers of African slaves, and this had a profound effect on their histories and their self-perception of race today. By 1791, the French had at least 500,000 slaves in Haiti, comprising 85 percent of the colony's population.[17] After winning independence, Haiti declared itself a black republic.[18] In the neighboring Dominican Republic, the Spanish had only 60,000 slaves; and despite intermarriage between the Spanish and the Africans, the people of the DR have historically emphasized their Hispanic identity.[19] In contrast to the Caribbean, greater numbers of Indians survived in the highlands of Guatemala and Mexico. Even in these two countries, where the indigenous people formed the majority of the population, they found themselves at the bottom of the new social hierarchy, which was dominated by the foreign colonists and their descendants.[20]

Independence Movements

In 1791, the Haitian slaves rebelled against the brutality of the French landholders and in 1804 achieved independence (being the second nation in the Western Hemisphere to do so). During the colonial period, Guatemala, El Salvador, Nicaragua, Costa Rica, and Honduras were governed by Spain as a unit, and in 1821 proclaimed their independence with almost no violence. There was a United Provinces of Central America, which dissolved in 1838 into five independent nations.[21] The political history from 1838 until 1945 was characterized by poverty for the majority and rule by a small elite class who maintained control of the government through civilian or military dictatorships.[22]

US Role in the Nineteenth Century

Scholars have written lengthy books on the role of the United States in Latin American history and foreign policy. Here we'll explore a few key points. In 1823, after nearly all the colonies had achieved independence from Spain and Portugal, the United States passed the Monroe Doctrine, which stated that further actions by Europeans to colonize land or interfere with states in the Americas would be viewed as acts of aggression requiring US intervention.[23] Despite the rhetoric of the Monroe Doctrine, the elites in LAC still looked to Europe for "culture" and technology. The poor—most often indigenous—were addressed by political and economic policies that aimed to modernize or protect them, depending on which was perceived as the best way to harness their labor or calm periodic uprisings.

US diplomacy combined goals of national security with protection of US interests and investment in Central America and the Caribbean. Starting in the 1890s, the United States advanced its own welfare by invoking the Monroe Doctrine to justify its interference in the internal affairs of the weaker, newly independent nations of Latin America.[24] After the Spanish-American War in 1898, the long list of US invasions and occupations includes Honduras, Mexico, Guatemala, and Costa Rica for short periods, with longer stays in Cuba, the DR, Haiti, Panama, and Nicaragua.[25]

US Role in the Twentieth Century

The Cold War, as a political and ideological contest between Western capitalism and Soviet communism, lasted from 1946 until 1991. This larger geopolitical conflict provided the framework for US interventions in LAC.[26] Throughout this period, the United States fought against democratic movements and in favor of the region's old regimes in Guatemala, Nicaragua, and El Salvador.[27] Potential Soviet threat and the Cold War were invoked in the 1980s by US president Ronald Reagan to justify aggressive yet covert military interventions against Central American democracies.[28] After successful revolutions by Cuba and then Nicaragua within its hemisphere, the United States sought to "draw the line against communism" and promoted "low-intensity conflict strategy" to attempt to destabilize and defeat the guerilla movements in El Salvador and the Sandinista government in Nicaragua (details follow in the chapters on these countries).

In 1999, US president Bill Clinton formally apologized for the role that the United States had played in backing the Guatemalan security forces in their brutal civil war that lasted thirty-six years (1960–1996). The apology shortly followed the report by the independent Commission for Historical Clarification (CEH) that detailed how the United States had provided military assistance by training Guatemala's military in intelligence and counterinsurgency techniques that they used against civilians in brutal atrocities, arbitrary executions and forced disappearances.[29] CEH asserted that 83 percent of those murdered were Maya indigenous, and that the state had committed hundreds of massacres of Maya communities, which has been described as genocide.[30]

Legacy of Civil Conflict

To understand contemporary politics in LAC today, it's important to recognize that in the last half of the twentieth century, there were three full-scale civil wars in Central America. The cumulative bloodshed is staggering, and the repercussions of the violence and turmoil are still felt today.[31] In Nicaragua 50,000 died in the revolution, plus 30,865 in the Counter-Revolutionary War (1972–1991).[32] In Guatemala 200,000 men, women, and children were killed, and the CEH report estimates that between 500,000 and 1.5 million were displaced internally or sought refuge abroad.[33] In El Salvador 75,000 were killed, 1 million fled, and 500,000 were internally displaced (1980–1992). Negotiated peace settlements between the government and the guerillas ended the war in El Salvador in 1992, and in Guatemala in 1996.[34] Global health workers need to be aware of the physical and emotional scars from these tragedies, as well as the resilience of the survivors.[35]

On January 1, 1994 (implementation day for the North American Free Trade Agreement [NAFTA]), in the state of Chiapas, a revolutionary group called Ejército Zapatitsta de Liberación Nacional (EZLN) occupied four major towns for several days. The Mexican army drove the Zapatistas out of the urban areas to the rural ones, where they have retained control in some of the towns. The Zapatistas spearheaded movements for indigenous rights and against corporate globalization. Though the Zapatistas are not a military force, at the time of this writing nineteen years later, they remain a political presence as an indigenous movement that emphasizes its autonomy or self-determination as coming from within, rather than being granted from an organization above.[36] The Internet has been vital to the movement's public communication and survival.[37]

Impact of Drug Trafficking

Mexico and Central America are situated between the world's largest suppliers and consumers of cocaine. Geography plays a key role in the northward passage of massive flows of drugs.[38] Both drug trafficking and the war on drugs have had profound effects on the region, and since the mid-2000s the crime situation has worsened significantly. Mexico's cartels have evolved into transnational organized crime syndicates involved in drugs as well as extortion and the human trafficking of undocumented migrants.[39] The violent struggles between and within the criminal organizations have led to a dramatic surge in the homicide rate. Drug traffickers smuggle cocaine from South America by boat on both sides of the isthmus. On the Pacific side, drugs move north into the Gulf of Fonseca, a saltwater bay bordered by Nicaragua, Honduras, and El Salvador. On the Caribbean side, the cartels have found the marginally populated, heavily forested, and weakly controlled coasts of Nicaragua and Honduras to be fertile grounds for landing planes and boats before moving north. The cocaine is then hidden in vehicles and driven across Central America to Mexico.

Transnational gangs, engaged in a violent fight to control the drug trafficking routes, use force to wield control over entire communities.[40] The movement of criminals and contraband within and between the nations of Central America has led to an escalation in violent crimes, murders, and kidnappings, as well as the growth of private security companies in response. Drug money perverts daily life in many ways—from the corruption of military and police officers, to the extortion of business owners required to pay for protection, to the constant fear of citizens living under the threat of crime. Arms trafficking and money laundering are related problems. Marijuana, heroin, and methamphetamines are also trafficked in addition to cocaine.[41]

The intentional homicide rate is generally considered to be a reliable indicator of the violent crime situation in a given country. In 2010 the murder rate in the United States was 5 per 100,000 people. In comparison, the rate was 7 in Haiti, 13 in Nicaragua, 18 in Mexico, 25 in the DR, 41 in Guatemala, 66 in El Salvador, and 82 in Honduras, which has now been labeled the world's most dangerous country.[42] Global health workers must be cognizant of the crime rates and consult with host organizations to take appropriate measures to minimize risks. In 2012, the Peace Corps pulled all of its volunteers out of Honduras,[43] and volunteers in Guatemala and El Salvador have since been provided with enhanced safety and security measures. The US State Department website provides comprehensive advice for safe travel abroad, including advisories about specific countries.[44]

In 2006, Mexico's president Felipe Calderón declared war on the nation's drug cartels. Over the next five years, more than 50,000 Mexicans were killed in drug-war-related homicides.[45] Although most of those killed were members of drug gangs, police officers, soldiers, and innocent civilians were also murdered. Journalists, human rights defenders, and migrants have been kidnapped, and have disappeared, with only a small percent of crimes investigated, tried, and sentenced.[46] The US Congress has provided extensive support to the LAC countries to try to eliminate the drug traffickers. Since 2007, the Mérida Initiative has provided Mexico with military equipment and services for the army, the police, and the intelligence agencies.[47] The more recent Central American Regional Security Initiative has expanded the geographic scope of the US interventions.[48] Critics have charged that a militaristic approach to the war on drugs has been counterproductive—it has reduced neither the flow of drugs nor the numbers of murders.[49] Some recommend that a more effective strategy would be to attack the root cause of the war on drugs by providing more drug treatment programs in the United States to reduce the demand for illegal substances.[50]

Social Determinants of Health

The *social determinants of health* refer to health inequities that arise from the societal conditions in which people are born, grow, live, work, and age. These have been described as the "causes of causes" of ill health.[51] Although it's now more than 500 years since the conquest, the historical roots of the LAC countries as hierarchies based on race and class have created persistent social and economic inequalities. Each nation has handled differently the tensions of social inequality inherited from 300 years of colonialism. Throughout the region there is a widespread economic gap between the populations of European descent compared to the indigenous and Afro-descendant people.[52]

To this day, Latin America as a region leads the world in terms of inequality, which has been intense and persistent due to low social and economic mobility and the "inequality of opportunities."[53] A small minority controls most of the resources and earns most of the income. The degree of inequality is hidden in statistics reported as averages. Although Guatemala is a lower-middle-income country, the average income masks very skewed income distribution. The urban nonindigenous people fare vastly better than the rural indigenous people, roughly 75 percent of whom live in poverty.[54] The Dominican Republic, an upper-middle-income economy, has one of the highest disparities in income distribution in the hemisphere, with the wealthiest 20 percent of the population receiving 53 percent of the country's gross income, while the poorest 40 percent receive only 14 percent, according to 2010 statistics.[55] In terms of resource distribution, even in low- or middle-income countries, the wealthy have access to comprehensive medical care while the poor are more likely to die of preventable diseases.[56]

As a result of the imperial system, there has been a concentration of land, wealth, and power by the large landowners or elites, while the majority of poor people own little or no land. Without access to sufficient productive land to sustain themselves, poor peasants are often forced to live on either riverbanks or bare hillsides, which have become over-farmed and deforested. The large landholders are more likely to grow commodities for export rather than consumer food staples such as corn, rice, and beans; this contributes to widespread food insecurity and malnutrition.[57]

Within LAC, many factors have led to the perpetuation of intergenerational inequality. Feeding children is a responsibility of families and society. Impaired growth in childhood has effects that last into adult life in the domains of cognitive development, school attainment, and wages.[58] Growth failure in children can affect both height and weight. *Stunting* is poor linear growth or low height; in LAC, stunting is more common than underweight (low weight for age) or wasting (low weight for height). The prevalence of stunting in children under age five ranges from 6 percent in developed countries to 19.2 percent in El Salvador to 54.5 percent in Guatemala.[59] Stunting cannot be reversed once it occurs, so prevention through early childhood nutritional interventions is crucial. The authors of the Guatemala chapter discuss a range of opportunities to improve the nutritional health of mothers and children at greatest risk, and the authors of the chapter on Mexico describe the successes of the conditional cash transfer program on the lives of poor families.

"Natural" Disasters

The landscape of LAC is stunning and diverse. As well as the coastal regions, the geography features rugged mountain ranges with fertile valleys and tropical rainforests. There is also a "dry corridor" that extends through parts of Guatemala, Nicaragua, and Honduras, where farmers cope with shallow, stony soils and droughts. Earthquakes and volcanic eruptions have caused countless deaths and destruction of vital infrastructure. Exposure to natural catastrophes in the absence of disaster reduction measures increases human vulnerability and can overwhelm local capacity to respond, leading to an outpouring of external assistance. The earthquake that devastated Haiti in 2010 was the worst natural disaster in the history of the Western Hemisphere: 250,000 deaths and more than 1.6 million left homeless.[60] In comparison, the Nicaragua earthquake of 1972 killed 6,000 people, the Guatemala earthquake of 1976 killed 23,000, and the Mexico City earthquake of 1985 led to 20,000 deaths.[61] Water disasters such as hurricanes, flooding, and landslides are common in LAC and can quickly devastate a community's infrastructure, disproportionately affecting the poor and vulnerable. In 1998, Hurricane Mitch killed 18,000 in Central America.[62] When flooding occurs, crops are destroyed, drinking-water sources become contaminated, and food shortages become acute. The consequences of these so-called natural disasters and the humanitarian responses are discussed in the individual chapters.

Economic Context for Healthcare

Given that poverty has such profound influences on health, it's important to take a look at some of the broad economic trends affecting Mexico, Central America, and the Caribbean. Ever since the Europeans exploited indigenous labor on the sugar and coffee plantations, the commodity trade has shaped history in this region.[63] By the late twentieth century, tourism and then remittances began to displace the central economic role of commodities. As a result of policy decisions and trade agreements in recent years, Central America and Mexico have experienced socioeconomic transformations including shifts from self-reliant food production (subsistence agriculture) to wage labor. When their countries become significant food importers, low-income households risk food insecurity when global food prices rise. Today, among the sixty-six low-income food deficit countries worldwide, the three in the Western Hemisphere are Haiti, Honduras, and Nicaragua.[64]

In the mid-1970s, rising oil prices led to a global economic crisis marked by high inflation, unemployment, and rising levels of foreign debt. Since the 1980s, the United States and the multilateral lending organizations, such as the International Monetary Fund (IMF) and the World Bank, have promoted economic models for underdeveloped countries that seek to balance trade and domestic budget imbalances through *structural adjustment* programs. Structural adjustment is done through a variety of activities following what is called the *Washington Consensus* or *neoliberalism* as a condition for poor countries to receive help to stabilize their economies.[65] The political and economic philosophy of neoliberalism emphasizes strong private property rights, free markets, and free trade.[66] Politicians and businesspeople have shifted economic control away from the public sector to the private sector. This neoliberal strategy is characterized by privatizing previously held public services such as telecommunications, utilities, education, and healthcare, as well as by reducing the numbers of public employees. Those who favor this philosophy and related policies say that a strong economy is the best way to help the poor. Those who disagree argue that the poor are excluded from the strong economy, and that underfunding key government programs hurts the poor disproportionately by widening the gap between how the rich and poor live, as well as by dismantling social and environmental protections.[67] The privatization of health services has impacted public health through reduction in the numbers of health providers and increased expenses for patients, because cost cutting and profit seeking are rarely compatible with covering the basic health needs of the population.

These structural adjustment programs generally seek to reduce imports and increase exports through trade liberalization. In 1994, the North American Free Trade Agreement was signed by Canada, the United States, and Mexico to lower trade barriers between them in order to promote increased economic activity. NAFTA opened up the Mexican markets to imports, ranging from corn to pork, from US companies. It also allowed transnational corporations to buy land in Mexico sold by many small-scale farmers because they could no longer make a living on it.[68] Mexico now depends on importing 42 percent of its food, and there is significant chronic malnutrition and food insecurity among the poor.[69] Trade agreements have changed the type of crops grown—from the basic grains that satisfy local demand to crops for export (such as counter-seasonal fruits and vegetables) and biofuel-producing crops (such as sugar cane and palm oil).[70] The chapter on Mexico describes the widespread consequences of NAFTA.

The Dominican Republic–Central America–United States Free Trade Agreement (CAFTA-DR) was formed in stages. El Salvador, Guatemala, Honduras, and Nicaragua joined in 2006, the Dominican Republic in 2007, and Costa

Rica in 2009. CAFTA-DR eliminates tariffs and other barriers to trade in goods, services, agricultural products, and investments. The treaty was intended to solidify democracy, encourage greater regional integration, and provide safeguards for environmental protection and labor rights.[71] Critics of these policies feel that they favor the profits of US corporations over the rights of LAC workers. They note that although exports have increased, the factories pay low wages that are insufficient to sustain a family, and that factories move from one country to another in search of the lowest possible minimum wage.[72]

The people of Mexico, Central America, and the Caribbean face many economic and political challenges. The waves of state terror and revolutionary insurrection that resulted in more than 300,000 deaths in the late twentieth century devastated the economies and the infrastructure. The neoliberal economic reforms have had significant human costs, including governments with fewer resources to respond to poverty and narcotic traffickers. One positive development is that civilian-led electoral democracies are in place. Though there are no active civil conflicts at the time of this writing, in June 2009 Honduras experienced a military coup when President Manuel Zelaya was ousted from the country (see the Honduras chapter for details). In response to the history of prior human rights violations, there have been truth commissions to promote reconciliation in El Salvador, Guatemala, Haiti, and Honduras.[73]

Millennium Development Goals

In 2000, the leaders of 189 countries signed the United Nations (UN) Millennium Declaration, a comprehensive vision of a future world with less poverty, hunger, and disease. Eight interdependent Millennium Development Goals (MDGs) were created, with the primary target of halving by the year 2015 the number of people who live on less than $1 US a day. This requires a comprehensive multi-sectorial approach based on sustainable economic growth, with a focus on the poor and on human rights.[74] There are eight MDGs with twenty-one core targets embedded within.

Goal 1. Eradicate extreme poverty and hunger.
Goal 2. Achieve universal primary education.
Goal 3. Promote gender equality and empower women.
Goal 4. Reduce child mortality.
Goal 5. Improve maternal health.
Goal 6. Combat HIV/AIDS, malaria, and other diseases.
Goal 7. Ensure environmental sustainability (targets includes basic sanitation, safe drinking water, increasing the proportion of land covered by forest, and improvements in the lives of slum dwellers).

Goal 8. Develop a global partnership for development (includes measures to make debt sustainable and to make essential medications affordable).

The nations pledged to meet the MDGs by 2015, and the actions taken so far have already had a significant impact worldwide in terms of reducing the proportion of people living on less than $1 a day. The UN publishes an annual *Millennium Development Goals Report* with country-specific profiles to mark the progress.[75] Within the LAC region, there is heterogeneity among nations, and persistent deficiencies have been identified.[76] Although wealthy countries have already attained the MDGs, less-developed countries already lag far behind, and some don't even have the statistical capabilities to measure the indicators. To achieve the MDGs, it is crucial that education, health, and the environment be addressed together—which means that multiple government sectors need to work cooperatively. MDG 3, the promotion of gender equity and the empowerment of women, acknowledges that in low-income countries women often experience discrimination throughout their lives, starting with less food for female children, then lower school enrollment for girls, and common experiences of violence against women.[77] Addressing the societal inequities that cause poverty in the first place is fundamental to the challenge of achieving the MDGs. Indeed, the measures to reduce child mortality are available to those who can buy them, but are not necessarily being delivered to the children most at risk: those who live in the poorest countries and in the most marginalized communities within those countries.[78]

Global Health and Globalization

Potential global health workers need to understand how global health is inextricably linked to social justice insofar as health inequities are symptoms of larger socioeconomic and political disparities.[79] Global health is

> an area for study, research, and practice that places a priority on improving health and achieving equity in health for all people worldwide. Global health emphasizes transnational health issues, determinants, and solutions; involves many disciplines within and beyond the health sciences and promotes interdisciplinary collaboration; and is a synthesis of population-based prevention with individual-level clinical care.[80]

Global health problems have ramifications that go beyond single countries; hence the need to consider the impact of globalization on health. Globalization has been defined by the World Health Organization (WHO) as the

> increased interconnectedness and interdependence of peoples and countries, and is generally understood to include two inter-related elements:

the opening of international borders to increasingly fast flows of goods, services, finance, people and ideas; and the changes in institutions and policies at national and international levels that facilitate or promote such flows. Globalization has the potential for positive and negative effects on development and health.[81]

Economic globalization has had a profound social impact. Practically speaking, while goods flow freely, people cannot. This limits migration and work opportunities and contributes to widening social and economic inequality. A positive result of globalization occurs when greater income improves access to food.[82] Potentially negative effects occur when financially strapped governments have limited resources to help all who are in need and to invest in public health, sanitation, and clean water.

Global Health Efforts on an International Scale

The International Federation of Red Cross and Red Crescent Societies (IFRC) was founded in Paris in 1919, following World War I, to improve the health of those in war-torn countries. The IFRC movement has expanded to 187 national societies that carry out relief operations and development work throughout the world. IFRC established a code of conduct to monitor its own organization with the hope that other agencies would adopt the same principles.[83] These serve as an ethical standard for guiding assistance efforts and are available in Spanish and French:

- The humanitarian imperative comes first. (Everyone has a right to receive humanitarian assistance to prevent and alleviate human suffering.)
- Aid is given regardless of the race, creed or nationality of the recipients and without adverse distinction of any kind. Aid priorities are calculated on the basis of need alone.
- Aid will not be used to further a particular political or religious standpoint.
- We shall endeavor not to act as instruments of government foreign policy.
- We shall respect culture and custom.
- We shall attempt to build disaster response on local capacities.
- Ways shall be found to involve program beneficiaries in the management of relief aid.
- Relief aid must strive to reduce future vulnerabilities to disaster as well as meeting basic needs.

- We hold ourselves accountable to both those we seek to assist and those from whom we accept resources.
- In our information, publicity and advertising activities, we shall recognize disaster victims as dignified human beings, not hopeless objects.

There are a number of key organizational actors in global health. The UN has spearheaded global health activities since its founding in 1945. In 1948, the World Health Organization was established as a specialized agency of the UN. WHO consists of 193 member countries with a mission to promote health development guided by the ethical principle of equity: "Access to life-saving or health-promoting interventions should not be denied for unfair reasons, including those with economic or social roots. Commitment to this principle ensures that WHO activities aimed at health development give priority to health outcomes in poor, disadvantaged, or vulnerable groups." WHO carries out its work in collaboration with partners including other UN agencies, international organizations, donors, and governments.[84] The following UN agencies fund substantial services in LAC: UNAIDS, the United Nations Children's Fund (UNICEF), the World Food Program (WFP), the United Nations Population Fund (UNFPA), as well as the Food and Agriculture Organization of the UN (FAO).

Founded in 1902, the Pan-American Health Organization (PAHO) is an international public health agency that seeks to improve health and living standards in the countries of the Americas, and is also a part of the WHO and UN systems. PAHO's activities include emergency preparedness for regional disasters such as hurricanes. In 1949, PAHO formed the Institute of Nutrition of Central America and Panama (INCAP) in association with the Central American Integration System (SICA). Headquartered in Guatemala City, Guatemala, INCAP is a regional organization that carries out groundbreaking research on nutrition and food security (described in the chapter on Guatemala). PAHO publishes *Health in the Americas*, a comprehensive two-volume work that monitors regional health conditions and trends; it is available online and in print, and is updated every five years. This reference is indispensable for health practitioners to learn about the health systems and the priority health concerns for each country.[85]

Since 1961, the United States Agency for International Development (USAID) has been the principal US agency providing assistance to developing countries. Foreign aid plays a vital role in advancing US national security and foreign policy in concert with the strategy that addressing poverty is a means to promoting peace and stability. USAID provides humanitarian aid and disaster relief such as support for the recovery process in Haiti. USAID also funds the types of healthcare improvement programs that help the nations of LAC meet their MDGs, with examples described in chapter 5 on Nicaragua.[86]

Partnerships with Nongovernmental Organizations

NGOs play a prominent role in virtually all of these countries and have a complex relationship with the delivery of health care, finances, and local health providers. These nonprofit agencies are organized outside of government and can range from small community-based grassroots organizations to large, institutional groups. The authors of the essays in this book share how they work closely with NGOs, and share as well the steps to avoid the potential danger of donor-driven projects that do little to build local capacity. (See table I.1 for a list of affiliated organizations).

The authors of the Haiti chapter discuss some of the problematic aspects of NGOs before and after the 2010 earthquake. They recommend that NGOs strive to train local providers and channel their support to strengthen local institutions and existing programs, rather than the NGOs creating parallel services under their own banner. Another valuable suggestion is for NGOs to leverage their effectiveness by cooperating and helping each other. The NGO Code of Conduct for Health Systems Strengthening has been developed with guidelines for NGOs to work collaboratively with governments and to limit their own potentially negative effects on the public health system. [87]

One of the challenges facing LAC today is that NGOs and private delivery systems need to be well articulated with the local social, cultural, and economic conditions to in order to develop sustainable health systems and to achieve the MDGs. It is unclear whether it will be possible to accomplish these objectives through a fragmented delivery system of subcontracted private organizations working under the umbrella of the country's Ministry of Health (MOH). For example, due to structural adjustment programs in Guatemala, government functions have been privatized and outsourced to a growing number of small local and foreign NGOs. A 2011 publication reports that patients there identified the importance of receiving high quality services rather than simply nominal coverage. Communities risk disillusionment when there is lack of coordination between NGOs.[88]

Health Systems Approach

One of the core values of global health stemming from the UN Universal Declaration of Human Rights is that access to healthcare is a universal human right. Leading global health physicians Paul Farmer and Jim Kim advocate for "a strong public sector [which] is the only guarantor of access to health care as

Table I.1 *Organizations with Which the Authors Partner*

Organization	URL	Countries
Partners in Health	www.pih.org	Mexico, Haiti
Doctors for Global Health	www.dghonline.org	Mexico, El Salvador
Wuqu' Kawoq	www.wuqukawoq.org	Guatemala
Nuestros Pequeños Hermanos™	www.nph.org	Honduras
Holy Family Surgery Center	www.holyfamilysurgerycenter.org	Honduras
Bridges to Community	www.bridgestocommunity.org	Nicaragua
Mayflower Medical Outreach	www.mmonicaragua.org	Nicaragua
Acción Médica Cristiana	www.amcenglish.org	Nicaragua

a human right."[89] An effective global health worker should understand the organization of the health system and the role of the public and private sectors. The health system of each country is linked to its value system and political structure. The essays in this book address the role of the Ministry of Health and its strategic plan. A well-functioning health system is essential to achieve the MDGs. WHO has identified six essential components: (1) service delivery, (2) health workforce, (3) financing, (4) medical products and technologies, (5) health information system, and (6) leadership and governance.

Specific public health interventions are often characterized by their structure as being *vertical, horizontal,* or *diagonal.* Some governments have established *vertical programs* that focus on preventing or treating individual diseases (such as malaria) or programs for distinct populations (such as children needing vaccinations); this is in contrast to horizontal efforts that focus on strengthening a health system to deliver comprehensive primary care. In general, vertical programs have an explicit outcome focus and are managed by a separate staffing and funding stream. Mexico developed an innovative diagonal approach that integrates vertical programs and bridges health clinics and homes, which has contributed to a sustained decline in under-5 mortality (MDG4).[90] This example illustrates that better health services as well as programs to address the social determinants of health are necessary in order to achieve the MDGs.[91]

Planning Your Experience

Global health volunteers need information from a broad variety of sources to plan an effective experience. This introduction includes a tool kit with country-specific information from a wide spectrum of organizations and

Table I.2 *Toolbox for Country-Specific Resources*

Source	URL	Key Information
US Library of Congress	http://lcweb2.loc.gov/frd/cs	Historical setting, social, economic, political systems
Central Intelligence Agency	www.cia.gov	*The World Factbook:* History, people, economy, government, geography
Pan American Health Organization	www.paho.org	*Health in the Americas Vol. I,* regional health; *Vol. II,* health conditions and health systems by country
World Health Organization	www.who.int	Country cooperation strategy and health profile
UN Millenium Development Goals	www.mdgmonitor.org	Data on progress toward reaching the MDGs
UN Development Program	http://hdr.undp.org	Human Development Index: a composite of health, education, income
US Department of State	http://travel.state.gov	Travel warnings, security information
US Centers for Disease Control and Prevention	www.cdc.gov	Travelers' health: vaccinations, tropical conditions, staying healthy
UNICEF	www.unicef.org	Health indicators focusing on women, children, adolescents

some suggested websites. In recent years some students and professionals have dedicated themselves to global health as an academic discipline and a career path. The Suggested Reading list includes a selection of textbooks that can provide background in public health for the general reader. The authors of *Caring for the World: A Guidebook to Global Health Opportunities* include an extensive directory of medical electives, research opportunities, language courses, and specific organizations. *Caring for the World* also addresses career development and has practical recommendations for trip planning, including cultural orientation, a suggested packing list, and a post-trip debriefing strategy.[92] The Consortium of Universities for Global Health (CUGH) and the Global Health Education Consortium have merged and are now one organization (CUGH). The website offers resources on a wide variety of topics including the extensive collection of global health education learning modules.[93]

The essays in this book provide the contextual background and cultural guidance for the reader to prepare his or her own global health experiences. For each country, we have included a section on history and politics, a case study, and examples of how organizations work to promote sustainable change. The importance of respectful collaboration, strategic alliances, and mutual learning is emphasized throughout. There are tremendous opportunities for volunteers to grow personally and professionally while aspiring to be global citizens.

Notes

1 David R. Welling, James M. Ryan, David G. Burris, and Norman M. Rich, "Seven Sins of Humanitarian Medicine," *World Journal of Surgery* 34.3 (2010): 466–70. John A. Crump, Jeremy Sugarman, and Working Group on Ethics Guidelines for Global Health Training, "Ethics and Best Practice Guidelines for Training Experiences in Global Health," *American Journal of Tropical Medicine and Hygiene* 83.6 (2010):1178–1182.

2 J. E. Heck, A. Bazemore, and P. Diller, "The Shoulder to Shoulder Model–Channeling Medical Volunteerism toward Sustainable Health Change," *Family Medicine* 39.9 (2007):644–650. P. Suchdev, K. Ahrens, E. Click, L. Macklin, D. Evangelista, and E. Graham, "A Model for Sustainable Short-term International Medical Trips," *Ambulatory Pediatrics* 7.4 (2007):3 17–320.

3 Booth et al., *Understanding Central America.* 69

4 Pan American Health Organization, *Health in the Americas, 2007* (Washington: PAHO, 2007), available from www.paho.org.

5 PAHO, "Human Rights & Health: Indigenous Peoples" (2008), accessed Aug. 5, 2012, available from www.paho.org. Jacob Kushner, "Haitians Face Persecution across Dominican Border," *NACLA Report on the Americas* 45.2 (2012):50–58.

6 Sarah Gammage, "El Salvador: Despite End to Civil War, Emigration Continues" (2007), accessed Mar. 9, 2012, available from www.migrationinformation.org.

7 Solomon R. Benatar, Abdallah S. Daar, and Peter S. Singer, "Global Health Ethics: The Rationale for Mutual Caring," *International Affairs* 79.1 (2003):107–138.

8 Laura Carlsen, "Beyond Solidarity" (2011), accessed Mar. 13, 2012, available from www.cipamericas.org.

9 Louise C. Ivers, Jean-Gregory Jerome, Kimberly A. Cullen, Wesler Lambert, Francesca Celletti, and Badara Samb, "Task-Shifting in HIV Care: A Case Study of Nurse-Centered Community-Based Care in Rural Haiti," *PLoS One* 6.5 (2011):e19276.

10 US Center for Citizen Diplomacy, "What is Citizen Diplomacy?" accessed Feb. 16, 2012, available from http://uscenterforcitizendiplomacy.org.

11 Jane Philpott, "Training for a Global State of Mind," *American Medical Association Journal of Ethics* 12.3 (2010):231–236.

12 Personal communication with Ryan Alaniz, 8-11-12

13 Green, *Faces of Latin America*, 14.

14 William Shawn Miller, *An Environmental History of Latin America* (New York: Cambridge University Press, 2007) 10.

15 Green, *Faces of Latin America*, 9.

16 Williamson, *The Penguin History of Latin America*, 141.

17 Laurent Dubois, *Haiti: The Aftershocks of History* (New York: Metropolitan Books, 2012) 4.

18 Green, *Faces of Latin America*, 148.

19 Ibid. 146.

20 Carmack et al., *The Legacy of Mesoamerica*, 182.

21 Booth et al., *Understanding Central America*, 50.

22 Ibid. 51.

23 Williamson, *The Penguin History of Latin America*, 323.

24 Ibid.

25 Grandin, *Empire's Workshop*, 18.

26 Ibid. 40.

27 Ibid. 82.

28 Ibid. 81.

29 Martin Kettle and Jeremy Lennard, "Clinton Apology to Guatemala," *The Guardian* (Mar. 11, 1999), available from www.guardian.co.uk.

30 Guatemalan Commission of Historical Clarification, "Guatemala: Memory of Silence" (1999), accessed Aug. 7, 2012, available from http://shr.aaas.org.

31 United Nations Office on Drugs and Crime, "Crime and Development in Central America: Caught in the Crossfire" (2007) 14.

32 Booth et al., *Understanding Central America*, 88.

33 Guatemalan Commission of Historical Clarification, "Guatemala: Memory of Silence."

34 Green, *Faces of Latin America*, 77.

35 Paul Dix and Pamela Fitzpatrick, *Nicaragua: Surviving the Legacy of U.S. Policy* (Eugene, OR: Just Sharing Press, 2011).

36 Carlsen, "Beyond Solidarity."

37 Carmack et al., *The Legacy of Mesoamerica*, 400.

38 UN Office on Drugs and Crime, "Crime and Development in Central America."

39 Nik Steinberg, "The Monster and Monterrey: The Politics and Cartels of Mexico's Drug War," *The Nation* (June 13, 2011).

40 Oakland Ross, "All Aboard the Cocaine Express: Deadly Cocaine Trade Reaches New Depths." *Toronto Star* (Jan. 21, 2012), available from www.thestar.com.

41 UN Office on Drugs and Crime, "Crime and Development in Central America."

42 UN Office on Drugs and Crime, "UNODC Homicide Statistics," accessed Feb. 28, 2012, available from www.unodc.org.

43 Elvin Sandoval, "U.S. Peace Corps Pulls Out of Honduras," *CNN U.S.* (Jan. 17, 2012), available from http://articles.cnn.com.

44 US Department of State, Bureau of Consular Affairs, "Tips for Traveling Abroad," accessed Mar. 8, 2012, available from http://travel.state.gov.

45 Christopher Reynolds, "Mexico, before and after Calderon's drug war." Los Angeles Times August 25, 2012 (latimes.com, accessed 11-14-12)

46 Laura Carlsen, "The Drug War's Invisible Victims" (2012), available from www.cipamericas.org.

47 Laura Carlsen, "Mexico's Spiraling Violence" (2011), accessed Mar. 16, 2012, available from www.cipamericas.org.

48 US Department of State, "The Central America Regional Security Initiative" (2012), accessed Feb. 16, 2012, available from www.state.gov.

49 Carlsen, "Beyond Solidarity."

50 Thomas B. Cole, "Mexican Drug Violence Intertwined with US Demand for Illegal Drugs," *JAMA* 302.5 (2009):482–483.

51 Michael Marmot, "Global Action on Social Determinants of Health," *Bulletin of the World Health Organization* 89 (2011):702.

52 Sara Kozameh and Rebecca Ray, "Surviving the Global Recession: Poverty and Inequality in Latin America," *NACLA Report on the Americas* 45.2 (2012):22–25.

53 United Nations Development Program (UNDP), *Regional Human Development Report for Latin America and Caribbean 2010: Acting on the Future: Breaking the Intergenerational Transmission of Inequality* (New York: UNDP, 2010), available from www.who.int.

54 US Global Health Initiative, "Guatemala," accessed Feb. 16, 2012, available from www.ghi.gov.

55 World Health Organization, "Dominican Republic Country Brief" (2012), accessed Aug. 7, 2012, available from www.who.int.

56 UNDP, *Regional Human Development Report for Latin America and Caribbean 2010*.

57 Booth et al., *Understanding Central America*.

58 Reynaldo Martorell, "Physical Growth and Development of the Malnourished Child: Contributions from 50 Years of Research at INCAP," *Food and Nutrition Bulletin* 31.1 (2010):68–82. Reynaldo Martorell, Bernardo L. Horta, Linda S. Adair, Aryeh D. Stein, Linda Richter, Caroline H. D. Fall, Santosh K. Bhargava, S. K. Dey Biswas, Lorna Perez, Fernando C. Barros, Cesar G. Victora, and Consortium on Health Orientated Research in Transitional Societies Group, "Weight Gain in the First Two Years of Life is an Important Predictor of Schooling Outcomes in Pooled Analyses from Five Birth Cohorts from Low-and Middle-Income Countries," *Journal of Nutrition* 140 (Feb. 2010):348–365.

59 Angela Cespedes, Aaron Lechtig, and Rachel Franchschi, "Social Protection Networks in Central America and the Dominican Republic: Do They Have a Nutritional Dimension?" *Food and Nutrition Bulletin* 32.2 (2011):171–180. Mercedes de Onis, Monika Blossner, and Elaine Borghi, "Prevalence and Trends of Stunting among Pre-school Children, 1990–2020 (2011), available from www.who.int.

60 US Department of State, "Haiti: Two Years Later," accessed Feb. 16, 2012, available from www.state.gov.

61 Miller, *An Environmental History of Latin America*, 119.

62 Ibid.

63 Eduardo H. Galeano and Cedric Belfrage, *Open Veins of Latin America: Five Centuries of the Pillage of a Continent*. London: Serpent's Tail, 2009.

64 Food and Agriculture Organization of the United Nations, "Low-Income Food-Deficit Countries (LIFDC)–List for 2012," accessed March 13, 2012, available from www.fao.org.

65 Birn et al., *Textbook of International Health*, 169.

66 David Harvey, *A Brief History of Neoliberalism* (New York: Oxford University Press, 2005), 2.

67 Birn et al., *Textbook of International Health*, 420–421.

68 David Bacon, "Mexico's Great Migration," *The Nation* (Jan. 23, 2012):11–18.

69 Laura Carlsen, "NAFTA is Starving Mexico" (2011), accessed March 13, 2012, available from www.fpif.org.

70 Carlos G. Aguilar, "Free Markets and the Food Crisis in Central America" (2011), accessed Mar. 13, 2012, available from www.cipamericas.org.

71 United States Department of Agriculture Foreign Agricultural Service. Fact Sheet on Dominican Republic-Central America-United States Free Trade Agreement 2009 [cited 14 November 2012], available from http://www.fas.usda.gov/info/fact sheets/CAFTA/CAFTA-DR0909.pdf.

72 Witness for Peace, "Fact Sheet: The 'Winners and Losers' of DR-CAFTA in Nicaragua's Free Trade Zones" (2012), accessed Feb. 16, 2012, available from www.witness forpeace.org.

73 Human Rights Watch, "World Report 2012: Honduras" (2012), accessed Aug. 9, 2012, available from www.hrw.org. Amnesty International, "Truth Commissions" (2012), accessed August 9, 2012, available from www.amnesty.org.

74 United Nations, "The Millennium Development Goals Report 2011" (United Nations, 2011), available from www.un.org.

75 UNDP, "MDG Monitor," accessed Feb. 16, 2012, available from www.mdgmonitor .org.

76 PAHO, *Health in the Americas*, 2007. A. K. Mitra and G. Rodriguez-Fernandez, "Latin America and the Caribbean: Assessment of the Advances in Public Health for the Achievement of the Millennium Development Goals," *International Journal of Environmental Research and Public Health* 7.5 (2010):2238–2255.

77 Skolnik, *Global Health 101*, 185–194.

78 UNDP, *Regional Human Development Report for Latin America and Caribbean 2010*, accessed Feb. 16, 2012.

79 Mark B. Padilla, Emily Pingel, Emily Renda, Armando Matiz Reyes, and K. Fiereck,

"Gender, Sexuality, Health, and Human Rights in Latin America and the Caribbean," *Global Public Health* 5.3 (2010):213–220.

80 J. P. Koplan, T. C. Bond, M. H. Merson, K. S. Reddy, M. H. Rodriguez, N. K. Sewankambo, and J. N. Wasserheit, "Toward a Common Definition of Global Health." *Lancet* 373 (2009): 1995.

81 WHO, "Health Topics: Globalization," accessed Feb. 16, 2012, available from www.who.int.

82 Meri Koivusalo, "The Impact of Economic Globalisation on Health." *Theoretical Medicine and Bioethics* 27 (2006):13–34.

83 International Federation of Red Cross and Red Crescent Societies, "Code of Conduct 2012," accessed March 14, 2012, available from www.ifrc.org.

84 WHO, "The Role of WHO in Public Health," accessed Feb. 16, 2012, available from www.who.int.

85 PAHO, *Health in the Americas, 2007*.

86 US Agency for International Development, "USAID Primer: What We Do and How We Do It," ed. USAID (Washington, 2006), available from http://transition.usaid.gov; and USAID, "The USAID Health Care Improvement Project FY2012 Activities," accessed Mar. 28, 2012, available from www.hciproject.org.

87 Health Alliance International, "The NGO Code of Conduct for Health Systems Strengthening" (2008 [cited 15 March 2012), available from http://ngocodeofconduct.org/.

88 Peter Rohloff, Anne Kraemer Díaz, and Shom Dasgupta, "'Beyond Development': A Critical Appraisal of the Emergence of Small Health Care Non-Governmental Organizations in Rural Guatemala," *Human Organization* 70.4 (2011):427–437.

89 Paul E. Farmer and Jim Y. Kim. 2008. "Surgery and global health: a view from beyond the OR." *World Journal of Surgery* no. 32 (4): 533–36.

90 Jaime Sepúlveda, Flavia Bustreo, Roberto Tapia, Juan Rivera, Rafael Lozano, Gustavo Oláiz, Virgilio Partida, Lourdes García-García, José Luis Valdespino. Improvement of child survival in Mexico: the diagonal approach. *The Lancet, Volume 368, Issue 9551 (2–8 December 2006): 2017–2027*.

91 K. Rasanathan, E. V. Montesinos, D. Matheson, C. Etienne, and T. Evans, "Primary Health Care and the Social Determinants of Health: Essential and Complementary Approaches for Reducing Inequities in Health," *Journal of Epidemiology and Community Health* 65.8 (2011):656–60, doi: 10.1136/jech.2009.093914.

92 Paul K. Drain, Stephen A. Huffman, Sara E. Pirtle, and Kevin Chan, *Caring for the World: A Guidebook to Global Health Opportunities* (Toronto: University of Toronto Press, 2009).

93 Consortium of Universities for Global Health. http://www.cugh.org/ accessed 14 November 2012.

Suggested Reading

Birn, Anne-Emanuelle, Yogan Pillay, and Timothy H. Holtz. *Textbook of International Health: Global Health in a Dynamic World*. 3rd ed. New York: Oxford University Press, 2009.

Booth, John A., Christine J. Wade, and Thomas W. Walker. *Understanding Central*

America: Global Forces, Rebellion, and Change. 5th ed. Boulder, CO: Westview Press, 2010.

Carmack, Robert M., Gasco, Janine L., Gossen, Gary H. *The Legacy of Mesoamerica: History and Culture of a Native American Civilization.* 2nd ed. Upper Saddle River, NJ: Prentice Hall, 2007.

Centers for Disease Control and Prevention. *CDC Health Information for International Travel: The Yellow Book.* New York: Oxford University Press, 2012.

Drain, Paul K., Stephen A. Huffman, Sara E. Pirtle, and Kevin Chan. *Caring for the World: A Guidebook to Global Health Opportunities.* Toronto: University of Toronto Press, 2009.

Grandin, Greg. *Empire's Workshop: Latin America, the United States, and the Rise of the New Imperialism.* New York: Metropolitan Books, 2006.

Green, Duncan. *Faces of Latin America.* 3rd. ed. London: Latin America Bureau; New York: Monthly Review Press, 2006.

Harvey, David. *A Brief History of Neoliberalism.* New York: Oxford University Press, 2005.

O'Neil, Edward, Jr. *Awakening Hippocrates: a Primer on Health, Poverty, and Global Service.* Chicago: American Medical Association, 2006.

Skolnik, Richard. *Global Health 101.* Edited by Richard Riegelman. 2nd ed. Essential Public Health Series. Burlington, MA: Jones & Barlett Learning, 2012.

Williamson, Edwin. *The Penguin History of Latin America.* New York: Penguin Books, 2009.

Suggested Websites

American College of Surgeons Operation Giving Back—Directory of resources for volunteer surgeons and other health professionals. www.operationgivingback.facs.org/.

Amigos de las Américas, an example of a service-learning program for high school and college students. http://www.amigoslink.org.

Consortium of Universities for Global Health. www.cugh.org.

Global Brigades www.globalbrigades.org.

Global Health Hub www.globalhealthhub.org.

Hesperian Health Guides www.Hesperian.org.

North American Congress on Latin America. www.nacla.org. Quarterly journal and source of news from other media outlets.

Building Partnerships in the Americas

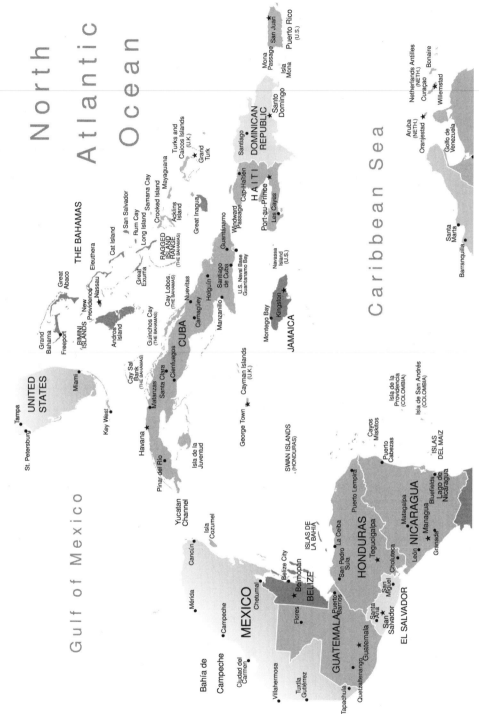

Mexico

Daniel Palazuelos and Linnea Capps

Mexico is a close neighbor of the United States and a major tourist destination. This can make the country seem familiar, but visiting beaches and colonial cities can't give a complete picture of the diversity of the land and people. This chapter concentrates on Chiapas, a poor state in southern Mexico, but the narrative of Chiapas can be told correctly only if the entire Mexican narrative is kept in mind. The story of Mexico is, among other things, a fascinating history of how cultures meet, compete, and meld; how countries develop; how democracies grow or falter; and how a people can maintain dignity despite incredible challenges. The story of Chiapas is a tale of how people on the periphery of a country, long marginalized and mostly forgotten, can reenter the national imagination and, in turn, renew its future.

This chapter attempts to use the trends illustrated by these narratives as a backdrop for discussing the problems faced by rural communities in one of the poorest states in Mexico. The people in these communities face many challenges, including geographic isolation, poor sanitation, food insecurity, and lack of access to services such as education and adequate healthcare. With these challenges in mind, we hope to explain how we have sought to partner personally and professionally with those most in need, to try to make a difference that we feel truly matters.

An Abbreviated History of Mexico

The point of this section is not to tell Mexico's full history in detail, yet we believe that the realities visible today have deep roots in the processes and themes of the past. We provide here a basic overview of historical periods in order to build a basic foundation on which any volunteer can continue learning and understanding. What follows is only one perspective of a multifaceted story. With this in mind, we recommend reading other renditions, starting with *The Discovery and Conquest of Mexico* by Bernal Díaz de Castillo, *Letters From Mexico* by Hernán Cortés, *The Broken Spears: The Aztec Account of the Conquest of Mexico* by Miguel Léon-Portilla, and *Open Veins of Latin America* by Eduardo Galeano. The US Library of Congress's Mexico country profile has a good basic inventory of the main events and the historical timeline.[1]

Mexico's history can be divided into the following historical periods:

Precolonial period, when sophisticated civilizations were thriving over a large geographic area

Colonial period, when Spain and the New World inhabitants were actively melting together into a new entity

Independence from Spain, when the new country attempted self-rule

French intervention, when that self-rule was challenged

Revolution, when class divisions erupted into violence

Post-revolution Mexico, when a single political party ruled with almost despotic control

Modern-day Mexico

We also include a side note discussing the implications of how Mexico's southern border was drawn.

Precolonial Period

In the precolonial period, indigenous people lived in a variety of ways throughout the Americas. Some developed impressive civilizations that can be counted as some of the truly greatest the world has ever known: examples include the Olmecs near the gulf; the Mayas in current-day southern Mexico, Belize, Guatemala, and Honduras; and the Aztecs in central Mexico. They built complex cities that certainly rivaled if not surpassed contemporary cities in Europe, and their scientific, cultural, and governmental achievements were staggering, especially when considering that the people had no beasts of burden and did not readily utilize the wheel. Other indigenous groups, such as those in the north of Mexico and current-day southeast United States, lived nomadic lives in a harsh desert terrain. All of this changed, however, once European explorers "discovered" the Americas.

To this day, the legacy of the indigenous is critical to how modern Mexicans envision themselves. And this portrait can be somewhat contradictory when it proudly admires the fantastic Maya ruins that soar over the thick rainforests, and simultaneously treats as foreigners entire impoverished populations who barely subsist on humble diets of beans and corn, and who continue to consider Spanish a second language.

Colonial Period

After the Spanish conquest of the few remaining Mayas and the many mighty Aztecs, the Spanish quickly worked to build a New Spain literally from the fallen stones of the indigenous temples they had razed to the ground. This was the traumatic birth of modern Mexico, in which the majority of the people are mestizo, a mixture of indigenous and European heritage. Octavio Paz, famous Mexican essayist and poet, describes the first mestizo birth as the product of a rape between the Conquistador Cortés and his translator, an indigenous princess now better known as La Malinche. La Malinche is a complicated figure in the popular Mexican imagination—she is both mother and traitor, both submissive and violated. Paz highlights how the word *chingar* (a complex word with multiple connotations) exemplifies the complicated role that the concepts of domination and power have taken on in popular Mexican culture.[2] Indeed, colonial society was structured along a rigid hierarchy, which was based on class, race, and gender, and to this day class divisions in Mexico tend to be cut across racial lines; one only needs to look at any Mexican television show or advertisement to notice that the faces of European descent continue to dominate the representation of wealth, commerce, and "high culture."

Independence from Spain

When New Spain joined the rest of the New World in seeking independence from their colonial rulers, some colorful figures emerged as great leaders. Their names are now almost impossible to avoid if one enters any public space or national area of interest: the priest Hidalgo, who issued the *grito*, or the famous call for rebellion; his student Morelos, who continued the struggle once Hidalgo was executed; the Spanish general Agustin de Iturbide, who defected and brought his army to the rebels. With such leadership and vision, the newly independent population should have gotten off to a great start. But unfortunately, the succeeding Mexican republic was plagued by revolts and consecutively disruptive changes in leadership. In fact, the presidency changed hands thirty-six times between 1833 and 1855. Much of the struggle was between liberals, who advocated for social reforms that would affect already powerful elites in the military and church, and conservatives, who favored maintaining these power differentials. Without good and constant leadership, the results were disastrous for a Mexico that at that time stretched from Canada to South America: in 1823, the United Provinces of Central America declared independence; in 1836, Mexico lost Texas to US settlers; in 1848, after the Mexican-American War ended with the Treaty of Guadalupe Hidalgo, Mexico lost almost one-half of its territory to the US occupiers (land that would later become the US states of California, Nevada, and Utah, and parts of Colorado, Wyoming, Arizona, and New Mexico). For many North Americans, the origin of these southwestern and western states may be only a historical footnote; for most Mexicans, it represents a great theft and serves as a reminder of the imperial aggression of the United States.

French Intervention and Mexico's Southern Border

In 1861, the liberals won the presidency with Benito Juárez, an indigenous Zapotec from Oaxaca. He pursued an agenda of economic and education reform. Though largely considered a relative golden age of leadership in Mexico, Juárez's reign was disrupted by the French occupation of Mexico City and by the installation of a Habsburg prince, Maximillian, from Austria to serve as emperor of Mexico. The prince's reign was short-lived, largely ineffective, and ended with his beheading in 1867 when Juárez was restored to the presidency. The French intervention and Maximillian's influence can still be felt today, not only in the European-styled avenues and parks in Mexico City, but also in the intolerance to foreign influence in Mexican internal affairs; foreigners may not participate in Mexican law or influence Mexican politics.

It's important to pause here for a side note about "La Otra Frontera"— that other (southern Mexican) border. This history of how Mexico defined its modern-day borders, and especially the southern border with Guatemala, helps to explain why it might seem that Chiapas is more like Central America than the rest of Mexico. Chiapas was historically isolated from the Spanish colonial authorities due in part to geography, but also because of its lack of mineral wealth or large areas of arable land. At the time of Mexico's independence from Spain, a group of merchants and ranchers tried to establish the Free State of Chiapas. During the next few years, several towns declared independence from Mexico, and some favored unification with Guatemala and the United Provinces of Central America. In 1824, a referendum was held, and the majority voted for incorporation with Mexico. Guatemala did not recognize the inclusion of all of Chiapas into Mexico until 1882, when the border between the two countries was finalized.[3]

Chiapas, as can be expected, has always shared many similarities with Central America. It has a large indigenous population that often feels a strong allegiance to its group. The people take pride in their storied past, and use these myths and stories of prior greatness to organize for future changes. The terrain on which they live is mountainous, similar to Guatemala's, and therefore poses significant infrastructure challenges that can only exacerbate existing social isolation. When hurricanes pass through Chiapas or Central America from the Caribbean, or earthquakes rumble in from the Pacific, livelihoods and communities are destroyed with equal abandon in any place unfortunately located in harm's way. The tradition of almost complete control of the local economy by a few local nonindigenous elites or foreign interests has sparked multiple social struggles that all too often have resulted in repression and bloodshed. The average people in both Chiapas and Guatemala share a common phenotypic appearance, and many will discuss at length their shared experiences with farming corn and beans on small plots, trying to get improved prices for their coffee crops, or the harsh conditions of work in the plantations running along the southern Pacific coast. Even a quick visit to either the capital city of Chiapas (Tuxtla Gutiérrez) or the capital of Guatemala City will probably have a soundtrack of Marimba music echoing through the city's central gardens.

Beyond these similarities, there is an important point of departure: the very simple reality that Chiapas is physically and logistically part of Mexico affords it a very different path on its way to development. Unlike many of the small and politically unstable countries in Central America, Mexico is a large and diverse country with increasingly democratic institutions, significant social investment programs by the government, and a growing economy that shapes and expands the common marketplace. The distant past may set up Chiapas to have a lot in common with its southern neighbors, but modern history has given Chiapas unique opportunities. When planning and implementing a global health project in Chiapas versus some other part of Mesoamerica, it would be shortsighted to see Chiapas as just an extension of Central America.

Revolution

When Juárez died in 1872, Porfirio Díaz was elected and ruled as a strong-arm dictator of Mexico for thirty-five years. His policies brought Mexico into the industrial age and launched public works projects, but banned political opposition, free elections, and a free press. Land, usually taken from peasant communal lands, accumulated in the hands of the small, mostly white elite. Díaz's political opponent Francisco Madero sparked the Mexican Revolution in 1910, but it was actually fought and invigorated by outraged *campesinos* (peasant farmers). In particular, the indigenous radical leader Emiliano Zapata captured the hopes of his followers with his battle cry "Tierra y Libertad! La tierra es de quien la trabaja" ("Land and Freedom! The land belongs to those who work it"). With another rebel leader, Pancho Villa, in the north and Zapata in the south, the revolution was a ten-year period of battles, shifting alliances, and many failed attempts to form a stable government; over 1 million people lost their lives in the conflict.

Post-Revolution Mexico

One of the most important documents to come out of the revolution was the constitution of 1917. Both an outline for how to run the country and a manifesto of the principles for which the revolution was fought, the constitution contained four key themes that would become recurrent narratives for Mexican policy in the twentieth century: land reform, rights and welfare programs, anticlericalism, and antiforeignism.[4] Not surprisingly, the period of reconstruction immediately following the revolution included building thousands of rural schools and redistributing some land from large landowners to peasants through the establishment of the *ejido* system (landholding cooperatives in which decisions about the land can be made only through consensus of all founding members). In Chiapas, some ejidos were established, but not enough to address the abject poverty in which many of the indigenous lived. Zapata's legacy, and the subsequent failure to realize Zapata's dream in Chiapas, would return to haunt Mexican politicians when the Zapatistas, a group of indigenous rebels, rose up demanding, among other things, that land continue to be redistributed in the state.

Lázaro Cárdenas was president during the 1930s, and part of his many social reforms included further land redistribution and the *expropriation* of foreign oil companies in Mexico to form PEMEX, the Mexican petroleum company. PEMEX would serve as one of the most important forms of revenue for the Mexican government during the twentieth century. It provided funding for improved public works and healthcare, but this "easy money" is also believed to have contributed to the creation of an impenetrable government bureaucracy and of nepotism as simply the way of doing business. This situation has been called the "resource curse," and many other countries have experienced the same fate once they found their revenue source deep in the earth instead of from taxes. Some predictions anticipate that without further investments or exploration for new deepwater reserves, Mexican oil could dry up within our lifetime. Whether this would reverse the curse by forcing the population to hold its elected leaders accountable once the government is forced to start collecting taxes in earnest, or would plunge Mexico into a nightmare of underfunding, is uncertain.[5]

Modern-Day Mexico

During the period around World War II, the Mexican economy expanded, and more conservative leaders governed the country. The party of Cárdenas was renamed the Partido Revolucionario Institucional (PRI, Institutional Revolutionary Party), and then governed Mexico for more than seventy years. Electoral fraud and strong-arm political tactics became routine; even though Mexico was considered a democracy, presidents could essentially handpick their successors through what was called the *dedazo* (*dedo* being the word for "finger," suggesting that this process was as easy as one person pointing a finger to the next). Starting in the 1940s, Mexico pursued the economic policy of *import-substitution industrialization* (in which imports are replaced by the local production of goods so as to minimize dependence on foreign markets). The result was sustained positive economic growth per year, leading some economists to proclaim "the Mexican Miracle!" In the 1970s, funds from a newly tapped oil reserve and inflated prices for oil due to the energy crisis in the United States helped fuel unprecedented spending and irresponsible governing. Once oil prices fell, however, the Mexican economy could not diversify quickly enough, and the economy fell into a tailspin of debt and inflation.

Structural Adjustment and NAFTA

In the early 1980s, in exchange for bailout loans, the International Monetary Fund pressured the Mexican government into undergoing major structural adjustment reforms in the government and economy. Also known as neoliberalism, this theory maintains that by decreasing government regulations, privatizing major sections of the economy, and decreasing government spending for social programs, the economy will grow. Though an argument can be made that this process stabilized the economy and contributed to economic growth, the undermining of important social safety nets magnified the already gaping socioeconomic inequalities in the society. The election of 1988 played out these tensions on the electoral front when Carlos Salinas de Gortari, proponent of the market reforms, came to power over Cuauhtémoc Cárdenas (son of the famous ex-president Lázaro Cárdenas), who led the charge against the neoliberal economic changes with the Partido de la Revolución Democrática (PRD, Party of the Democratic Revolution). The tale commonly told is that on election night, when it seemed that Salinas might be defeated, a mysterious electrical failure occurred. Once the lights finally came back on, Salinas held the majority of votes by only a small margin. For many Mexicans, this disputed election is proof positive of just how corrupt Mexican democracy can become.[6]

Once in power, Salinas took neoliberalism to a new height. He considered his major achievement to be the North American Free Trade Agreement, signed by Canada, the United States, and Mexico, to pursue policies that would favor commerce between the three countries. As explained in the section on NAFTA later in this chapter, the effect on Mexico of the neoliberal reforms in general, and NAFTA in particular, has been profound.

The Zapatista Uprising

However, Salinas did not conclude his term on the high note he had anticipated, because on January 1, 1994, the day that NAFTA took effect, a previously unrecognized rebel group in the southern state of Chiapas—the Zapatistas— began an uprising in defense of the rights of indigenous people. It was fitting that this revolt began in Chiapas, as this state is unique in many ways: it has much in common historically and culturally with Guatemala, and only a few years earlier, Guatemala had fought one of the longest and bloodiest civil wars in Central America's history for many of the same issues that inspired the Zapatistas. Chiapas also has a wealth of natural resources that are in large measure exported to other states, making Chiapas a sort of colonized territory within Mexico's borders. In addition, a commonly quoted phrase is "the Mexican Revolution never came to Chiapas," meaning that the benefits of the revolution, such as land redistribution, were not enjoyed equally by the poor of Chiapas. All these elements created a rich powder keg from which a revolution exploded, when given some external ignition.

When the spark finally came, a charismatic hooded Zapatista leader, Subcomandante Marcos, became the iconic spokesman for why the revolution was necessary. His many writings proclaimed with great passion and eloquence that poverty, discrimination, poor education, the unfair distribution of land, the lack of true participatory democracy, and inadequate health services were among the underlying causes that prompted the revolt. The Zapatistas were not fighting to secede from Mexico and join their cousins in the south; instead, they wanted to more fully be recognized as a part of Mexico and to receive the benefits promised by the revolution of 1910. Inspired by the rebel leader Zapata, who fought for land reform during the Mexican revolution, the Ejército Zapatista de Liberación Nacional (EZLN, Zapatista National Liberation Army) was composed mostly of impoverished indigenous rebels who came to international attention when they declared war on the federal government and took over several towns in an area called "the highlands."

Many saw the EZLN as a movement that was taking up arms in order to call attention to the plight of all the poor and marginalized who stood to be even further abused by the neoliberal reforms in Mexico. The fighting was intense in a few areas of Chiapas for twelve days in January 1994, but the struggle quickly evolved into a low-intensity conflict that has continued now for more than eighteen years. (It's important to note that as of 2012, Chiapas is a relatively safe destination for tourists and volunteers as long as the usual precautions are taken.) Negotiations during the early years after the rebellion resulted in the San Andrés Accords in 1996. This agreement would have allowed for more autonomous community decision-making and redistribution of land in the conflict zones, but it was never converted into law. In response, the Zapatistas declared the Mexican government the "Mal Gobierno" (Bad Government) and vowed to continue building their new society "in resistance," which means refusing all government services, including education and healthcare, in favor of creating independent structures. There continues to be a large military presence in parts of Chiapas to monitor (and many say intimidate) the Zapatistas.

The Zapatistas Today

The Zapatista communities have worked to build their autonomous institutions since 1994. They created Juntas de Buen Gobierno (JBG, Good Government Councils), each of which functions as the governing body of several autonomous municipalities. Some of these councils have been able to perform such functions as maintaining a census, birth and death records, and a judicial system. Families do not send their children to public schools, and many Zapatista communities have their own schools with volunteer teachers who have been trained by Zapatista indigenous teachers or by volunteers from other parts of Mexico and the world. In some of the larger communities, there are now secondary schools. The autonomous communities have also avoided using Mexican government healthcare and have developed their own system that includes many essential elements: vaccination campaigns and other public health measures, simple clinics run by health promoters, and a few more sophisticated clinics and hospitals.[7] There have been important successes: vaccine coverage, for example, is excellent in many of the communities. The challenge for all of these initiatives is that many of the Zapatista communities are very small and geographically isolated. Teachers and health promoters are volunteers who also must care for their own families and their corn or coffee crops. Healthcare is especially expensive, and the communities can't pay the costs of even some of the simplest medical treatments. For many, the Zapatistas provide an example of how a rebel group can successfully build and maintain autonomous structures; visiting Zapatista communities will quickly show just how hard it is to maintain those structures at a level that consistently addresses the deep needs of poverty.

Contemporary Politics

The Zapatista uprising may have been only a small peasant revolt in one corner of the republic, but it ended up influencing Mexico in profound and far-reaching ways. Many have called it a "postmodern revolution" because the real damage done was not on the battlefield, but in the press when an international eye turned to Mexico's internal affairs and forced its leaders to reflect deeply about the face they were showing. It is no coincidence that only six years later, in 2000, Mexico celebrated its first true democratic presidential election when PRI lost for the first time in seventy years. The winner was Vicente Fox of the right-of-center Partido Acción Nacional (PAN, National Action Party). This was the first peaceful regime change in Mexico's history. As

Fox's term came to an end in 2006, PAN collaborated with PRI to try to derail the election of the popularist PRD candidate, Andrés Manuel López Obrador; PAN's candidate, Felipe Calderón, won the presidency in a very close election, but the election was followed by large protest demonstrations by those who thought López Obrador had actually won.

Impact of Drug Trafficking

Modern-day Mexico continues to struggle with other very real challenges. Drug trafficking and the associated violence, for example, have plagued the country. After a crackdown by the United States on shipments from Colombia during the 1980s, more drugs began to be shipped from Colombia through Mexico. In the late 1990s, President Zedillo brought the military into the fight against drug cartels. Several border cities, especially Tijuana and Ciudad Juárez, began to suffer from a rapidly increasing murder rate. In the early 2000s, President Fox made some attempts to eliminate the corruption in the anti-drug police forces, but by then more than 90 percent of cocaine entering the United States was coming through Mexico.[8] Since the beginning of the war on drug traffickers by President Felipe Calderón (which some feel he started in order to strengthen his mandate to rule after barely winning the heavily contested presidential election in 2006), many parts of Mexico, especially in the north along the US border, have experienced violence because the attempt to control the powerful drug-trafficking gangs has sparked police-gang and inter-gang warfare. More than 15,000 organized crime killings occurred in 2010 alone, with some sources reporting the death toll at over 40,000 since 2001.[9] All this has begun to cause social unrest and more tension in relations with the United States, which many Mexicans feel should be doing more to reduce the key factors adding to this serious problem: illicit drug consumption in the United States and the illegal trafficking of American arms to drug cartels in Mexico.

The presidential election of 2012 was seen by many as a referendum on the PAN war against the drug cartels. The PRI political party regained control of the presidency with the victory of Enrique Peña Nieto. This was a critical moment in Mexico's history, and only time will tell where it is heading.

Mexico Today

Indeed, there are many ways in which modern-day Mexico is rapidly changing. New processes are influencing many of the realities that have long characterized and structured daily life. Although the Catholic church, along with the worship of the Virgin of Guadalupe, has been central to Mexican culture for centuries, Protestant missionaries have successfully converted large percentages of some populations (especially in Chiapas) and are changing the way converts think of themselves and society.[10] The Mexican economy has long relied on products produced locally and allowed few imports, but NAFTA has almost overnight changed the Mexican marketplace, often with far-reaching consequences. Economically, Mexico has become one of the world's larger economies, the average standard of living is gradually improving, and an important, newly formed middle class is growing in size and influence. The lives of the extremely poor, on the other hand, are improving at a much slower pace, and some still live as if it were the "old Mexico" where women had many babies only to see a good percentage of them die young. Immigration of large numbers of Mexicans to "the north" continues as always; more than 11 million were living in the United States as of 2010, yet the absolute number of those crossing the border has decreased, probably due to the severe recession of 2008 that resulted in decreased job opportunities for migrant workers.[11]

Chiapas
Geography and Population

Chiapas is located in southeastern Mexico, bordering the states of Tabasco, Veracruz, and Oaxaca, with the Pacific Ocean to the south and Guatemala to the east. Chiapas is the eighth largest of the thirty-one Mexican states, with a territory of 74,415 square kilometers. The state has a complex geography with several distinct regions.

The twentieth century has seen major population growth in Chiapas. In 1940, there were fewer than 1 million inhabitants. By 2010, the population of Chiapas had grown to 4,796,580, making it the eighth most populous state in Mexico. This has changed the environment in Chiapas, and the life of Chiapanecans, in important ways. For example, the population of the Lacandon forest was only 1,000 in 1950, but by the mid-1990s it had increased to 200,000. When the rainforest in the eastern part of the state was subject to land reform in 1940, cattle ranchers, loggers, and subsistence farmers migrated into the area from the overcrowded highlands. The environmental and cultural impact has been intense. Although Chiapas has some of the greatest biodiversity on the planet, whole forests of virgin jungles are rapidly disappearing as the land strains under the weight of a population explosion. It's important to remember that it isn't only the campesinos' usage of the land for farming that makes Mexico a country with one of the fastest rates of deforestation in the world; logging and agriculture entrepreneurs have equally as disastrous an impact.[12] The unsustainable usage of Chiapas's natural heritage is concerning to most. How do we get beyond this initial shock and begin to address, if not reverse, the root problems involved? This is paramount. And to do it, we must further understand the nature of inequality. We will explore the multiple facets of this question in the following sections.

Socioeconomic Inequality

Mexico is a rich country. It has a wealth of natural resources, a hardworking populace, and a vibrant cultural history. Unfortunately, the majority of Mexicans are poor. How these two realities can exist in the same country has a lot to do with the way that wealth is unequally distributed. One measure of inequality, the Gini index (see *Gini coefficient* in Glossary), ranks Mexico in the middle of all Latin American and Caribbean countries in terms of income inequality. However, Latin America is the world's most unequal region, and Mexico has a much higher level of income inequality than many countries in Asia and Eastern Europe.[13] The richest man in the world as of this writing, Carlos Slim, is Mexican, and he was able to amass huge wealth through a monopolistic control of telecommunications in the country.[14] On the other hand, nearly half of Mexicans live in poverty, and up to 10 percent live in extreme poverty.[15] The rich and the poor may pass each other casually on the street, but they don't live side by side. As in the United States, another very unequal country, the rich live in pockets of wealth and enjoy a lifestyle that rivals the best in the world, while the poor live in rural areas or urban shantytowns that are plagued by illness and violence.

Chiapas, in spite of its impressive natural resources, is one of Mexico's most economically impoverished states. It also has the highest proportions of indigenous people among the Mexican states, and the two go hand in hand; 27% of Chiapas's population is indigenous, and nearly one-third of them are unable to communicate in Spanish.[16] In some of the municipalities in the highlands of Chiapas, more than 80 percent of the population is indigenous, and in some communities, up to one-half of the population does not speak Spanish. Another measure of Mexico's highly unequal distribution of income and wealth is the Indices of Marginalization published by the Mexican government agency CONAPO (Consejo Nacional de Población). These statistics show that Chiapas has the second-highest level of socioeconomic inequality among all of Mexico's states.[17] In 2012, billboards in Chiapas trumpeted the headline "We are no longer first in societal disadvantage," but despite incremental progress, Chiapas continues to fall behind the rest of the country on key health and poverty indicators.

Poor, illiterate, marginalized populations often have few opportunities to control the processes that decide their fate. If these processes are left unchecked, the marginalized may suffer great injustices and disproportionate ill-health.[18] There are many ways to combat this. One strategy is to focus on the structures and processes that produce the injustices, what have been called the social determinants of health or the *upstream* factors. This is usually not an easy fight because it often touches the special interests, who may be profiting personally from the status quo. Another strategy is to also focus on helping the people who suffer the damages one sees *downstream*, such as the illness and violence that has become an all-too-common part of being poor in the modern world. Clearly, healthcare is one very powerful mechanism by which to accomplish this second strategy. We have found that when talking about healthcare, it is wise to first discuss how much money is budgeted for the services, and how those services are to be delivered.

Spending for Healthcare, and Healthcare Reform[19]

Mexico is considered a middle-income country and is a member of the Organization for Economic Cooperation and Development (OECD). According to 2010 OECD data, Mexico's spending for healthcare is 5.9 percent of gross domestic product (GDP). This places it last among all the other OECD members, who put an average of 9 percent of their GDP into healthcare spending. Around one-half is out-of-pocket spending, meaning the patient pays for the care directly without any help from other sources, such as an insurance plan. It is interesting to note that both Mexico and the United States rank lowest in how much government funds contribute to total spending for healthcare, even though they occupy the two ends of the spectrum in terms of total spending (with the United States spending far more than any other country).[20]

A fractured care delivery system, inadequate funding, and weak stewardship are all issues that have long plagued the Mexican healthcare system. After the PAN won over the PRI in the presidential election of 2000, one of the key issues that the party hoped to address was the lack of access to quality healthcare services by about one-half of the population. The minister of health at the time, Julio Frenk, and his team developed an important healthcare financing solution: Seguro Popular (SP, Popular Insurance). Before SP was implemented, approximately 40 percent of Mexicans had access to care through the IMSS system (Instituto Mexicano del Seguro Social); this is a national healthcare system, managed by the government and funded by government revenues (mostly taxes and profits from oil) as well as contributions from patients and employers. Only those with salaried jobs in the formal economy had access to this service. A smaller percent of workers and their families had access to similar insurance programs linked to specific government sectors (for example, the Institute for Social Security and Services for Civil Servants (ISSSTE) or expensive private insurance.

This left 50 percent of the population without access to health insurance, which often meant lack of access to comprehensive healthcare. Their only care options included traditional medicine in their communities (for example, herbs and home remedies, traditional folk healers such as *curanderos* or *hueseros*, and faith-based healing); drugs purchased over the counter at pharmacies or grocery stores; private doctors who often charged high prices on a fee-for-service schedule; and the safety-net government system run by the individual state governments, called Secretaría de Salud (SSA, Secretary of Health). Some Mexicans still refer to this system as *Salubridad*, a name it once had. In the SSA system, funding was minimal, and patients were often expected to *cost-share*, or pay for part of their treatment at the *point-of-care*, with prices adjusted per a socioeconomic sliding scale. It was primarily through this SSA system that SP would direct its new funding.

Overall, SP is a national insurance program that was designed to combine federal funds, state contributions, and family premiums in a way that could potentially cover all of the uninsured patients while also increasing the quality of care received in the SSA system. In the spirit of equity, Chiapas, a poor state with a high burden of disease and marginalization, was slated to get a proportionally higher state distribution. How much the states would continue to receive, however, was pegged to how many patients stayed enrolled. The hope was that this would create an incentive for the system to keep patients satisfied and enrolled by providing them with higher-quality care. In addition, patients were used to paying their out-of-pocket costs only after they were sick, but this new model asked that they pay an insurance premium beforehand to create a culture of "pre-payment" that, it was hoped, would improve the quality of care because patients would, in theory, start demanding better care.

Now, more than a decade after its inception, the experience with SP has been mixed. Although it has achieved near universal enrollment of all eligible families,[21] not enough pay their premiums,[22] and state governments inconsistently pay their share. This threatens to keep SP underfunded. In addition, Mexico has a *decentralized* healthcare system, which means that each state has considerable freedom to roll out SP as it sees fit; the quality of the management of SP, therefore, differs significantly from state to state.[23] This sometimes unanticipated lack of funding means that even though SP promises a minimum package of services to enrollees, the average patient continues to encounter inadequate options at the moment when they're needed most. In addition, SP, as a mere funding mechanism, has not done enough to assure that the various delivery systems (IMSS, ISSSTE, the private doctors, SSA) coordinate care among themselves; this lack of coordination can only lead to duplicated services, thwarted follow-up for chronic diseases such as diabetes and tuberculosis (TB), and ultimately, wasted resources.

It's interesting to note that at the same time when the government was reforming its system, the Mexican pharmaceutical industry was also undergoing a big change. One can't walk more than a block in any Mexican city without seeing a pharmacy, and the Farmacias de Similares, with its iconic Dr. Simi mascot dancing to blasting techno music outside the pharmacy, has been a major addition to the healthcare landscape. With Dr. Simi, any patient has access to a diagnosis and a drug, usually at a fraction of the cost of any other private provider, and without having to wait for hours in a government waiting room. Most medicines in Mexico are over-the-counter, which means that anyone can buy them without a prescription, although antibiotics have recently been added to the list that requires a prescription. The whole point of SP was to develop a national insurance program that would control the healthcare costs that Mexicans would pay once they got sick; the private pharmaceutical market, on the other hand, came up with its own unique solution at the same time.

Nevertheless, with SP, catastrophic spending for healthcare (defined as the money a family pays to care for an ill family member that ultimately ends up impoverishing the family) has decreased.[24] Mexico is indeed on the path toward healthcare coverage for all—meaning that all citizens will, in theory, have access to some form of service—though the actual state of health of the general population continues to tell a much deeper story.

Health Outcomes and Disparities

Social inequality occurs when certain segments of a population don't have the same access to opportunities or resources as compared with other segments of society. There may be many reasons for this, such as where people live, who they are, or what they believe. Either way, societal inequality often generates the social determinants of health, as mentioned earlier. These are the processes and risk factors that determine which populations get sick and become further impoverished, and which will stay well and thrive.

There are many ways to measure just how healthy or unhealthy a population really is, and each measurement offers another insight into what processes might be making people sick. The government-reported statistics of 2008 begin to tell the story. Compared to those who live in Mexico City, Chiapanecans simply live differently; they have higher rates of illiteracy (21.3 percent versus 2.6 percent), are less likely to live in houses with plumbing (71.7 percent versus 98.1 percent), and more likely to have a dirt floor (30.1 percent versus 1.0 percent). These factors suggest a poverty that is unhealthy, and the canary in this coal mine is the children. Chiapanecans in general have higher infant mortality (21.0 per 1,000 live births versus 11.4 in Mexico City), higher perinatal mortality (96.8 per 1,000 live births versus 52.9 in Mexico City), and higher total mortality in all children under age five (24.9 per 1,000 versus 14.1 in Mexico City).[25] (See section "An Exploration of Mexico's Improving Child Health.")

A 2006 Physicians for Human Rights (PHR) study of predominately indigenous communities found that the statistics for the indigenous communities were even worse than those for the state of Chiapas as a whole.[26] The study found that 23 percent of children had not completed their immunization schedules, even though officially reported vaccination rates are greater than 95 percent for the state. The poor vaccination coverage was attributed to lack of access to health services and, in some communities, to distrust of government health services. Stunting was found in 54.7 percent of the children, indicating chronic malnutrition.[27] In assessing maternal health, the study documented eight maternal deaths in the prior two years. The estimated maternal mortality rate was 607 per 100,000 births, a level that was seven times the national rate. Only 16 percent of all deliveries occurred in hospitals or healthcare facilities. Traditional birth attendants were present at 74 percent of the deliveries, and family or neighbors at another 7 percent. This study shows that although government-reported state and national averages are helpful, certain pockets of society suffer in very different ways from others. Some populations are so marginalized or isolated that they might not even be counted. And if they are counted, their suffering may simply be averaged in, and therefore somewhat hidden.

Fecundity, and the Politics of Wombs

Fecundity refers to the number of children women are having; it is decreasing overall in Mexico, with a national average of two children per couple, similar to the US average. This should be seen, in general, as a positive trend because of the individual and societal benefits of having fewer children. The women in many poor and marginalized populations, however, continue to have on average three to four or more children. This reproduction rate contributes to a population explosion that many believe threatens Mexico's future as resources become scarce, and as the society struggles to find a place for all of these people, who may live until their late seventies. Although it has been well studied that factors such as the mother's education and her ability to make decisions for herself contribute to how many babies she will decide to have, a dominant Mexican theme has been to focus on pressuring at-risk women to simply have fewer children—instead of developing strategies to empower women to make this decision for themselves.[28] In the poor communities of

Chiapas, where grossly unequal power relations often structure society, even the forced sterilization of indigenous women has been documented.[29]

Through our conversations with poor women in Chiapas, we have learned that they are often fully aware of the challenges of having many children. Yet they continue to do so because they don't feel they have a choice beyond what their husbands want, they don't have access to affordable contraception options, or they feel that a large family is the only form of social protection available when they reach old age and are unable to work. Having more family members in a poor family expands the number of people available to do necessary labor. Also, the family's economic base is diversified when different members can do a variety of jobs to bring in money when work is scarce or irregular. We've seen that by forcing family planning on poor families, instead of addressing gender inequality and the precarious financial systems on which poor people depend, this skewed emphasis might actually intensify the sensation of being disadvantaged, and in turn, potentially exacerbate a root cause of the poorest families having so many babies in the first place. In the less marginalized sections of society, where the dominant message of "smaller families are happier families" has taken hold, an argument can be made that it was an improved decision-making capacity, and not only the truth behind the message, that led these families to implement the advice.

Diseases Associated with Poverty

Tuberculosis

Tuberculosis is a disease that is preventable and curable. It can be fatal if not properly treated. Many developed countries have achieved low rates of pulmonary TB. This was done primarily by testing high-risk populations and family members of individuals with active disease, and then providing adequate treatment for all infected individuals. Because the treatment for TB is a mixture of multiple medicines given for six months or longer, an adequate treatment usually follows the DOTS (directly observed therapy, short-course) protocol, in which patients are watched in government clinics as they take their medicines daily. It is now well recognized that all programs should also include access to second-line regimens for multidrug-resistant tuberculosis (MDR-TB). In addition, studies have shown that patient-centered initiatives, such as the practice of having other community members *accompany* patients through their treatment, dramatically increases compliance rates.[30] Although Mexico has made significant strides toward eliminating TB overall, the disease continues unabated in many sections of society, especially among the indigent, poor indigenous, and increasingly, poor diabetics.

To explain why TB persists in Mexico, it's important to understand not only the pathophysiology of the disease, but also the factors that put certain people at risk, and what happens when they fall ill. TB is much more likely to be transmitted among people living in dark and poorly ventilated homes. Many poor families live in overcrowded houses, often with more than five people living in one or two rooms. Even though many people are exposed to TB, the majority will have the *latent*, or dormant, form in which people harbor the bacteria in their lungs and never actually develop the active form of the disease. Once active, TB produces a chronic cough, occasionally generating bloody sputum; fever; and weight loss. Any disease process that weakens the immune system, such as malnutrition, AIDS, and even diabetes (all diseases associated with poverty), may spark the conversion from latent to active TB.[31]

Those with active disease are highly contagious, and each will go on to infect multiple other people.[32] They may or may not seek care, but because the symptoms are so nonspecific, it's easy for a clinician to miss the diagnosis. The test to diagnose TB, a sputum sample collected in the morning that is then analyzed with a microscope to see if bacteria are present, is notoriously insensitive. If the sputum is not collected correctly, or if the lab technician is not careful, it's easy to miss the bacteria. Even if the patient is properly diagnosed, he or she must take the cocktail of prescribed medicines faithfully, daily for at least six months. This can be difficult, and in practice, many Mexican patients in Chiapas are not carefully followed to assure that they are taking each pill correctly; the burden of following up with the doctor falls on the patients, even though the cost of transportation to the DOTS clinic may be prohibitive. Adherence to the treatment regimen is considered the patient's responsibility, although the clinics may occasionally run out of medicines. Patients who stop taking their medicines are considered "abandoners" and are often quickly dismissed as "bad patients," even when the side effects were not well explained or treated with other readily available medicines.[33] Dr. Flores (see box, "Working in Middle-Income Latin America") explains some of the sociopolitical factors that he sees working behind the scenes.

Working in Middle-Income Latin America: The Burden of Structural Mediocrity

DR. HUGO ERNESTO FLORES NAVARRO, Director, Compañeros en Salud–México

Lucía is a twenty-eight-year-old woman who has been coughing since she was fifteen. Recently, she began to cough up blood. She lost a sister to tuberculosis, and two of her brothers-in-law, with whom she has lived, have also been diagnosed with the disease. Lucía even had a chest x-ray

BUILDING PARTNERSHIPS IN THE AMERICAS: A GUIDE
FOR GLOBAL HEALTH WORKERS; ED. BY MARGO J.
KRASNOFF.   Paper   265 P.
HANOVER: DARTMOUTH COLLEGE PRESS, 2013

ED: GEISEL SCHOOL OF MEDICINE AT DARTMOUTH.
ON OPPORTUNITIES FOR SERVICE IN CENTRAL AMERICA.
LCCN 2013-4432
  ISBN 161168420X   **Library PO#** FIRM ORDERS

	List	35.00	USD
8395 NATIONAL UNIVERSITY LIBRAR	**Disc**	5.0%	
App. Date 4/16/14 SHHS 8214-08	**Net**	33.25	USD

SUBJ: POOR--MEDICAL CARE--DEV. COUNTRIES.

CLASS RA418.5   DEWEY# 362.1   LEVEL ADV-AC

YBP Library Services

BUILDING PARTNERSHIPS IN THE AMERICAS: A GUIDE
FOR GLOBAL HEALTH WORKERS; ED. BY MARGO J.
KRASNOFF.   Paper   265 P.
HANOVER: DARTMOUTH COLLEGE PRESS, 2013

ED: GEISEL SCHOOL OF MEDICINE AT DARTMOUTH.
ON OPPORTUNITIES FOR SERVICE IN CENTRAL AMERICA.
  LCCN 2013-4432
  ISBN 161168420X   **Library PO#** FIRM ORDERS

	List	35.00	USD
8395 NATIONAL UNIVERSITY LIBRAR	**Disc**	5.0%	
App. Date 4/16/14 SHHS 8214-08	**Net**	33.25	USD

SUBJ: POOR--MEDICAL CARE--DEV. COUNTRIES.

CLASS RA418.5   DEWEY# 362.1   LEVEL ADV-AC

done that showed signs indicative of TB, yet today she was discharged from a district hospital with a diagnosis of an "atypical pneumonia" and a prescription for clarithromycin, an antibiotic that is not effective against TB. The reason: the only sputum sample that Lucía gave during her three-day hospitalization—the only study that was performed on her—did not show the TB bacilli. No plan to see if she gets better was put into place. When I asked the other clinicians whether this was satisfactory, I was met with more shoulder shrugs than data.

I chose this case because it illustrates many of the challenges of working in the parts of Mexico that remain neglected, with people who remain underserved by the current systems. I call this "the forgotten Mexico," though I know that the situation is similar in many other parts of Latin America. After years of work in this context, I realize more and more how the problem is structural.

THE NOBODIES

Why has Lucía been coughing for thirteen years and yet never been properly diagnosed or treated?

Mexico, like most of the countries in Latin America, is very heterogeneous. The quality of services available for different segments of the population varies greatly depending on socioeconomic status. In effect, this distribution of resources creates and reinforces an already solid caste system. The wealthy have access to a world-class education and healthcare, and in general enjoy a high quality of life; on the other hand, the poor, who often live in the same cities, cannot read—and die of treatable diseases simply because they lack access to existing resources.

Lucía lives in one of the communities served by the Partners in Health project in the state of Chiapas. The people in this area have been forgotten by society, and have never enjoyed the partial progress that other sectors of society have achieved. Given that Mexico is a middle-income country that already has medical systems in place, our work has focused not on creating parallel systems of care that obviate the responsibility of the government to provide medical care. Instead, we live alongside the people in their environment and work with them and with the government to negotiate improved systems that are community-based and responsive to the real needs of the people.

Several factors have contributed to Lucía's ongoing illness. First, the clinic in the community where she lives is seriously understaffed and often lacks even basic supplies. It is very difficult to find doctors who want to work and live in isolated communities that lack many of the modern amenities we take for granted, such as telecommunications and hot water on demand for bathing. When a doctor is assigned to these clinics, she or he often strives to be there for as little time as possible—a couple of days, or a month maximum. Almost all of the assigned doctors I have met said they viewed the assignment as a burden, counting the days on the calendar until they could return to their private practices in the city.

Second, official guidelines are only as good as their execution. The Ministry of Health considers TB a priority, and has established official guidelines for its diagnosis and management. These guidelines insist that all patients with a chronic cough should be screened for TB. A case is considered positive not only if there is a positive bacilloscopy (a microscopic examination of a sputum sample, which is a notoriously insensitive test), but also if there is clinical, radiologic, and epidemiologic evidence that is backed up by a physician. Under these criteria, Lucía could and should have been diagnosed and treated years ago, given that she had the characteristic symptoms, contact with other infected people in her family, and a suggestive x-ray.

Third, a weak laboratory system weakened the quality of an already inadequate test. The few sputum samples that Lucía was able to give in her local clinic came back negative. Many TB cases are missed because an individual sputum sample produced a false-negative result. Perhaps it was due to the shortcuts taken by the doctors collecting the sample, such as dividing a single sample into three specimens instead of taking three consecutive samples? Perhaps Lucía's samples were not appropriately managed—waiting on a shelf for two or three weeks before being analyzed? Perhaps the technician who looked at her sample stained it incorrectly, or looked at it for only a few seconds and then quickly gave up looking for the microbes because he was overworked or simply inattentive? These are all important operational reasons for the false-negative test, but for me, the issue goes even deeper.

For diseases like TB that speak of poverty and neglect, it is more convenient to *not* find cases than to find them. It looks better for the health system to conclude that Lucía does not have TB, and then go along with business as usual. Thus, no efforts were ever made to thoroughly investigate her chronic bloody cough; no importance was given to the fact that her sister had died of TB; and Lucía never got sent from her community clinic to get an x-ray or further studies (the x-ray she received was from a private doctor). If these efforts had been made, and the case had been accurately diagnosed as TB, the system would have been obliged to apply the lab resources, medicines, and personnel necessary to solve it, using a strict DOTS protocol. This is more expensive than doing nothing, and it requires a medical infrastructure that is missing in Lucía's neck of the Sierra Madre Mountains. So instead, a negative sputum result was an easy justification to deny her condition in a bureaucratic system where the patient sometimes matters less than the official statistics.

THE VULTURES

So what are the options for a patient like Lucía?

Pain and disease are a reality for everybody at some point in life, but pain and disease with general despair, with no means of relief, is a reality for billions of people in the world. The right to receive medical care must be universal, because the alternative of denying medical care for economic reasons to those who need it most—but cannot pay for it—leaves people to suffer and die needlessly. For me, this is indeed one of the worst forms of what has been termed *structural violence*, which means that the way structures in society are set up translates into a form of violence on people.[34] Having seen someone die needlessly, one feels deeply just how cruel structural violence can be. As a physician working for the poor, I see this too often, and it never ceases to amaze me how brutal the world can be.

Forgotten populations are neglected not only in healthcare, but also in education. Without the education to navigate medical bureaucracies, people are often ill equipped to question doctors, interpret medical advice, and advocate for themselves. Without understanding, how can they make informed life-or-death decisions?

This neglect by the system leaves marginalized populations at the mercy of medical con men, charlatans, snake oil salesmen, unregulated private doctors, and pseudo-doctors. In our area, this can take many forms. It could be another poor community member who tries to earn a living by selling fictitious "miracle" products, such as high-priced vitamins claiming to cure paralysis. It could also be a fee-for-service, fully licensed doctor who owns the pharmacy connected to his clinic and, perhaps due to poor training, poor ethics, or simply perverse incentives, will charge patients unreasonably high fees for inadequate care, and will order unnecessary studies and treatments. (I was amazed to once see the report of an ultrasound for *herpes zoster*, and another ultrasound report for earwax.) These treatments often add up to obscene prices, sometimes up to $500 US, which can be up to 50 percent of a family's yearly income! All of these people knowingly take advantage of the poor, whose need and also the lack of basic health literacy leaves them vulnerable to such criminal acts. The government has few mechanisms to regulate and supervise private healthcare. Through the years, Lucía had numerous encounters with these types of providers, taking different and irregular treatments, which may have left her TB bacilli resistant to the antibiotics that she received incorrectly.

THE SYSTEM: AN ABYSS OF BUREAUCRACY

In various interviews, government officers from the Ministry of Health at the local level have told me that they are well aware of these phenomena, but are "unable to proceed" because citizens have made no formal complaints. Taking into consideration that these citizens often do not know they are being deceived, that they do not know the formal mechanism through which to file a complaint, that the offices are usually hours away from their homes, and that their previous experiences with the government have not resulted in anything positive, this perspective can be viewed as passively abdicating the need to help. The government officer, my colleague, is right that democracy works best when engaged citizens dialogue with responsive government staff. I'm afraid that this dialogue doesn't happen because the two groups can never actually sit at the same table.

To date, Lucía has remained invisible—but we are trying to shed some light on her situation. We work with local partners, including both community and government groups, to strengthen the availability and quality of local services. On paper, the Mexican healthcare system is great—it provides free care to the poorest and aims for 100 percent coverage. The group of people with whom I work, Compañeros en Salud, believes that if this free and patient-responsive care actually gets to the poorest, then many injustices will be corrected. We work hard every day to ensure that this happens, but Lucía's story shows us just how difficult this can be sometimes. Part of the challenge of working in a country like Mexico is that everybody has done enough to meet the minimum requirements for their job, but nobody was incentivized to see that the sum of their actions actually achieved a good outcome for the patient. Once I hear Lucía tell me that she is back to health, I'll know that we've truly done our job. It will be a result of which we can all be proud—no one should accept the idea that mediocrity is enough for the poor and sick.

In the highly marginalized Chiapanecan communities where we work, the situation is difficult. The 2006 PHR survey conducted in indigenous communities included a question about chronic cough to screen for the possibility of active TB. The researchers then collected sputum samples from those over age fifteen who had chronic cough. In the forty-six communities studied, 29 cases of active TB were found, of which only 13 had previously been detected by health services. This rate of detection is far below the World Health Organization recommendation of 75 percent for adequate control of the disease. The data also suggest an extremely high rate of TB in these communities, more than ten times the reported rate for the country as a whole. Of the 29 cases, 4 had not received any medical care. Of those who did receive medical care, only 13 had been diagnosed with TB. Of those 13, only 6 were receiving appropriate treatment.[35] A follow-up study in similar communities found a rate of secondary MDR-TB of 29.2 percent, an alarmingly high percentage.[36]

Although the Mexican TB system has made significant efforts to address the problem, these facts suggest that the number of TB cases detected does not appear to be falling in the most affected and neglected populations. This situation will remain as long as physicians and other frontline health workers continue to experience systemic barriers to treating patients. These barriers include the occasional shortages of medications, the difficulty in ordering more sophisticated laboratory tests to make a diagnosis accurately or to detect drug resistance, and the inability to easily reach out to patients who have been "lost to follow-up."

Chagas Disease

A second example of a disease almost entirely associated with poverty and poor housing in Chiapas is Chagas disease. Also called *American trypanosomiasis*, the disease is caused by a blood-borne parasite, *Trypanosoma cruzi*. The reduviid bug, which lives in houses made of thatch, palm leaves or mud, transmits it. A small proportion of cases are transmitted in childbirth or by blood transfusion. Most new infections are in children, and in the vast majority of cases, there are no symptoms in the early phase of the infection. In a substantial proportion of those infected, the parasites slowly damage the heart or the gastrointestinal system and begin to produce symptoms twenty to thirty years later. In Mexico, the manifestations are almost entirely related to heart damage. Those affected begin to have signs of heart failure often as young adults (ages thirty to forty). The heart failure can, over several years, become completely disabling, with patients unable to do even minimal physical work. There is no cure, and almost everyone with this type of *cardiomyopathy* will eventually die of the disease.

Chagas disease is a classic example of a *neglected tropical disease* because relatively little research money is dedicated to finding a cure or improving treatment. Diseases such as this remain neglected probably because the people who get them are not involved in the political and economic processes that determine how research money is spent, and won't be able to pay for treatment even if available.

Nevertheless, Chagas disease can be prevented by a combination of insecticides and improved housing. South America, for example, has made great strides in controlling the disease using these methods.[37] Mexico has begun some control efforts since the early 2000s with a specific program committed to epidemiologic vigilance and promotion of better housing. However, these efforts have not reached all communities at risk for transmission; studies from 2001 of the prevalence of positive blood tests for infection with trypanosomiasis have shown high proportions of infection in several highland and jungle areas of Chiapas.[38] A small study of the patient population of the Doctors for Global Health–supported hospital in Altamirano has suggested that Chagas disease is likely to be the most common cause of heart failure in some of the indigenous populations in Chiapas.[39] Although the Secretary of Health may be making valuable efforts to combat Chagas disease and ensure that it doesn't enter the blood available for transfusions,[40] Chagas is still significant in Chiapas, as poverty continues to be a major reality in many people's lives.[41]

Modern and Traditional Medicine[42]

Framing Illness in Mexico: Hot and Cold

Many foreign clinicians, and even some Mexican clinicians who grew up in urban environments, are perplexed by the way many Mexican patients describe their symptoms and what they believe to be the cause. Several disease theories are part of the "folk knowledge" one encounters throughout Latin America. For example, disease states such as *susto* and *nervios* are blamed for one's poor health. Symptoms are described as *dolor de los riñones* or *de los pulmones* (kidney or lung pain) to locate the pain, but the pain may actually have no relation to these organs. Symptoms may be due to *aire* (air), and pain may move around the body like a scampering animal. Foods, medicines, and the environment are described as either *caliente* (hot) or *frío* (cold), with often confusing inconsistencies. (Most medicines are believed to be *caliente*, which explains why they cause side effects, but a cool glass of water in the wrong situation can cause serious diseases).

The hot-cold dichotomy is probably the most common and essential to understand. It would be a mistake, however, to think that these beliefs are "wrong," and to simply dismiss them as folk medicine. Instead, they represent a complex system of understanding and interacting with the world that has been influenced by history, and is reinforced daily though important social relations. Though it defies easy definition, the belief system is largely based on the principle that health is maintained when the body is both internally balanced and externally harmonized with the natural world and society. Anthropologists have studied the origin of these ideas, and the most powerful influence seems to be the Hippocratic-Galenic humoral theory of medicine that came to the New World with the Spanish; this is in opposition to the idea that the belief system is an indigenous tradition that has persisted despite the conquest, though its almost immediate adoption suggests that it probably did reinforce some already key indigenous concepts. Some pre-Columbian practices, such as the traditional ceremonial steam bath, continue to be used by contemporary indigenous populations to manipulate body temperature for therapeutic ends.* This practice dates back thousands of years, suggesting that, as in much of Latin America, what we see today is an inextricable combination of influences from Amerindian and European cultures; although not all Mexicans use steam baths, many even nonindigenous Latin Americans will describe their health in terms of the balance between hot and cold influences.

Perhaps what makes the logic of the contemporary hot-cold system so complex for novices is that it is not necessarily a way to diagnose and treat, but rather it serves as a method of validating traditional remedies. In this way, information about which herb, pill, or food is recommended for various symptoms is passed along via word of mouth. The patient will take the prescription and pay close attention to its effect in the body. Whether the prescription has worked will be rationalized through the principles of hot and cold ("yes, this herb worked because it was cold and the disease was very hot"). For each individual, family, and group, consensus on the issue is built and rebuilt with each new experience. This consensus might differ within families, from family to family, or from one village to the next. But some rules are hard and fast, and will even maintain striking similarities across different Latin American countries.

The reason for the persistence of these belief systems is probably that the basic principles are simple and easy to understand, but the infinite permutations allow for considerable discussion and consensus building. In our experience, we have seen how this discussion builds community and fortifies relationships. It can also cause considerable strife between those who are dogmatic about their disagreement. For the neophyte, it's better to enter these conversations with an open ear and an inquisitive mindset—this might be a way to get deeper into people's lives and build trust on their own terms.

NOTE

* K. Groark, "Vital Warmth and Well-being: Steambathing as Household Therapy among the Tzeltal and Tzotzil Maya of Highland Chiapas, Mexico," *Social Science and Medicine* 61 (2005):785–795.

An Exploration of Mexico's Improving Child Health

For decades, the death rate for Mexican children has been dropping. Reducing mortality in children is MDG 4, and Mexico is one of the few countries on track to meet the set goal by 2015.[43] Because children are such a vulnerable population, especially newborns and children under age five, their death rate is a major indicator of a variety of factors ranging from the strength of the public health system to the degree of overall poverty in certain segments of the society.

Under-five mortality encompasses three main indicators: (1) newborns who die within a few weeks of being born, (2) infants who die within the first year of life, and (3) toddlers who die before their fifth birthday. Each group of children is more likely to die of different causes: newborns and infants are most likely to succumb to complications resulting from a traumatic birth, low birth weight, congenital abnormalities, or infections; older children under age five are more likely to succumb to pneumonia, diarrhea, vaccine-preventable diseases if they are not immunized, and malnutrition. To save the oldest children, we must provide services such as antibiotics, oral rehydration solution (ORS), immunizations, improved nutrition, and vitamins—all relatively possible with only minor investments and crucial changes in the economy. To save the youngest children, including newborns, we must improve the health of pregnant women, improve the options that pregnant women have when giving birth, and provide access to cesarean sections and neonatal care—all relatively complicated and expensive interventions.

Some Mexican professionals ascribe much of the improvement in childhood mortality to key interventions implemented by the government health system. Influenced by the principles of *selective primary healthcare* (SPHC),[44] the interventions have centered on the GOBI-FFF strategy: first, GOBI (growth monitoring, ORS for diarrhea, breastfeeding exclusively in the first six months of life, immunizations) and then FFF (family planning, female education, feeding programs for malnourished children). This is in opposition to the strategy of *comprehensive primary healthcare*, as advised at the famous WHO meeting at Alma Ata in 1978 and best exemplified by the successes of the Cuban and Costa Rican health systems.[45] To say it simply, selective primary healthcare does the minimum necessary to achieve key aspired outcomes for priority diseases while controlling costs in the process; comprehensive primary healthcare focuses on the broader risks and processes involved in keeping people and communities sick or healthy, and then considers the investments needed to achieve priority goals.

Nevertheless, one curious observation is that the decline in childhood mortality in Mexico began years before even the first selective intervention was put in place, and some interventions, such as the immunization campaigns, came only after crises such as the epidemic outbreak of measles in the late 1980s. What other factors were playing a role? This is interesting to consider because it allows us to reflect on the general societal and economic processes that are also critically important to keeping people healthy.

Perhaps being Mexican has something to do with it? Some anthropologists point to the positive attributes of Mexican culture, especially the strong family unit and self-care practices, and think that these might explain the *healthy migrant effect* observed in the United States (where Mexican immigrants are healthier than other minority groups in similarly poor socioeconomic situations).[46] It's easy to see how these cultural practices might also benefit a child's health while still in Mexico. Yet these practices are likely centuries old, and child mortality only began to decrease decades ago. Culture is important, but the probable reality that culture was beneficial for many years before children started surviving longer makes it difficult to say that culture *caused* the improvements in child survival.

It's unclear how much of an impact the oil boom and subsequent increase in government spending during the 1970s affected the health of Mexico's children. Nevertheless, even after the neoliberal structural reforms of the 1980s gutted the public health institutions, the improvements in child mortality persisted. In addition, with the neoliberal reforms also came a concurrent widening of the gap between the richest and the poorest, as evidenced by Mexico's worsening Gini coefficient that increased until it peaked in the late 1990s.[47]

Although it is generally accepted that inequality drives disparities in health outcomes, not even worsening inequality would stop the improvements in childhood mortality. This suggests that some other safety valve, some other process, was giving sick and impoverished babies a fighting chance.

Conditional Cash Transfer Programs and Remittances

Certainly important to note is Mexico's experience with a *conditional cash transfer program* called Oportunidades (originally called Progresa). In this program, poor women are given monthly stipends in return for adherence to key indicators centered on health and human development: attending health talks, going to regular primary care visits, allowing their children to get the health interventions mentioned earlier, and keeping their children in primary school.[48] Though some find this program paternalistic,[49] most evidence suggests that it does empower the women[50] and benefit their children.[51] One study in particular found less anemia and improved growth in children of families enrolled in the program.[52] Indeed, it makes sense to assume that women who receive monthly stipends and participate in government health programs will have healthier and less malnourished children. But this program did not reach a large population until around the late 1990s, so this is only a recent benefit that still doesn't tell the entire story of improved child survival in Mexico.

From years of spending time in rural impoverished communities, we've seen that the remittances sent home to families from immigrant relatives who are working in the United States serve as another potentially important safety valve. We have heard farmers in our project sites refer to these remittances as "unconditional love cash transfers," a humorous term in opposition to the logic implicit behind the Oportunidades program. The statistics show a significant truth behind this phrase: remittances are often sent to the poorest families, and the money is often used on daily expenses such as food, clothing, and healthcare.[53] A dramatic increase in remittances occurred during the 1990s, rising from under 1 billion dollars total in 1984 to over 5.8 billion dollars in 2000.[54] Again, this doesn't provide the whole story, but it gives us another possible explanation.

Overall, it may simply be that as Mexico has developed and its economy has grown, Mexican children on average have benefited in a variety of ways. Some Mexican families, little by little, have probably had more options for first preventing illness in their children (for example, through an improved diet, improved hygiene practices, improved public services and sanitation, and completion of full vaccination regimens); and then more options for caring for their children if they did get sick (for example, through giving ORS or antibiotics). These numbers are averages, however, and do not reflect the reality that many of the most marginalized sectors of society have not benefited as much as others.

Epidemologic Transition

One factor in particular, the improved diet, deserves special mention because malnutrition of every kind has indeed decreased in Mexico,[55] and the greatest strategy to keep children healthy is to keep them well fed. But the Mexican diet is changing to one now high in fat and sugar. Long ago considered rare treats, cheap *chatara* (junk food) is often the main form of sustenance available to the poor. As a consequence, the once healthy *gordito* (chubby child) is now becoming obese and stunted.[56] The current generation of children, as it grows older, may unfortunately die younger than its parents' generation, from diseases such as diabetes and heart disease. This frightening phenomenon replays the inequalities that have always distinguished the health of the poor and rich, and it brings into question the very nature of what we consider progress and development. Even worse, these chronic noncommunicable diseases are coming before the classic infectious pandemics of the poor, such as infectious diarrhea, have receded. The shift from infectious to noninfectious diseases has been called the *epidemiologic transition*;[57] Mexico may have gotten better at saving kids' lives, but unfortunately, the kids then got stuck in an epidemiologic overlap.[58]

NAFTA and Associated Health Consequences

One of the most powerful influences on the Mexican diet and lifestyle has been the macroeconomic changes the country experienced with the adoption of neoliberalism and its flagship policy, the North American Free Trade Agreement. Despite the concerns expressed by many and the resistance demonstrated by groups such as the Zapatistas, the passing of NAFTA has allowed US products to flood into Mexico at reduced cost. The effects have been staggering. US chain stores are now in every major Mexican city, and US-owned brand names can be found in even the most isolated communities. US-style pop music tops the charts, and Hollywood movies can be viewed in large, plush Cineplexes. Obesity, especially childhood obesity, is skyrocketing. Many Mexican immigrants, returning home after working for years in the United States, have brought with them a desire for US products and have in turn influenced their neighbors' tastes. This, along with a growing desire to become a "first-world country" like the United States and European countries, has created a ripe market of consumers for many previously unavailable products.

To fully understand the impact of NAFTA on Mexico, one needs to understand that the way NAFTA was written and implemented favored the United States. Under NAFTA, unlike the free trade agreements in Europe, only goods and services, not unskilled labor, were included. This meant that although US products could freely enter Mexico, Mexican unskilled workers were given no new special contracts to work legally in the United States.[59] But the US economy relies heavily on the Mexican workforce, so without appropriate systems to monitor employment practices, most Mexican workers could easily get a job once they reached US soil. This usually meant having to pay elevated fees to smugglers to enter into the United States as undocumented laborers. This has been the status quo for years, and it is estimated that as of 2010, more than 11 million undocumented immigrants are living in the United States.[60] Despite their labor, however, few of these workers receive concurrent rights or benefits, even though usually over one-half contribute to US federal and state income taxes, social security taxes, and Medicare taxes. They pay into these programs because many purchase fake social security numbers in order to secure a job. Few questions are asked until later, when their salary deductions are flagged and put into a special category for all the other mismatched tax forms, called the Earnings Suspension File. It is impossible to know how many of the workers in this file are illegally in the United States.[61] Overall, it is estimated that illegal immigrants contribute up to $7 billion US to social security alone each year.[62]

Another example of how NAFTA has been unfavorable to Mexico is that US policy did not anticipate the consequences of key decisions on the Mexican economy. Free trade theoretically abolishes *levies*, or taxes on imports, as well as *subsidies*, or government aid to businesses. But the United States never stopped subsidizing US farmers. This created a skewed system in which cheap, subsidized US corn flooded Mexico and destabilized the Mexican corn industry. The country that first domesticated corn, and continues to use it as a staple food, suddenly became dependent on US corn imports.[63] When corn was later used to make biofuel, food prices soared, and many poor Mexicans were suddenly struggling to afford their daily tortillas.[64]

Indeed, the story of multinational corporations in Mexico is extremely relevant to the health trends being observed in modern Mexico. Coca-Cola, for example, is a major part of Mexican life today, as Mexicans are the second-largest consumers of the ubiquitous sweet drink (second only to consumers in the United States).[65] Though many Mexicans still live in poverty, the price of cola is usually well within reach of almost all segments of society. In many areas, it is actually cheaper and more readily available than purified water. Mexico is home to a wealth of natural freshwater springs and rivers that could conceivably provide potable tap water for large segments of society. Chiapas, for example, enjoys deep freshwater aquifers. Yet the main extraction of water in the colonial tourist town of San Cristobal is controlled by Coca-Cola, which received federal permits during the presidency of Vincente Fox (himself a former chief executive officer of Coca-Cola in Mexico) to pump at will for its bottling plant and pay no taxes or other compensation to the local government.[66] Because of the low price and agreeable taste, and due to the lack of fresh tap water, it's now common to see Mexican children drinking Coca-Cola for breakfast. It shouldn't be any wonder that in 2006, 24.3 percent of all young Mexicans between ages two and eighteen were classified as either obese or overweight.[67] As this generation ages, it risks record rates of obesity-related chronic diseases, such as diabetes, kidney disease, and heart disease. Diabetes in particular, if uncontrolled, is very debilitating and leads to complications that are expensive to treat. The costs are going to be a serious challenge for an already struggling medical system.

Nongovernmental Organizations

Since the Zapatista uprising in 1994, many NGOs have become involved in Chiapas doing a wide spectrum of work. This includes leading educational trips and exchanges, as well as advocating for human rights, social and economic justice, women's rights, and nonviolent conflict resolution. In 2006, EZLN formed La Otra Campaña to strengthen its ties to other parts of civil society in Mexico, especially human rights advocates, trade unions, and students' and women's rights groups. There are also many organizations and individual supporters of the Zapatista communities, other indigenous communities, and poor and isolated nonindigenous communities.

The international opinion about NGOs is varied, and runs the gamut of those who consider them agile and free-moving entities that can serve the neediest populations when governments fail to do so,[68] to those who blame NGOs for a neocolonial manipulation of vulnerable segments of the society for their own personal, selfish, even imperialist agendas.[69] All NGOs behave in different ways, and may even behave in varied ways within a single organization, depending on the community or the initiative. Although no clear guidelines exist concerning what constitutes a "good" or "bad" NGO, there are a few key principles to which all organizations should adhere. Websites such as charitynavigator.com will help in sorting out which NGOs are worthy of your partnership, and which are mere "beltway bandits." This is a descriptive, derogatory term reserved for groups that sometimes have offices in the beltway around Washington, DC, and receive large amounts of US foreign aid money that was given in goodwill, but then was squandered on high overhead costs, lush office spaces, and disproportionate salaries for expatriate staff. Such behavior historically has translated into little benefit for the poor people who appear in the classic NGO "glossy reports."[70] A "good" NGO not only will receive a high rating from independent evaluators like Charity Navigator, but also will be involved in activities that maximize benefit for people on the ground instead of for staff.

We will now give more details on two NGOs with which we currently work in healthcare, in two very different communities in Chiapas. Although no group is perfect, we are proud of the work of these NGOs, and we want to discuss why we feel they make a difference.

Doctors for Global Health

Doctors for Global Health works in the municipality of Altamirano with Hospital San Carlos (HSC). DGH supports the community health program of the hospital and also sends volunteers to work in the hospital and the communities. HSC was founded in 1969 by American nuns in order to serve the local population of indigenous Mayas, and was handed over shortly afterward to Mexican nuns of the Daughters of Charity of St. Vincent de Paul. The hospital is located in the town of Altamirano, which encompasses a population of approximately 10,000 people, but patients usually come to the hospital from more than 400 surrounding villages. HSC has twenty-four to thirty beds each in its adult and pediatric wards, in addition to a six-bed labor and postpartum ward. There is an adult isolation unit and a two-bed pediatric isolation unit for patients with active TB who need to be isolated from other patients to avoid infecting them. The outpatient clinic sees about 1,000 to 1,200 visits per month.

Several years ago, the Mexican government built a public hospital in Altamirano, but indigenous patients are often unwilling to use government facilities because of the lack of available interpreters (many of the indigenous patients seen in Altamirano speak Tzeltal, Tzotzil, Tojolabal, or Chol exclusively, although some are bilingual in Spanish). In addition to these concerns, many potential patients say they avoid the Mexican state hospital system because of their doubts about the quality of care delivered in these facilities.

DGH supports the community health program of HSC, which works in five of the autonomous Zapatista municipalities. The goal of the program is to train village health workers (health promoters) who do preventive care including vaccination campaigns, prenatal care, and treatment of minor illnesses. The Mexican physician who directs this program is training and supervising approximately 100 health promoters among these municipalities. Because these communities are "in resistance" and do not accept healthcare from the Mexican public health system, the health promoters and the physician do most routine medical care with backup from HSC. (The box "Putting Liberation Medicine into Practice" describes in more detail how DGH works with the

Zapatista communities). These communities have a very strong autonomous governing structure, the Junta de Buen Gobierno, and all of the training and health work is approved by the JBG. Volunteers who want to work in the communities must be aware of the cultural issues and linguistic barriers, and any new project must be formally presented to the JBG and be approved before any work in the community can start.

Putting Liberation Medicine into Practice
DR. JUAN MANUEL CANALES, Community Physician

In the construction of autonomous communities, health plays a strategic role in protecting the rights of everyone, whenever they have been—and are being—violated and ignored by past and current governments in Mexico. The indigenous people in Chiapas took up arms in December 1994 against the marginalization and discrimination they had been suffering since colonial times. Their actions brought attention to the theft of their lands and the looting of natural resources. Yet the people continue to live in extreme poverty eighteen years after the armed uprising. They achieved partial recovery of their lands and forced the government to respect their rights; however, the current government continues to disregard the agreements of San Andrés Larráizar signed by President Ernesto Zedillo (1994–2000).

The government continues to make war in a different manner, using social programs supported and financed by the World Bank, the International Monetary Fund, and various United Nations organizations such as the World Health Organization and the UN Development Program. The funds that come from these programs are often used to reward supporters of the party in power, who are the first to benefit from loans for businesses and projects to improve housing. Development projects promoted by the federal government and the state of Chiapas, such as ecotourism projects and healthcare initiatives, are often designed in offices of development officials without much input from the communities that will be directly affected. These programs may provide individual assistance but don't actually empower communities. They are perceived by the people as violating the right to health and education, and as showing a lack of respect for their customs and ability to organize their own communities.

This situation is complicated by the federal government's war on drug trafficking, supported and financed by the US government, which is being

used to intimidate and terrorize communities and to demobilize any social movement that is struggling to resist militarization of civilian life and
the loss of the sense of ownership of the lands inherited from their ancestors. These factors make it difficult to construct autonomous communities, but we have chosen to accompany them in their struggle because we
know that their demands are just.

HOW WE SUPPORT AND ACCOMPANY THE AUTONOMOUS
HEALTH SYSTEM AND PRACTICE LIBERATION MEDICINE

We do this through medical education and the practice of community
medicine. We train and accompany health promoters (men and women);
we accompany them in their effort to build what *they* want, not what *we*
want. As health professionals, we believe in medical science and the scientific method, but we also break with some of the paradigms of medicine, and discover new ones as we think together as a group in search
of the common good. We share our accumulated knowledge. We learn
from practical experience, through observation and common sense, and
popular action.

We have many problems, including the threats of paramilitary groups,
and difficulties with local governmental authorities and the Mexican army.
There is government persecution, repression, and imprisonment of activists who are trying to develop their autonomous municipalities. We also
face the lack of material resources, medications, classrooms for teaching,
books, and housing, and sometimes water shortages. We don't let these
create obstacles to educating people about health. We use participatory
methods of teaching to work with people who barely read and write, and
who speak another language (Tzeltal and Tojolabal). This is not a major
obstacle, because the real barriers of inequality and social injustice are
being broken by all of us. We, the outsiders, identify with their demands
for justice, freedom, and democracy. We unite with them to strengthen
their struggles to defend their culture. We support them in defending
their territory, disobeying, and resisting. Much of this support is simply
being there, eating and sleeping in their homes, and talking with them
about their daily lives—how they plant corn and beans, or harvest coffee.
We know their families; we know why they are often ill with problems that
don't affect more prosperous communities. We see how much more difficult than ours their life is.

The health promoters choose topics for training classes, and design
the construction of the autonomous model of health. We can suggest

and propose, but we do not impose our will. Over the years that we have been accompanying the people, they have constructed, deconstructed, and reconstructed again, but have never stopped looking for new forms to advance their work. They continue to find ways to deliver basic preventive and curative care without forgetting the traditional medicine passed down from their ancestors.

At times, we feel we can see the results of popular education in health. We watch the promoters confronting health problems in their communities with humility, patience, calm, and confidence, trying to help people who come to seek relief. It strengthens us and encourages us to continue supporting and accompanying them in this effort to share experiences and wisdom.

One particular initiative deserves mention. We have continued to report new cases of TB. The number during the year 1997 was 125, and ranged from 47 to 127 in the subsequent years from 1998 to 2010. The number of new cases does not appear to be decreasing. This represents only the patients who are able to come to the hospital. The expense of transportation from their isolated communities prevents people from seeking medical care and returning to the hospital for follow-up visits. During the late 1990s, approximately 40 percent of patients did not complete treatment. As explained earlier in the section on TB, DOTS is the recommended strategy for treating and following patients, but this has not been possible because of lack of resources for long-term community-based projects. In addition, many patients come from very small, isolated rural communities. In 2000, Doctors of the World Switzerland began a project to help patients pay the cost of diagnostic tests and transportation to return for follow-up visits. Much more investigation of contacts was done too, causing the number of documented new cases to increase in 2005. Also, the rate of patients' not completing treatment fell to 6.5 percent.

Partners in Health

Partners in Health has been supporting work in Chiapas since the early 1980s, when one of the founders, Paul Farmer, still a student at Harvard Medical School, was introduced to an NGO working to help Guatemalan refugees who had fled into Chiapas to escape the genocide in their home country. For decades, PIH continued to support the work through financial and technical assistance. In 2005, Hurricane Stan devastated the communities in the southeastern part of Chiapas. In response, PIH gave renewed attention to marginalized communities in this area, the Sierra Madre Mountains. The villages in this area are small (with an average of only 50 to 100 families per community) and boast several health facilities, but they have only precarious mountain dirt roads as the main route of transport. People live in this inhospitable area because when land reforms after the Mexican revolution opened the territory for the formation of ejidos, many people came flooding in from the coffee plantations on the coast. They were once part of the Mam indigenous group, but now they speak only Spanish after a policy of forced "Mexicanization" during the 1930s. This process occurred when the Mam peasants were forced to burn their traditional clothing, and vow never again to speak Mam, in exchange for food and education. The Mam were targeted because they occupied both Mexican and Guatemalan territories; when the southern Mexican border was finally drawn in 1882, decisions were made concerning how the resources would be divided among the ruling elite and landholders, without considering how or where the indigenous majority lived. Making the Mam Mexican was just another way to seal the southern border.[71]

Because of the area's remoteness and low population density, the PIH project has focused on a model of patient-centered care that is based in the community. In addition, as its name implies, PIH is always looking for partners in building ever-stronger efforts. In Chiapas, the local PIH chapter Compañeros en Salud–Mexico (CES) is working to strengthen existing government clinics in remote areas by improving staffing, assuring a consistent supply chain, and engaging in participatory community outreach. CES is also partnering with Mexican medical schools to recruit social service–year physicians and provide them with a unique package of training and support throughout the year that sets them up to succeed in serving patients.

Another key way that PIH partners with communities is through hiring and training community health workers to build strong linkages between community members and the local clinic. CHWs are leaders selected by their community who are tasked with accompanying patients living with chronic diseases such as diabetes, hypertension, epilepsy, asthma, and mental health disorders. CHWs conduct regular home visits, and often accompany patients on their visits to the clinic. Project physicians, nurses, and *acompañantes* work together as a clinical team, each contributing crucial tasks and insights to a patient's care. When on-site, everyone eats the same meals (usually only black beans and tortillas) and uses the same quality of resources (bathrooms, sleeping arrangements, and so on). With this structure, the clinical team management is truly horizontal, meaning that every contribution is valued and decisions about strategy are made as a group. At best, this model allows the team to be a nimble, conscientious, responsive entity that seeks to strengthen the social safety net. The site is also a clinical training site for talented medical students and residents from both Mexican and US medical schools.

Final Thoughts and Advice

Mexico is a profoundly diverse, complicated country that defies easy categorization. One of the main challenges, and great pleasures, of working in Mexico is this very reality. As a final piece of advice, we offer this rule of thumb: when in Mexico, assume that what you are seeing is more complex than it appears, and assume that you don't know the whole story. Mexicans have become accustomed to foreigners who confidently and arrogantly act as if they already understand Mexico. To these visitors, Mexico will stay hidden. By assuming that you don't know, you will learn more. Listen before you speak, and speak less than you normally would; your Mexican colleagues will appreciate you for it. Whether this is your first trip or one after many, the richness of Mexico should always be a source of fascination, and the people may become some of the truest friends you've ever had.

Notes

1 Library of Congress–Federal Research Division, "Country Profile: Mexico" (July 2008), accessed Dec. 9, 2011, available from http://lcweb2.loc.gov/frd/cs.

2 O. Paz, *The Labyrinth of Solitude: The Other Mexico, Return to the Labyrinth of Solitude, Mexico and the United States, the Philanthropic Ogre* (New York: Grove Press, 1985).

3 *Enciclopedia de Los Municipios y Delegaciones de México Estado de Chiapas* (Mexico: INAFED Instituto para el Federalismo y el Desarrollo Municipal/SEGOB Secretaría de Gobernación, 2010), accessed Aug. 3, 2012, available from www.e-local .gob.mx.

4 D. M. Coerver, S. B. Pasztor, and R. Buffington, *Mexico: An Encyclopedia of Contemporary Culture and History* (Santa Barbara, CA: ABC-CLIO, 2004).

5 J. Gledhill, "'The People's Oil': Nationalism, Globalization, and the Possibility of Another Country in Brazil, Mexico, and Venezuela," *European Journal of Anthropology* 52 (2008):57–74.

6 A. Reding, "Aztec Sun Rising: The Cárdenas Challenge," *World Policy Journal* 14.3 (1997):63–70.

7 D. Earle and J. Simonelli, *Uprising of Hope* (Lanham, MD: Altamira Press, 2005).

8 S. O'Neil, "The Real War in Mexico: How Democracy Can Defeat the Drug Cartels," *Foreign Affairs* 88.4 (2009):63–77.

9 V. Ríos and D. Shirk, "Drug Violence in Mexico: Data and Analysis through 2010, Special Report" (San Diego, CA: Trans-Border Institute, Joan B. Kroc School of Peace Studies, University of San Diego, Feb. 1, 2011), available from http://justice inmexico.files.wordpress.com.

10 V. G. Burnett, "Protestantism in Latin America," *Latin American Research Review* 27.1 (1992):218–230.

11 J. S. Passel and D. Cohn, "Unauthorized Immigrant Population: National and State Trends, 2010" (Pew Hispanic Center Publications, 2011), accessed Dec. 23, 2011, available from http://pewhispanic.org.

12 T. Rudel and J. Roper, "The Paths to Rain Forest Destruction: Crossnational Patterns of Tropical Deforestation, 1975–1990," *World Development* 25 (1997):53–65; and J. Alix-Garcia, A. De Janvry, and E. Sadoulet, "A Tale of Two Communities: Explaining Deforestation in Mexico," *World Development* 33.2 (2005):219–235.

13 United Nations Development Program, *Regional Human Development Report for Latin America and the Caribbean 2010: Acting on the Future: Breaking the Intergenerational Transmission of Inequality* (New York: UNDP, 2010), accessed Dec. 23, 2011, available from http://hdr.undp.org.

14 D. Luhnow, "The Secrets of the World's Richest Man," *Wall Street Journal* (Aug. 4, 2007), available from http://online.wsj.com.

15 World Bank, website, accessed December 1, 2012, http://data.worldbank.org/country/mexico.

16 Instituto Nacional de Estadística y Geografía, "Pérfil Sociodemográfico de la Población que Habla Lengua Indígena" (2009), accessed Dec. 23, 2011, available from www.inegi.org.mx.

17 Consejo Nacional de Población, "Indices de Marginación 2005" (monograph, D.F. México 2006), accessed Dec. 23, 2011, available from www.conapo.gob.mx.

18 P. Farmer, *Pathologies of Power* (Berkeley, CA: University of California Press, 2005).

19 J. Frenk, E. Gonzalez-Pier, O. Gómez-Dantés, M. A. Lezana, and F. M. Knaul, "Comprehensive Reform to Improve Health System Performance in Mexico," *Lancet* 368.9546 (2006):1524–1534.

20 Organization for Economic Cooperation and Development, "OECD Health Data 2012: How Does Mexico Compare" (2011), accessed Dec. 9, 2011, available from www.oecd.org.

21 Knaul, Felicia Marie, Eduardo González-Pier, Octavio Gómez-Dantés, et al., "The Quest for Universal Health Coverage: Achieving Social Protection for All in Mexico," *Lancet* 380.9849 (2012):1259–1279.

22 J. Lakin, "The End of Insurance? Mexico's Seguro Popular, 2001–2007," *Journal of Health Politics, Policy and Law* 35.3 (2010):313–352.

23 N. Homedes and A Ugalde, "Twenty-Five Years of Convoluted Health Reforms in Mexico," *PLoS Medicine*, 6.8 (2009):e1000124.

24 O. Galárraga, S. G. Sosa-Rubí, A. Salinas-Rodríguez, and S. Sesma-Vásquez, "Health Insurance for the Poor: Impact on Catastrophic and Out-of-Pocket Health Expenditures in Mexico," *European Journal of Health and Economics* 11 (2010):437–447.

25 Organización Panamericana de la Salud, "Indicadores Básicos de Salud 2000–2008," Secretaría de Salud (SSA), Subsecretaría de Innovación y Calidad, Dirección General de Información en Salud, D.F. México, accessed Dec. 23, 2011, available from http://new.paho.org/mex.

26 Physicians for Human Rights, "Excluded People, Eroded Communities: Realizing the Right to Health in Chiapas, Mexico" (2006), accessed Dec. 9 and 23, 2011, available from www.phr.org.

27 H. J. Sánchez Pérez, M. Hernán, A. Ríos-González, M. Arana-Cedeño, A. Navarro,

D. Ford et al., "Malnutrition among Children Under Five Years of Age in Conflict Zones of Chiapas, Mexico," *American Journal of Public Health* 97.2 (2007):229–232.

28 G. S. Laveaga, "'Let's Become Fewer': Soap Operas, Contraception, and Nationalizing the Mexican Family in an Overpopulated World," *Sexuality Research and Social Policy* 4.3 (2007):19–33; A. Nazar-Beutelspacher, D. Halperin-Frisch, and B. Salvatierra-Izaba, "Effectos de las Practices Anticonceptivas sobre la Fecundidad en la Región Fronteriza de Chiapas, Mexico," *Salud Pública de México* 3.8 (1996):13–19; and A. Nazar-Beutelspacher, D. Molina-Rosales, B. Salvatierra-Izaba, E. Zapata-Martelo, and D. Halperin, "La Educación y el No Uso de Anticonceptivos entre Mujeres de Bajo Nivel Socioeconómico en Chiapas," *Perspectivas Internacionales en Planificación Familiar* 1999:9–15.

29 J. D. Kirsch and M. A. Cedeño, "Informed Consent for Family Planning for Poor Women in Chiapas, Mexico," *Lancet* 354.9176 (1999):419–420.

30 D. C. Mitnick, S. S. Shin, K. J. Seung, M. Rich, S. Atwood, J. Furin et al., "Comprehensive Treatment of Extensively Drug-Resistant Tuberculosis," *New England Journal of Medicine* 359 (2008):563–574.

31 TB can also present as an enlarged lymph node commonly called *scrofula*, or in a variety of other extrapulmonary presentations (outside of the lungs), but these are much less common. Although most Mexicans receive a vaccine for the disease, called the BCG vaccine, this doesn't protect them from either the latent or active form of the disease. The vaccine probably only decreases the chance of the active disease going to the central nervous system and causing meningitis.

32 M. de Lourdes Garcí-García, A. Pance-de-León, M. E. Jiménez-Corona, A. Jiménez-Corona, M. Palacios-Martínez, S. Balandro-Campos et al., "Clinical Consequences and Transmissibility of Drug-Resistant Tuberculosis in Southern Mexico," *Archives of Internal Medicine* 160 (2000): 630–636.

33 I. Reyes-Guillén, H. J. Sánchez-Pérez, J. Cruz-Burguete, and M. Izaurieta-de Juan, "Anti-Tuberculosis Treatment Defaulting: An Analysis of Perceptions and Interactions in Chiapas, Mexico," *Salud Pública de México* 50.3 (2008):251–257.

34 P. Farmer, "On Suffering and Structural Violence: A View from Below" *Daedalus* 125.1 (1996):261–283.

35 Physicians for Human Rights, "Excluded People, Eroded Communities."

36 H. J. Sánchez-Pérez, A. Díaz-Vázquez, J. C. Nájera-Ortiz, S. Balandrano, and M. Martín-Mateo, "Multidrug-Resistant Pulmonary Tuberculosis in Los Altos, Selva and Norte Regions, Chiapas, Mexico," *International Journal of Tuberculosis and Lung Diseases* 14.1 (2010):34–39.

37 Y. Yamagata and J. Nakagawa, "Control of Chagas Disease," *Advances in Parasitology* 61 (2006):129–165.

38 M. A. Mazariego-Arana, V. M. Monteón, M. A. Ballinas-Verdugo, N. Hernández-Becerril, R. Alejandre-Aguilar, and P. A. Reyes, "Seroprevalence of Human Trypanosoma Cruzi Infection in Different Geographic Zones of Chiapas, Mexico," *Revista de Sociedad de Medicina Tropical* 34.5 (2001):453–458.

39 L. Capps and B. Abad, "Chagas Cardiomyopathy and Serology in a Small Rural Hospital in Chiapas, Mexico," *Pan American Journal of Public Health* 15.5 (2004):337–340.

40 A. Attaran, "Chagas' Disease in Mexico," *Lancet* 368.9549 (2006):1768; and R. T. Conyer, "Chagas' Disease in Mexico–Response from the Mexican Ministry of Health," *Lancet* 368.9549 (2006):1768–1769.

41 P. J. Hotez, M. E. Bottazzi, C. Franco-Paredes, S. K. Ault, and M. R. Periago, "The Neglected Tropical Diseases of Latin America and the Caribbean: A Review of Disease Burden and Distribution and a Roadmap for Control and Elimination," *PLoS Neglected Tropical Diseases* 2.9 (2008):e300, doi:10.1371/journal.pntd.0000300.

42 G. M. Foster, *Hippocrates' Latin American Legacy* (Langhorne, PA: Gordon and Breach, 1994); and A. J. Rubel, C. W. O'Nell, R. Collado-Ardón, and A. Susto, *Folk Illness* (Berkeley, CA: University of California Press, 1984).

43 J. Sepúlveda, F. Bustreo, R. Tapia, J. Rivera, R. Lozano, G. Oláiz et al., "Improvement of Child Survival in Mexico: The Diagonal Approach," *Lancet* 368.9551 (2006):2017–2027.

44 J. A. Walsh and K. S. Warren, "Selective Primary Health Care: An Interim Strategy for Disease Control in Developing Countries," *New England Journal of Medicine* 301.18 (1979):967–974.

45 K. S. Warren, "The Evolution of Selective Primary Health Care," *Social Science and Medicine* 26 (1988):891–898.

46 A. Waldstein, "Popular Medicine and Self-Care in a Mexican Migrant Community: Toward an Explanation of an Epidemiological Paradox," *Medical Anthropology* 29.1 (2010):71–107.

47 Sepúlveda et al., "Improvement of Child Survival in Mexico," 2023.

48 Tina Rosenberg, "A Payoff Out of Poverty?" *New York Times* (Dec. 21, 2008), Section MM, 46.

49 V. Smith-Oka, "Unintended Consequences: Exploring the Tensions between Development Programs and Indigenous Women in Mexico in the Context of Reproductive Health," *Social Science and Medicine* 68 (2009):2069–2077.

50 S. L. Barber and P. J. Gertler, "Empowering Women to Obtain High Quality Care: Evidence from an Evaluation of Mexico's Conditional Cash Transfer Programme," *Health Policy and Planning* 24.1 (2009):18–25.

51 L. C. H. Fernald, P. J. Gertler, and L. M. Neufeld, "10-Year Effect of Oportunidades, Mexico's Conditional Cash Transfer Programme, on Child Growth, Cognition, Language, and Behaviour: A Longitudinal Follow-up Study," *Lancet* 374.9706 (2009):1997–2005.

52 J. A. Rivera, D. Sotres-Alvarez, J. Habicht, T. Shaman, and S. Villalpando, "Impact of the Mexican Program for Education, Health, and Nutrition (Progresa) on Rates of Growth and Anemia in Infants and Young Children: A Randomized Effectiveness Study," *JAMA* 291.21 (2004):2563–2570.

53 G. A. Zarate-Hoyos, "Consumption and Remittances in Migrant Households: Toward a Productive Use of Remittances, *Contemporary Economic Policy* 22.4 (2004):555–565.

54 J. Airola, "The Use of Remittance Income in Mexico," *International Migration Review* 41.4 (2007):850–859.

55 Sepúlveda et al., "Improvement of Child Survival in Mexico," 2021.

56 L. C. Fernald and L. M. Neufeld, "Overweight with Concurrent Stunting in Very

Young Children from Rural Mexico: Prevalence and Associated Factors," *European Journal of Clinical Nutrition* 61 (2007):623–632.

57 A. R. Omran, "The Epidemiologic Transition: A Theory of the Epidemiology of Population Change," *Milbank Memorial Fund Quarterly* 49.4 (1971):509–538.

58 S. C. Martínes and F. G. Leal, "Epidemiological Transition: Model or Illusion? A Look at the Problem of Health in Mexico," *Social Science and Medicine* 57 (2003):539–550.

59 World Bank, "Global Economic Prospects 2005: Trade, Regionalism, and Development" (monograph, Washington, DC: World Bank, 2005), 116, accessed Dec 9, 2011, available from http://books.google.com.mx.

60 Passel et al., "Unauthorized Immigrant Population."

61 The White House, "Economic Report of the President" (Washington, DC: US Government Printing Office, 2005), 107.

62 E. Porter, "Illegal Immigrants Are Bolstering Social Security with Billions," *New York Times* (Apr. 5, 2005), accessed Dec. 23, 2011, available from www.nytimes.com.

63 "Mexico Condemns Increase in US Agricultural Subsidies," *Mexico Economic News and Analysis on Mexico* (May 22, 2002), accessed Dec. 23, 2011, available from www.allbusiness.com.

64 W. Bello, "Manufacturing a Food Crisis," *The Nation* (June 2, 2008), accessed Dec. 23, 2011), available at www.thenation.com.

65 C. L. Gutiérrez-Ruvalcaba, E. Vásquez-Garibay, E. Romero-Velarde, R. Troyo-Sanromán, C. Cabrera-Pivaral, and O. Ramírez-Magaña, "Sweetened Beverages as a Risk Factor for Adolescent Obesity in Guadalajara, Mexico," *Boletín Médico del Hospital Infantil de México* Nov-Dec 2009:60.

66 J. Nash, "Consuming Interests: Water, Rum, and Coca-Cola from Ritual Propitiation to Corporate Expropriation in Highlands Chiapas," *Cultural Anthropology* 22.4 (2007):621–639.

67 J. A. Rivera, L. M. Irizarry, T. González-de Cossío, "Overview of the Nutritional Status of the Mexican Population in the Last Two Decades," *Salud Pública de México* 51.4 (2009): S645–S656.

68 D. C. Esty, "Non-Governmental Organizations at the World Trade Organization: Cooperation, Competition, or Exclusion," *Journal of International Economic Law* 1 (1998):123–147.

69 T. Nolutshungu, "Why I Am Bothered by Neo-colonialist NGOs," *Arusha Times* (May 3, 2008), available at www.arushatimes.co.tz; and I. Illich, "To Hell with Good Intentions" (speech, Cuernavaca, Mexico: Conference on InterAmerican Student Projects [CIASP], Apr. 20, 1968).

70 K. Day, "Riding Herd on the Bad Guy Image of 'Beltway Bandits,'" *Washington Post* (Feb. 9, 1994), B1.

71 R. A. Hernández Castillo, *Histories and Stories from Chiapas: Border Identities in Southern Mexico* (Austin, TX: University of Texas Press, 2001).

2 Guatemala

Peter Rohloff and Anne Kraemer Díaz

Diverse in language, culture, and landscape, Guatemala is an authentic blend of the modern and the ancient. Traditional and modern ways of life are constantly negotiated in crowded markets, on busy streets, and among small farm plots that dot the countryside. Guatemala is a common vacation destination and also a travel hub for Spanish learners, lovers of archaeological ruins, and volunteers. At the same time, for the indigenous Maya who constitute the majority of Guatemala's population, day-to-day life is often a struggle to put food on the table, to find access to healthcare, and to provide a steady income for the family.

In this chapter, we describe the difficult and complex historical and sociological features that determine the healthcare landscape in Guatemala, with a special focus on the needs of the country's Maya population. In particular, we use cases studies in chronic child malnutrition and adult type 2 diabetes to explore how effective healthcare programming can address the needs of indigenous people in Guatemala today.

Geography and Population

Guatemala is defined geographically by mountainous terrain in the central and western highlands. To the east and north, the landscape transitions to a lowland limestone plateau. Bordering Mexico to the north, the Pacific Ocean to the west and south, El Salvador to the southeast, and Honduras, Belize, and the Gulf of Honduras to the east, Guatemala is slightly smaller than the state of Tennessee at 108,890 square kilometers.[1]

The lowlands to the east and both coasts have a tropical climate. The highlands, on the other hand, range from warm to cool during the day and can be quite cold at night. There are two seasons: rainy from May to October, and dry from November to May. Four active and more than twenty dormant volcanoes span the Sierra Madre Mountains running north-south through the country. Rich biodiversity in flora and fauna is found throughout more than twenty different ecological zones. Because of such great ecological diversity, a wide range of cash crops and subsistence crops are grown in Guatemala. The main cash crops are coffee, sugar, bananas, cotton, cardamom, and cacao;

the main subsistence crops are corn, beans, fruits, and vegetables. As of this writing, broccoli, asparagus, spices, snow peas, and cauliflower are increasing as export crops. Coffee and sugar account for almost 50 percent of the labor demand in Guatemala, and coffee alone generates almost one-third of Guatemala's foreign exchange.[2] Tourism is also a large and growing industry, and is probably the most important segment of the economy in the highlands and core archeological region. Additionally, remittances sent from immigrants in the United States home to their families in Guatemala made up 10 percent of GDP in 2008, although these numbers may currently be waning because of recent, more aggressive US immigration and deportation policies.[3]

Guatemala is one of the most populous countries in Central America, with over 14 million people. However, the GDP per capita is only about one-half of the regional average for Latin America and the Caribbean.[4] More than half of Guatemala's population lives below the national poverty line, and extreme poverty disproportionately affects the country's indigenous population.[5] The major population centers are found in the highlands. Guatemala City, the capital, is the largest city, with over 2.5 million inhabitants in the metropolitan area. Quetzaltenango is the second-largest city, with about 200,000 inhabitants.[6] Guatemala is divided into 22 departments, 331 municipalities, and 20,485 towns and villages.[7] Some 48 percent of the population lives in urban centers, with the remainder living in rural communities.[8] Internal migration hovers around 10 percent, and migration out of Guatemala is high. Overall, the country's population is rapidly growing at a rate of about 2 percent per year.[9]

Guatemala is rich in cultural, ethnic, and linguistic diversity. The population is divided primarily into indigenous, mestizo (mixed indigenous-European), and European-descendant sectors. Guatemala has one of the highest proportions of indigenous people in the hemisphere, who consist primarily of the Maya, but also the Xinka and Garifuna peoples. According to recent figures, about 40 percent of the population is indigenous, but this is highly contested as a low number.[10] The mestizo population is locally known by the term *Ladino*. Most of the indigenous Maya population live in rural areas, where almost 44 percent are monolingual in one of the twenty-one Mayan languages.[11] The official language of Guatemala is Spanish, but the twenty-one Mayan languages, along with Xinca and Garifuna, are recognized as co-official in the communities where they are spoken.

Religious practices in Guatemala include Catholicism, Protestantism, and traditional Maya religion. Interestingly, charismatic Protestantism is rapidly expanding in Guatemala, which now has one of the highest proportions of Protestants in Latin America.[12]

Brief History

The Mesoamerican Region

The territory of Guatemala was previously part of a pre-Columbian cultural area known as Mesoamerica.[13] Mesoamerica was distinct from the southwest United States and Northern Mexico cultural areas, and it formed a region spanning present-day Central and Southern Mexico, Guatemala, Belize, Honduras, and El Salvador. After 3000 BC, several societies flourished in this region, sharing ethnic, architectural, agricultural, and technological features.[14]

In Mesoamerica, intensive agricultural techniques produced corn, beans, squash, chili peppers, and cacao, which fostered a robust agricultural trade economy through a network extending from Central Mexico to Honduras. Bartering and trade likely took place in large, specialized markets, which could often feature thousands of vendors selling not only agricultural goods, but also the many tools and technologies of the day.[15] Civilizations in the region also shared common architectural features, such as corbelled vaults, plazas, ball courts, stepped pyramids, and extensive roads made of stone. Construction was typically with stone, mortar, and plaster. Buildings and pyramids were decorated with facades depicting rulers, deities, ceremonies, and hieroglyphic texts (written in the Maya, Mixtec, Aztec, or Mixe-Zoquean writing systems, depending on the exact location and time period). Professional scribes wrote on stone, pottery, and books made of bark paper or deerskin folded accordion style. The books described genealogical records, history of rulers, and calendars with important dates (such as wars or successions of power) as well as cosmology and astronomical observations.

The calendrical system in Mesoamerica was particularly involved, and relied on a vigesimal number system, which used a base count of 20 rather than 10, to tell time. There were actually three major calendar systems used in Mesoamerica. The first of these was a 260-day ritual calendar, the Tzolk'in,[16] comprising 13 months of 20 days. This calendar was used alongside a 360-day calendar, the Haab', with 18 months of 20 days (and 5 extra monthless days to correct for the solar cycle). Together, the Tzolk'in and Haab' formed a "calendar round," which repeated a complete cycle approximately every 52 years. To track time over longer periods, a Long Count calendar was used; one of the larger units of measure was the b'ak'tun, a cycle of 144,000 days or 394.5 solar years.[17] Recently, the fact that the thirteenth b'ak'tun of the Long Count ended on December 21, 2012—marking the beginning of another cycle of 144,000 days—generated a great deal of apocalyptic interest.[18]

Mesoamerican religion was complex and pantheistic. Individual gods had defined and unique roles, such as bringing the rain or causing disease. The ball courts were an important social space, where a ritual ball game was used to reenact the interactions between the living world and Xibalba, the underworld. Throughout the region, human sacrifice, ritual cannibalism, and auto-sacrifice through bloodletting were at times used to communicate with the deities.[19]

The Maya and the Spanish Invasion

Mesoamerica was inhabited at least 13,000 years ago, but Maya civilization in Guatemala did not begin to flourish until around 2000 BC. The period between 2000 BC and 250 AD is known as the Preclassic Period in Maya civilization.[20] During this period, small villages and agricultural communities coalesced into concentrated settlements throughout Guatemala. The last few centuries of this era witnessed the rise of cities such as Tak'alik' Abaj, Chocolá, and Kaminaljuyu in the Guatemalan highlands, with pyramids, inscribed stone monuments, and complex hydrologic systems. This period also saw the emergence of Maya ceremonialism based on the observation of celestial events at sites such as Uaxactún and El Mirador.[21]

The Classic Period, 250–900 AD, when Maya civilizations flourished, saw the rise of the large Maya Lowland cities including Tikal, Quirigua, and Calakmul. At this time, dynastic records using Long Count dates also first appeared, along with a boom in stone sculpture, architecture with corbelled vaults, elaborate polychrome ceramics, and finely crafted jades. The Postclassic Period, from 900 AD until the arrival of the first Spanish conquistadors, was marked by a decline in the lowland city centers and an increasing population in the highlands. Highland cities included Kumarcaaj (Utatlán), Iximché, and Mixco Viejo, which were the capitals of the K'ichee', Kaqchikel, and Pok'omam Maya, respectively, at the time of the Spanish conquest.[22]

The arrival of Spanish commander Pedro de Alvarado in 1524 changed Guatemala forever. Alvarado overtook the Kaqchikel capital of Iximché, renaming it Cuauhtemalan ("the place of trees" in the Nahuatl language spoken by some of Alvarado's guides from Central Mexico); it became the first European settlement in Central America.[23] Due to heavy resistance fighting around Iximché, the Spanish moved their capital to Santiago de los Caballeros (now present-day Ciudad Vieja) in 1527. This settlement was destroyed by an earthquake, resulting in relocation yet again of the capital into the Panchoy Valley, at the site of present-day La Antigua, in 1543.[24] The capital was moved one final time to its current location in Guatemala City in 1773 following a large earthquake that destroyed much of La Antigua.[25]

Beginning with but continuing after Alvarado, the Spanish imposed their rule of law and way of life over the indigenous population. An *encomienda* system was put into place, which gave grants of land, as well as indigenous people to work that land, to the *encomenderos*, or Spanish conquistadors.[26] In 1549 Spanish law made slavery illegal, effectively ending the encomienda system. But this was replaced by a system of *repartimiento*, or forced labor, whereby indigenous people were obligated to work either for free or for minimal wages for a specific number of weeks or months each year on Spanish-owned farms and mines.[27]

In colonial Guatemala, political structure and social organization was driven in part by a caste system organized around origin. Those who were born in Spain, the Peninsulares, were the highest ranking, typically semidetached from local politics, and interested mainly in turning a profit. Creoles were of direct Spanish descent, but born in the Americas and therefore of a lower status than the Peninsulares, and less well supported by the Spanish crown. Mestizos, those of mixed indigenous-European descent, were barred from owning land and could not hold positions of power; they often served as intermediaries between the higher social classes and the indigenous population. Indigenous Maya, as well as a small number of African slaves, occupied the lowest rungs of the social ladder.[28]

Independence from Spain and Rise of the Nation

Freedom from Spain grew out of an independence movement from 1810 to 1821, spearheaded by largely wealthy creoles who sought economic independence. On September 15, 1821, Guatemala, El Salvador, Nicaragua, Costa Rica, and Honduras proclaimed independence from Spain and formed a new unified entity, United Central America. This union dissolved rapidly, however, and Guatemala emerged as an independent state in 1840.[29] Subsequently, for the next several decades, the Ladino (mestizo) sector of the population grew rapidly through intermarriage, as indigenous people migrated into urban areas in search of economic advancement. This emerging Ladino working and middle class endeavored to imitate and emulate elite lifestyles in urban centers. Paradoxically, therefore, despite the indigenous roots of the Ladino class, its expansion led to a deepening rift between urban centers of power and rural indigenous communities.[30]

From the 1890s until the 1940s, Guatemala struggled to adapt to the modern industrial world by encouraging infrastructural growth and trade. In particular, Guatemala became an agricultural powerhouse, although this was in large measure under the direct control of foreign interests such as the US-based United Fruit Company.[31] Guatemala held its first democratic elections in 1945, ushering in a democratic window known as the Ten Years of Spring under the presidencies of Juan José Arévalo (1945–1951) and Jacobo Arbenz Guzmán (1951–1954). Both presidencies were characterized by attempts to implement substantial social reforms, especially land and agrarian reform. In particular, Árbenz's platform emphasized land redistribution because by the early 1950s, much of the country's land as well as its railroad and electrical utilities were controlled by foreign business interests, chief among them the United Fruit Company. Under Árbenz's Agrarian Reform Law of 1952, uncultivated land on estates larger than 672 acres was to be redistributed to individual families, with compensation given to landowners.[32] Árbenz's policies angered foreign business interests and also stirred up anticommunist Cold War sentiments, resulting in the overthrow of his government in 1954 in a coup d'état directed in part by the Central Intelligence Agency of the United States. "Liberation fighters" installed the formerly exiled Guatemalan army leader Carlos Castillo Armas as president, and he immediately reversed a decade of socioeconomic, educational, labor, and political reforms.[33]

Civil War

At least partially in response to the overthrow of the Árbenz presidency, and as a reaction to the subsequent repressive policies of the new military government, a grassroots leftist guerilla movement gained steam slowly beginning in the early 1960s, at first largely among Ladino inhabitants in the eastern portions of the country and in Guatemala City. But beginning in the 1970s, the movement rapidly expanded throughout the indigenous highlands. The military government responded with predictable brutality: abductions, disappearances, violence, mutilations, and public disposal of bodies were common. The conflict reached its peak in 1982, when General Efraín Ríos Montt took power following a coup, dissolved Congress, and declared a state of emergency. He launched a coordinated, systematic scorched-earth campaign among indigenous communities in the highlands, which resulted in the destruction of hundreds of communities, tens of thousands of deaths, and over 1 million refugees.[34]

In 1983, Ríos Montt was removed from power in yet another coup, but he resurfaced years later to form a powerful political party, the Guatemalan Republican Front (FRG). He was elected president of Congress in Guatemala in 1995 and 2000, and even made an electoral bid for the presidency in 2003.[35] Three decades after the genocide, Ríos Montt and several of his military aids have been brought to trial for crimes against humanity and genocide. Congressional immunity ended for Ríos Montt on January 14, 2012; and on January 26, 2012, Judge Carol Patricia Flores placed the eighty-five-year-old Ríos Montt under house arrest and set bail at 500,000 quetzales ($65,000 US).[36] In May 2012, Judge Flores charged Ríos Montt for a second genocide because of his role as general during the massacre at Dos Erres, Petén.[37] As of this writing court proceedings are pending. The formal end to the thirty-six-year armed conflict occurred in 1996, with the signing of peace accords between the representatives of the guerilla organization Unidad Revolucionaria Nacional Guatemalteca (URNG) and the Guatemalan military.

In 1998, just a few years after the signing of the peace accords, the Human Rights Office of the Archdiocese of Guatemala published an extensive report documenting the abuses of the Guatemalan military during the civil war. Just a few days after the publication of the report, its principal author, Bishop Juan José Gerardi, was brutally assassinated in his home.[38] A second report on the war, the United Nations-supported Commission for Historical Clarification,[39] was published in 1999; the report found that, over the course of the conflict, some 200,000 people were killed, of whom 83 percent were indigenous Maya. The report also concluded that 93 percent of the human rights violations during the conflict were perpetrated by the Guatemalan military, not by the guerilla resistance.[40]

Post–Civil War Society

The signing of the peace accords in 1996 and the end of the civil war provided hope for peace and prosperity in Guatemala. However, since 1996 the government has increasingly grown weaker while organized crime and urban violence are on the rise.[41] Neoliberal policy, as exemplified by treaties such as the Central American Free Trade Agreement (CAFTA-DR), ratified in 2006, has had far-reaching and destabilizing consequences.[42] For example, once the granary of Central America, Guatemala now relies on food imports to supply some basic staples. The influx of food products such as yellow corn from the United States further deters local agriculture, as small farmers cannot compete in a market flooded with the highly subsidized grain products.[43] As a result, fluctuations in grain prices can no longer be buffered by domestic production capacity, leading to further dependence on foreign foods and contributing to chronic food insecurity.[44] International mining companies have also caused a series of problems for local water sources, further affecting agricultural production.[45]

Price increases in the basic food basket have risen dramatically since the mid-2000s. In September 2011, the basic food basket was estimated at 80 quetzales ($10 US) per day for the twenty-six basic food items;[46] but daily wages are generally only 40 to 60 quetzales (the minimum wage was set at 56 quetzales in 2010[47]) for the head of the household in rural families. It is estimated that more than one-half of the total population in Guatemala cannot afford the basic food basket.[48]

President Álvaro Colom took office in 2007, promising to provide healthcare, education, financial opportunities, and development in rural areas. But his presidency was largely ineffectual,[49] in part because of pressures from the global financial recession as well as the "war on drugs," which has Mexican drug cartels pouring into Guatemala. In response to this new violence, vigilante justice and lynchings have risen in rural communities. Outside observers have called present-day Guatemala a failed state because of the increased violence,[50] especially against women (feminicide), and the overall lack of government control. The November 2011 election of General Otto Pérez Molina as president was made possible because of his *mano dura* (iron fist) platform, which promised better policing and other solutions to tackle drug and urban violence. But critics have accused Pérez Molina of human rights abuses committed under his command during the civil war.

Growth of the Nongovernmental Civil Sector

The rapid explosion of the civil sector in Guatemala began in the 1960s with two events. First was a US initiative to support community cooperatives and projects as part of US President John F. Kennedy's Alliance for Progress.[51] Second was the increase in rural community organizing by movements such as Catholic Action. Organized as a secular movement in the Catholic Church, Catholic Action was led by foreign priests who came to Guatemala on the invitation of President Castillo Armas following the 1954 coup.[52] In 1976, a large earthquake caused widespread destruction in the highlands, prompting the quick arrival of many small international organizations to provide relief, which further cemented the system of interaction between local, state, and foreign actors shaping the nongovernmental sector in Guatemala.[53] During the 1980s, the most violent period of the civil war, the growth of the nongovernmental sector slowed, but then exploded again following the 1996 peace accords.[54]

As mentioned earlier, the post–peace accords era in Guatemala has not brought about the long-awaited thriving of democratic involvement as was hoped, but rather it has been characterized by an increasingly weakened state apparatus controlled by neoliberal interests. This has allowed a massive and unregulated influx of foreign aid organizations.[55] Today in Guatemala, the nongovernmental sector is flourishing with little to no oversight by national or local entities, leading to an ever-expanding collage of overlapping organizations. Recent estimates have suggested that as of this writing, more than 10,000 NGOs are operating in Guatemala.[56]

Language and Indigeneity

A large proportion of the population of Guatemala is indigenous Maya, although the exact number is disputed. In the nearly two centuries since Guatemalan independence, various shades of national integrationist discourse have had a vested interest in underestimating the true size of the indigenous presence. Therefore, despite the fact that global fecundity rates remain much higher for indigenous communities than for nonindigenous communities, the official percentage of the population that is indigenous has tended to decrease steadily over the years. Based on 2008–2009 statistics, it officially sits at 38 percent, a decrease of 11 percent from 1999.[57] Naturally, these official statistics are disputed, often hotly, by various independent observers and pro-indigenous organizations, whose own estimates vary widely from 50 to 80 percent.[58]

Mayan Languages Today

Regardless of the exact percentage of the population that is indigenous Maya and the precise proportion of this population that maintains use of Mayan languages, the fact remains that the Mayan languages remain an important mode of communication and the most important index for cultural or ethnic identity throughout most of Guatemala, especially in rural areas.[59] In fact, for most Maya intellectuals and community leaders today, the issue of Mayan language sovereignty is nearly synonymous with the overall cause of Maya populations. For example, Demetrio Cojti, who is Kaqchikel Maya and probably the most prominent Maya intellectual alive today, roundly denounces all attempts to define the plight of Maya along other than ethnolinguistic lines as "glottophagy" (the devouring of languages).[60] Indeed, for centuries the suppression and displacement of Mayan languages has been the key strategy in the efforts of state actors and civil sector elites to *blanquear* (whiten or sanitize) the Maya population.[61] There are twenty-one Mayan languages spoken in Guatemala, and the four largest of these (Kaqchikel, K'ichee,' Q'eqchi,' and Mam) each have more than 500,000 speakers.[62]

Since the signing of the peace accords in 1996, Mayan languages have achieved notable gains on the national stage. For example, bilingual Spanish-Mayan education in public schools has flourished under a special branch of the Ministry of Education, DIGEBI (Dirección General de la Educación Bilingüe), and a Maya Education Movement, under the direction of the Committee for Mayan Education (CNEM, Comité Nacional de Educación Maya), has greatly influenced both public and private primary school education.[63] Further, the signing of a new National Language Law (Ley de Idiomas Nacionales) in 2003 guaranteed co-official status with Spanish for Mayan language in each of the communities where the languages are spoken, with special legislative mention being made of the right of all citizens to access public health, legal, and police services in their native language—although, of course, the practical manifestations of these provisions still lag far behind their legislative reach.[64]

Table 2.1 *Major Mayan Languages and Regions Where They Are Spoken*

Language	Number of Speakers	Departments Where Spoken
Chuj	38,000	Huehuetenango
Ixil	69,000	El Quiché
Kaqchikel	476,000	Baja Verapaz
		Chimaltenango
		Escuintla
		Guatemala
		Sacatepéquez
		Sololá
		Suchitepéquez
K'ichee'	922,000	Chimaltenango
		El Quiché
		Huehuetenango
		Quetzaltenango
		Retalhuleu
		Sololá
		Suchitepéquez
		Totonicapán
		San Marcos
Mam	520,000	Huehuetenango
		Quetzaltenango
		San Marcos
Popti'	38,000	Huehuetenango
Poqomchi'	70,000	Alta Verapaz
		Baja Verapaz
		El Quiché
Q'anjob'al	99,000	Huehuetenango
Q'eqchi'	727,000	Alta Verapaz
		Baja Verapaz
		Petén
		El Quiché
		Izabal
Tz'utujil	48,000	Sololá
		Suchitepéquez

Note: The ten Mayan languages with the largest number of speakers are represented in the table.

Source: Data are adapted from M. Richards, *Atlas Lingüístico de Guatemala* (Editorial Serviprensa: Guatemala City, 2003).

From the standpoint of the prospective healthcare volunteer investigating a stay in Guatemala, learning a Mayan language has never been easier. Thanks to the tireless work over the past few decades of Mayan linguistics and language rights organizations such as the Proyecto Linguistico Francisco Marroquin, the Academy of Mayan Languages, and Oxlajuuj Keej Maya' Ajtz'iib', grammars and dictionaries are readily available in nearly all Mayan languages. Formal language instruction in K'ichee' and Kaqchikel Maya also can be obtained at language schools in the major tourist centers of Quetzaltenango and Antigua, and intensive field schools sponsored by universities and NGOs also exist.[65]

Language Barriers and Disparity

It is a well-established fact that disparities in healthcare outcomes and economic well-being in Guatemala map closely to indigeneity. For example, according to the World Bank, although 55 percent of the general population of Guatemala lives in poverty and 15 percent in extreme poverty, for the indigenous subsection of the population these numbers are 80 percent and 30 percent, respectively.[66] The under-five child mortality rate for the nonindigenous population is 36 per 1,000 live births, but it remains at 55 per 1,000 live births for the indigenous sector.[67] Similarly, in primarily indigenous provinces of Guatemala, maternal mortality rates are often twice those of primarily nonindigenous provinces.[68]

What is not often appreciated, however, especially in the case of healthcare, is how closely these disparities are tied to language barriers. As we have discussed, most urban Maya are fully bilingual with Spanish or, in some cases, may even be losing their fluency in their native Mayan language. But the situation is markedly different in rural communities, where 75 percent of Guatemala's population still resides.[69] Based on our own experiences developing child nutrition programs in central Kaqchikel-speaking regions of the country, it is not uncommon for more than 50 percent of rural women to have no real functional fluency in Spanish.

Unfortunately, although recent legislative advances do technically guarantee the right to healthcare in one's maternal language, this is generally not actually the case. An extremely small number of practicing physicians have any working knowledge of a Mayan language; even physicians who come from an indigenous background tend to abandon or lose their ability to use their maternal language, mostly because of a general disdain for indigenous languages in the Guatemalan medical community. Even among NGOs, with an ostensible commitment to grassroots organizing, it is uncommon for anyone except low-level staff to have any proficiency in Mayan languages.[70]

The misapprehensions and misunderstandings that result from being unable to converse freely about illness in one's language of choice leads to the prevailing notion among many indigenous communities of "not being attended"[71] by the medical establishment. This mistrust and apprehension by indigenous patients, in our experience, is a major determinant of the underutilization of healthcare services, much more so than rural geography and lack of proximity to healthcare infrastructure.[72]

Healthcare System

The Guatemalan public healthcare system is composed of two major systems. First is the Ministry of Public Health and Social Assistance (MSPAS), which provides a complete range of government-subsidized healthcare services throughout the country. The system is hierarchical, with smaller and more rural communities covered by health posts (Puestos de Salud), which are typically staffed by an *auxiliar de enfermería* (auxiliary nurse, the equivalent of a licensed practical nurse in the United States) or medical student.[73] Larger municipalities have larger posts (Centros de Salud), which offer more complete services and usually have a full-time physician on staff. Each Centro de Salud is responsible for managing referrals from various Puestos de Salud in its region. Farther up the referral chain are the regional or provincial hospitals and, finally, two large quarternary referral centers, the Hospital San Juan de Dios and the Hospital Roosevelt, both located in Guatemala City. Technically speaking, all services provided by MSPAS are free or heavily subsidized. But in reality, many essential medications and most laboratory or diagnostic services are outsourced to private enterprise, so most patients do accrue significant and often insurmountable expenses when navigating the system.[74] The MSPAS system is supplemented by a second major system, the Guatemalan Social Security Institute (IGSS). IGSS is an entirely separate healthcare system, also hierarchically organized, that provides health coverage only to individuals who are employed by a corporation that pays a social security tax. Because a majority of all employment outside Guatemala City is informal, IGSS is essentially an urban healthcare system to which very few rural inhabitants have access.

There are large disparities in the distribution of MSPAS healthcare resources. For example, 80 percent of all Guatemalan physicians work in Guatemala City, and the poorest 40 percent of citizens—largely rural—account for only one-quarter of national healthcare expenditure.[75] Because of this infrastructural disparity, many people seek healthcare services from a patchwork array of laboratories, pharmacies, and private hospitals (*sanitarios*). Indeed, in one rural community where we work, we surveyed healthcare utilization patterns and discovered that two-thirds of individuals sought medical advice and treatment directly from pharmacies rather than through physician consultations.

Since the signing of the peace accords and the end of the civil war in 1996, the political response to the lack of public healthcare services in rural areas of Guatemala has been the System for Social Assistance (SIAS). SIAS began in 1997 with funding from the Inter-American Development Bank,[76] and is essentially an outsourcing plan whereby MSPAS contracts with numerous NGOs to provide basic healthcare services in rural areas not served or underserved by public infrastructure. Although critics of SIAS note that it has perpetuated a programmatic focus on quantity (*cobertura*, or coverage) over quality, and that it has often undermined local community authority structures,[77] SIAS has undoubtedly been successful on its own terms, providing new services to an additional 3.2 million people from 1997 to 2002 alone.[78] Another important result of SIAS has been that in recent years, NGOs have in effect become the de facto primary providers of healthcare services for much of rural Guatemala.

It's also important to note the extent to which other forms of public-private partnerships and international collaborations have transformed the quality and extent of specialist medical services available to the public, although these are generally concentrated only in Guatemala City. For example, founded in 1994 as a collaboration between MSPAS and the Fundación Aldo Castañeda,[79] the Cardiovascular Surgery Unit (UNICAR), is a state-of-the-art cardiovascular surgery center, the most advanced in all of Central America. Nevertheless, due to a lack of robust systems for the detection and referral of congenital heart disease in rural areas, the center operates considerably below capacity.[80]

Community Health Workers

No discussion of the healthcare system in Guatemala would be complete without a look at the community health worker; in this community-based model for healthcare, laypeople with basic training in public health and preventive medicine self-organize for the sake of their own communities. Guatemala was the first country in the world to train and deploy CHWs, largely because of the efforts of one pioneering public health worker, Dr. Carroll Behrhorst, who developed the first CHW programs in the Department of Chimaltenango in central Guatemala in the 1960s.[81] His model of *comprehensive primary healthcare* was subsequently hailed by multiple international polities and widely adopted worldwide.[82] During the peak years of violence during the civil war, CHWs were often targeted for assassination or disappearance due to their important role as community leaders and organizers. To date, CHW programs remain a vital part of the primary health landscape in many rural, indigenous communities. Several regional and national organizations seek to coordinate and advocate for the work of CHWs, including the Asociación de Servicios Comunitarios de Salud (ASECSA), which was formed in 1978 and today has a membership of dozens of different CHW organizations spanning the majority of departments in Guatemala.[83]

Recently, however, several factors have contributed to a sharp decline in the importance of CHW programs as providers of healthcare. First, the SIAS program mentioned earlier has considerably reworked the role of the CHW under a new title, the *guardián de salud* (health guardian), who is less independent and serves mostly as a point person for referrals to higher-level Ministry of Health facilities; because many former CHWs now work as *guardiánes de salud*, they have seen their former authority and autonomy sharply curtailed. Second, there has been an immense boom in a new health profession, the *auxiliar de enfermería*. *Auxiliares de enfermería* are a more professionalized and highly trained healthcare workforce, and in many communities, they now outnumber CHWs and command higher salaries.[84] Indeed, in our experience, many former CHWs have retrained as *auxiliares de enfermería*. Third, the last several decades have seen increased training and licensing opportunities for lay midwives; the increased professionalization and organization of lay midwives has also led to their assuming many of the public health responsibilities formerly conducted primarily by CHWs.[85]

Child Malnutrition in Guatemala

Of particular importance as a health indicator in Guatemala is the rate of child malnutrition. Guatemala has one of the highest rates of stunting in the world, and 56 percent of all malnourished children in Central America reside in Guatemala.[86] In a 2008–2009 national survey,[87] 43 percent of children between ages three months and sixty months were stunted, a statistic that masks the considerably worse outcomes that prevail in the rural, primarily indigenous central highland regions of the country. Indeed, in the rural communities where we work, we routinely encounter rates of child stunting upwards of 70 percent, and the World Bank estimates that the rate of stunting in indigenous children is twice that in nonindigenous children.[88] The causes of the malnutrition disparity in the indigenous population are complex and multifactorial, and include food insecurity, poverty, lack of access to healthcare facilities in rural settings, inadequate agricultural land holdings, and unequal access to education and economic opportunities.

The INCAP Trial

Child malnutrition research in Guatemala is well known worldwide, mainly due to the efforts of a single large study, the Institute of Nutrition of Central American and Panama (INCAP) cohort trial. INCAP is a nongovernmental research unit, based in Guatemala, that has been setting standards for nutrition research in underdeveloped countries for decades.[89] In the cohort study, INCAP's largest study to date, four villages were randomized to receive two cups a day of either *Incaparina* (a vegetable protein, milk, and micronutrient mixture) or a control drink containing only sugar, flavoring, and micronutrients. The intervention continued for eight years (1969–1977), and rigorous data was collected to determine the effects of the supplementation on all pregnant and lactating women, and on children under age seven years.[90] Following this intervention, an impressive, sustained follow-up allowed for many repeat analyses, both on the recipients of the supplement and on three subsequent generations. This wealth of nutritional data has been published in over 200 scientific manuscripts to date.[91] Further, Incaparina has become one of the most popular nutrient supplements for children in Guatemala over the last several decades, still controlling a large market share today.

Among the key findings of the study has been the discovery that a relatively brief period of high-quality caloric supplementation (and not just micronutrient supplementation) can have positive effects on the wellness of populations. Beneficial growth effects were observed not only in supplemented individuals, but also in subsequent generations. Other benefits of supplementation included improved school performance and higher adult wages.[92] The study also demonstrated definitively that child malnutrition in Guatemala was primarily a problem of stunting (low height-for-age), rather than wasting (low weight-for-height) or underweight (low weight-for-age).[93] Finally, the study showed that the principal causes of growth failure in children were exposure to chronic infectious disease (for example, diarrhea) and low-quality foods, and that growth failure in childhood predicted functional deficits in adulthood.[94]

At the same time, there have been important secondary consequences of the INCAP cohort trial. Due to logistical considerations (language barriers, for example, and proximity to Guatemala City), indigenous communities were excluded from the trial.[95] Previously, INCAP had conducted several important studies in indigenous communities.[96] But following the success of the trial, much effort was refocused on follow-up analyses of the cohort. As a result, there has been a paucity of sustained, high-quality investigation of malnutrition in indigenous regions of Guatemala since the 1960s. In some ways, therefore, the INCAP cohort trial represents the crystallization within the academic sphere of a larger ideological problem of the chronic social abandonment of indigenous populations in Guatemala.

School Nutrition

Even though the INCAP cohort trial demonstrated unequivocally that the growth faltering of children in Guatemala occurs early, often in the first year of life,[97] the majority of Guatemala's official nutrition policy has remained focused on school nutrition programs, such as the School Cookie program of the 1980s–1990s and the Glass of Milk program of the 2000s.[98] The historical roots of this emphasis on school nutrition date to the 1950s and parallel efforts by wealthier countries to develop school-based programs. For example, by the early 1900s, school feeding programs were popular in many European countries, and the National School Lunch Act was passed in the United States in 1946.[99] Because much of the early funding for nutrition programs in Guatemala came from agencies based in these countries, such as the United Nations Children's Fund (UNICEF) and USAID,[100] the emphasis was likely a reflection of program and funding priorities at the time. Additional impetus was provided by technical advisors from INCAP, who had close ties to academic nutrition centers in the United States, and who formulated several nutritional products suitable particularly for consumption by school-age children.[101]

The innumerable small NGOs working throughout Guatemala have largely followed the governmental institutes and large international agencies in matters of nutritional policy. This means that, in large measure, most nongovernmental efforts to combat malnutrition have also been historically efforts directed at school-age children. This has been a natural extension of the fact that the majority of NGOs working on child nutrition have been, first and foremost, education assistance organizations, working to improve scholarship and retention and graduation rates among the rural poor. Indeed, improvements in school retention rates simply from providing hot school lunches are often marked.[102] However, taken together, these historical factors have all meant that, until very recently, articulated policies and strategies for more effectively and specifically targeting malnutrition earlier in life—in infants and young children—have been lacking.

New Policy Developments and Technologies in Child Nutrition

Since 2008, nutrition policy in Guatemala has finally begun to swing away from school-only programming toward more preventive and comprehensive interventions in early childhood. These policy changes have come on the heels of strong policy statements by USAID and the World Food Program (WFP) in favor of early childhood and preventive nutritional programs.[103] These conceptual shifts in nutrition policy have been favorably received in the Guatemalan media, which has rapidly adopted the concept of "first 1,000 days" of life, from conception to age two years, as a critical window for nutritional intervention.[104] Further, the newly elected government of Otto Pérez Molina has made the prevention and treatment of early childhood malnutrition a priority, and has drafted and disseminated a new multilevel strategic plan called Hambre Cero (Zero Hunger),[105] although this has not yet been substantively implemented.

Since 2007, the spectrum of nutritional products that are available in Guatemala and suitable for infants and young children has increased. By far, the nutritional product most commonly used remains Incaparina, the vitamin-fortified vegetable protein and milk "gruel" discussed earlier, which is fully marketized and readily available. Incaparina is now in competition with several other similar brands, some of which are available on the market (for example, Bienestarina) and others that are distributed only by NGOs (for example, WFP's Vitacereal). All of these products have two distinct disadvantages that can make their use challenging in small children, although with proper planning and monitoring, these challenges can be largely overcome. First, the products must be cooked by adding the dry supplement powder to hot water, which introduces the possibilities of contamination with non-potable water and improper preparation. Indeed, in our experience, most caregivers tend to prepare these products with a very thin consistency, which dilutes their nutritional impact and can be harmful if they satiate the child and displace breast milk and other foods in the diet. Second, these products are extremely popular with all members of the family, and the ration intended for the at-risk child is often shared among multiple family members, further diminishing its intended impact.

However, organizations working to prevent child malnutrition in young children are no longer limited only to Incaparina and similar products when designing nutritional programs. For example, micronutrient powders that are mixed directly into food—known internationally as Sprinkles and locally as Chispitas—are available on the local market. This product has been found in multiple countries to be effective in treating iron deficiency anemia. In some countries, it has also been shown to lower rates of acute illness and chronic malnutrition.[106] The effectiveness of Chispitas in treating anemia has been evaluated locally in Guatemala, although these results have not been published. The Ministry of Health provides Chispitas in periodic supplementation campaigns, and in our own work we have also independently verified that they are both effective and well liked by most recipients and their caregivers.[107]

Another class of nutritional products that are new to Guatemala are the ready-to-use supplementary foods (RUSFs); these products include Plumpy'Doz™ and Nutributter®, developed by the French nutritional company Nutriset. RUSFs have several theoretical advantages over Incaparina (because they do not require cooking and cannot be diluted) and Chispitas (because they contain calories in addition to micronutrients). In addition, data worldwide have shown that these products can significantly reduce rates of chronic malnutrition.[108] The major disadvantage of RUSFs is that they are currently available in Guatemala only by importation, which raises questions of both cost and sustainability. Still, exciting initiatives are currently underway to produce RUSFs on-site in Guatemala using locally sourced ingredients.[109]

Effective Child Malnutrition Interventions: Practical Reflections

Our own work on child malnutrition has been in the context of our efforts with Wuqu' Kawoq, one of several NGOs committed to finding effective solutions to child malnutrition in Guatemala. In the rural Kaqchikel and K'ichee' speaking communities where we work, we routinely encounter rates of chronic child malnutrition that exceed 70 percent of children under age five. Wuqu' Kawoq's commitment in these settings has been to develop collaborative, community-based solutions to malnutrition that increase awareness about the problem as well as empower communities to act on their own behalf.

When we began working on child malnutrition, our programs focused on using a network of CHWs to identify and treat cases of malnutrition. Treatment included coordinating medical care and simultaneously providing supplementary fortified foods. But we quickly realized that although these programs were successful in their own way, they did not address the larger challenge of preventing malnutrition in the first place.

Looking back at our child growth data from these programs, we noticed that most infants were born at normal weights and heights and grew well for the first six months of life. But between six and nine months, we noticed nearly universal growth failure; in particular, although children maintained relatively normal weights, their heights began to suffer. That is, they began to become stunted, or to suffer from chronic malnutrition. This window in child development between six and nine months corresponds closely with the time at which a child should begin to receive *complementary foods*—mashed vegetables and fruits, small amounts of protein, and finger foods.[110] Through a series of intensive interviews with mothers of these small children, we discovered that poverty and food insecurity, coupled with lack of knowledge about appropriate infant feeding techniques, were the primary culprits. Faced with limited food resources, mothers were choosing to continue exclusively breast-feeding their infants so that food could be allocated to other family members. When food was finally introduced to children, often not until after age nine months, it typically was in nutrient-poor forms, such as thin soups and other liquids. Families in which growth failure did not occur were more likely to include men with more stable employment or who did not suffer from alcoholism.[111]

Based on these findings, we modified our nutrition programs to include a larger emphasis on the prevention of malnutrition. Currently, therefore, all pregnant and lactating mothers receive supplementary nutrition and, beginning at six months, all infants automatically begin fortified nutrient supplementation as well. We couple universal nutritional supplementation with educational segments on breast-feeding, malnutrition, and infant feeding practices; the segments are delivered by trained CHWs and reinforced by periodic checkups with pediatricians. These methods seem to be effective; in one community, for example, we saw a 50 percent reduction in the rate of malnutrition in a little less than two years. Currently, we focus our efforts on consolidating these gains, by continuing to train community leaders and parents to run their own nutritional programs, and by collaborating with other like-minded NGOs to increase the scale of programs and share lessons learned.

Noncommunicable Disease in Guatemala

Guatemala has a relatively low burden of infectious diseases. For example, the rate of HIV infection in Guatemala is only around 1 percent,[112] and the TB prevalence is around 110 per 100,000, which is in the middle of the range for the Latin American region.[113] Similarly, in 2009 there were only 7,000 confirmed cases of malaria.[114] So Guatemala is prototypical for a developing country undergoing the transition from a high proportion of disease burden caused by infectious diseases to a high proportion of disease burden caused by chronic and noncommunicable diseases.

Indeed, it is well known that the growing burden of NCDs in low-income countries is one of the most pressing global health problems today. For example, in 2008 it was estimated that over 60 percent of all global deaths were due to NCDs.[115] And although we typically think of NCDs as being diseases of developed countries, in fact a larger proportion of the NCD burden now falls on lower-income countries; as much as 80 percent of the global burden of deaths due to cardiovascular disease and diabetes now occur in developing countries.[116] Although the Guatemalan Ministry of Health has developed norms for the diagnosis and treatment of NCDs in its rural health posts,[117] in practice these norms are rarely successfully implemented. The major barriers are a lack of essential medications and minimal staff competencies in the management of these conditions at the rural health posts. Although there is little population-based data for the prevalence of these conditions, extrapolation from hospital-based data at least allows us to draw the conclusion that rates of NCDs in Guatemala are rising rapidly.[118]

Diabetes in Guatemala

Diabetes is a prototypical NCD. Nearly 350 million people globally suffer from diabetes, and most of them live in low- or middle-income countries.[119] The number of deaths from diabetes worldwide is projected to double by 2030.

In Guatemala, a recent statistical modeling effort estimates that the prevalence of diabetes from 1980 to 2008 has increased from 8.9 to 11.5 percent in men and from 8.0 to 14.0 percent in women.[120] In a sample of urban-dwelling Guatemalans found to have a diabetes prevalence of 8.4 percent, only 50 percent were previously known to have diabetes, and the rates of other comorbid risk factors, such as obesity and hypertension, were also high.[121]

Unfortunately, we have no precise data on the burden of diabetes in rural indigenous populations. But in our own patient population served by Wuqu' Kawoq, diabetes is one of the most common reasons that adults seek medical attention, and there is considerable interest at the community level for better management of the condition. There are several plausible explanations for why indigenous populations in Guatemala might be especially vulnerable to the effects of diabetes. First, given their rural and marginalized position in society, they have little access to healthcare systems. In particular, most healthcare services for rural populations are provided by the Ministry of Health's SIAS program, which focuses on vaccination and maternal-child health; diagnosis and treatment for diabetes and other NCDs are not included under the SIAS mandate. Second, in many indigenous communities, an increase in sedentary lifestyle and the erosion of traditional diets and agricultural ways of life predisposes to the emergence of obesity and other risk factors for diabetes.[122] Finally, there is compelling evidence from other regions of the world that chronic undernutrition in childhood might predispose to the emergence of diabetes, obesity, and cardiovascular disease in adulthood.[123] So we can speculate that a direct line can be drawn between the overwhelming rates of indigenous child malnutrition in Guatemala and the emergence of diabetes and other chronic diseases in indigenous adults. This further underscores the pressing social need to definitely address child malnutrition and also to provide expanded support for the management of NCDs in adults who were malnourished as children.

Diabetes in Indigenous Populations: Needs Assessment

Since 2008, we have been involved in running a pilot community-based program for the management of adult type 2 diabetes, which has about 100 patients enrolled as of this writing. In the run-up to the program, we conducted extensive interviews with diabetics and health practitioners to determine the needs of this patient population. We give an overview of these findings here, and we have also summarized them in more detail elsewhere.[124] Given the highly fractured and diversified healthcare landscape in Guatemala and the lack of a coherent public sector plan for the management of diabetes, patients are at the mercy of a confusing array of therapeutic options: public clinics (which do not have medications), private physicians and clinics, health promoter associations, and herbal practitioners. It's common for patients to "resource shop"—bouncing back and forth among these various options in search of an affordable and coherent treatment plan, generally expending large amounts of money and time in the process.

The cost of diabetes medication is usually prohibitive. At effective doses, generic medications for diabetes often cost around 200 quetzales ($25 US) per month, which might represent 25 percent of the monthly income in some impoverished rural communities. Because these medications are not routinely available at public health posts, most patients have no choice but to seek healthcare from private physicians, where costs are even steeper: consult fees are typically $5 to $10 US per visit, and most private physicians have close relationships with name-brand pharmaceutical companies, meaning that medication costs are often three to four times the generic rate. Therefore, it's typical for patients to take medications intermittently for just a few weeks until their savings run out, or to seek help directly from less-well-trained venues. For example, in our survey sample, a majority of patients sought to save costs by skipping medical consultations and purchasing medications directly from private pharmacies, which are typically not run by licensed or trained pharmacists. Many patients also seek help from herbalists, where costs, surprisingly, are often not any lower than pharmaceuticals, given that most herbalists aggressively market their own proprietary blends of medicinal plants.

Pilot Program for the Community-Based Management of Diabetes
Based on these findings, we felt that it was essential to develop a medical home for diabetic patients, where they could obtain longitudinal and consistent care for their diabetes. Our model program has two components.

The first component is an educational arm. Each patient is assigned to a health promoter or auxiliary nurse, who is responsible for coordinating that patient's care. In biweekly or monthly meetings, the health promoter or nurse provides diabetes-related educational content to the patient, focused on reinforcing and discussing strategies for adhering to a diabetic dietary regimen; reviewing results of blood sugar tests (each health promoter is equipped with a fingerstick blood glucose machine); and assessing for medication side effects, as well as ensuring adherence to the prescribed medication regimen.

The second component of the program is regular contact with a medical provider, who acts as the patient's primary care doctor. These visits occur two to four times per year, and they are conducted collaboratively with the participation of the health promoter or nurse assigned to the patient. At these visits, medication dosages are adjusted, and close attention is paid to the diagnosis and treatment of other comorbid medical conditions, such as kidney disease, high blood pressure, and obesity.

The program has been highly successful in terms of improving blood glucose control for enrolled patients. Also, patients rate the program very positively, and return rates are high. In particular, patients have expressed appreciation for the continuity of care the program offers; each patient develops a lasting relationship with his or her health promoter and physician, thus promoting trust and improving adherence to a lifelong medication regimen. And because all medical consultations and health promoter visits are conducted in Kaqchikel, patients endorse improved comprehension of their disease process, of proper use of medications, and of the importance of dietary restrictions.

Effective Diabetes Care in Guatemala: Practical Reflections

In our work with adult diabetics in Guatemala, the program component that has most overwhelmingly contributed to improved diabetes control has been the provision of free medications to all patients. As discussed earlier, diabetes medications are prohibitively expensive for most of our patients. Without access to free medications, most patients will take medications only intermittently, or at reduced, nontherapeutic doses. To improve the sustainability of these efforts, we have had to work closely with the generic pharmaceutical industry in Guatemala to ensure a firm supply chain for low-cost medications. This has been successful, and our current programmatic costs for a typical diabetic patient run around $25 to $75 US per year, depending on medication dosages and comorbid medical conditions.

In addition, the importance of a longitudinal educational component and support network cannot be underestimated. Health promoters and nurses assigned to each patient have been invaluable in improving dietary and medication adherence. Health promoters also are able to educate families of diabetic patients, which has dramatically improved their willingness to support the dietary and lifestyle needs of their relatives.

Another major programmatic innovation has been the universal implementation of glycosylated hemoglobin measurements in all patients. When we began the program, we relied heavily on the measurement of fasting fingerstick blood glucose to assess disease control. But this proved to be an impossible logistical barrier because most patients had work restrictions, which prevented measurement of their blood glucose while they were fasting. Further, some people would take their medications only in the few days prior to their health promoter visit, resulting in an inaccurate assessment of their overall blood glucose control. Glycosylated hemoglobin measurements permit a more accurate assessment of blood glucose levels over the three months preceding the test (in effect, they provide an "average" blood glucose reading), so they are the standard of care for monitoring diabetes in developed countries. Although glycosylated hemoglobin measurements are not routinely used in Guatemala, point-of-care testing kits for this measurement are now available at a reasonable cost. In keeping with these market developments, WHO has recently, after much debate, recommended the use of these measurements in developing countries.[125]

Finally, we emphasize the need for the involvement of primary care physicians and other highly trained medical providers in the management of diabetes in Guatemala. Given the fractured healthcare landscape, most patients in our program present relatively late in the course of the disease, already with multiple diabetes complications and other related medical problems, such as severe high blood pressure, peripheral nerve damage, eye disease, foot ulcers, and kidney disease. Given the advanced stage at presentation, we advocate for a strong and collaborative role for health promoters with medical supervision in the diagnosis and management of diabetes.

Conclusions
Global Health Work in Guatemala

Medical and volunteer work in Guatemala is challenging. Practically, the fact that sociopolitical stability after the peace accords has not really materialized is of prime importance. The rise in violent crime, drug trafficking, and political corruption requires that close attention be paid to personal safety. Fortunately, in most rural areas of Guatemala, security issues are not as prominent as in the major urban areas such as Guatemala City.

The rapid growth of the NGO sector is another perplexing issue. There have been few effective efforts to coordinate among various NGO activities, although recently several Internet-based efforts at coordination have emerged that might serve as an initial starting point for people seeking work opportunities.[126] Also, we have been involved in the development of a networking conference series, Collective Futures (Futuros Colectivos), which represents a novel effort to foster dialogue and collaboration among NGOs.[127] Elsewhere, we have proposed minimum criteria for evaluating the effectiveness of NGOs working in rural Guatemala; these include an emphasis on the decentralization of NGO infrastructure (no "NGO compounds"), limiting the role of elite management and salary disparity in favor of engaging local community leadership, and developing real accountability structures within target communities.[128] We suggest that, when choosing any potential work arrangement, these factors should be taken into account.

Finally, acquiring relevant knowledge about Maya culture and basic skills in a Mayan language should be considered a prerequisite for work in rural Guatemala, although by no means do we wish to suggest that these are the only skills necessary for work in the field. The Proyecto Lingüístico Francisco Marroquín, based in Antigua, Guatemala, runs an excellent language school that offers instruction in many Mayan languages. Similarly, university- and NGO-affiliated field schools currently offer instruction in Kaqchikel and K'ichee' and are authoritative resources on the subject.[129]

Providing Direct Aid to Indigenous Communities

Florencio Calí is a native Kaqchikel speaker and lifetime resident of Tecpán, located in the central Kaqchikel-speaking region of Guatemala. He has a background in tourism and microfinance work, but since 2008 he has been working as a program manager for Wuqu' Kawoq.

Florencio first began working for Wuqu' Kawoq in the wake of a large natural disaster in Guatemala. He was discouraged by the inefficiency and disorganization that he saw in disaster relief efforts, and he was interested in working with an organization that was providing direct aid to rural communities. He was also excited to be able to provide services in Kaqchikel, his native language.

Currently, Florencio's primary activities include coordinating multiple child nutrition programs. He works with local groups of women and other community leaders to develop integrated approaches to nutrition work, and he oversees other staff as they collect data to ensure that programs are effective and of high quality.

Since 2010, Florencio has also devoted considerable energy to developing a referral network in Guatemala City, which allows him to quickly facilitate high-level medical care for patients that he encounters in rural communities who have complex medical problems and require emergency care.

"I am happy to be working in this job," he says, "because I see that the things I do go directly to the communities I work in and have an immediate impact."

Notes

1 Instituto Nacional de Estadística de Guatemala (INE).
2 COVERCO and International Labor Rights Fund, "Labor Conditions in the Guatemalan Sugar Industry" (2005), available from www.dol.gov; and Pan American Health Organization, *Health in the Americas, 2007* (Washington: PAHO, 2007).

3 R. Vargas-Lundius, G. Lanly, M. Villarreal, and M. Osorio, *International Migration, Remittances and Rural Development* (International Fund for Agricultural Development, 2008).

4 World Health Organization, "Basic Indicators: Guatemala 2006."

5 WHO, "Basic Indicators: Guatemala 2006."

6 INE (Nov. 15, 2011), available from www.ine.gob.gt.

7 PAHO, *Health in the Americas, 2007*. Guatemalan Congress (2011), available from www.congreso.gob.gt.

8 PAHO, *Health in the Americas, 2007*. WHO, "Basic Indicators: Guatemala 2006."

9 Metz, *'Ch'orti'-Maya Survival in Eastern Guatemala*. CEPAL, Impacto del Tratado de Libre Comercio de Centroamérica en la agricultura y el sector rural en cinco países centroamericanos (2007).

10 PAHO, *Health in the Americas, 2007*.

11 Programa de las Naciones Unidas para el Desarrollo. "Diversidad étnico-cultural y desarrollo humano: la ciudadanía en un Estado plural," Ciudad de Guatemala, Documento oficial P964 (Informe Nacional de Desarrollo Humano: Guatemala, 2005).

12 K. O'Neill, *City of God: Christian Citizenship in Postwar Guatemala*, The Anthropology of Christianity Series (Berkeley, CA: University of California Press, 2009).

13 P. Kirchoff, "Mesoamerica," *Acta Americana* 1.1 (1943):92–107.

14 M. Coe, *The Maya* (London: Thames and Hudson, 2011).

15 Kirchoff, "Mesoamerica," 92–107; Coe, *The Maya*. J. Gasco, M. Masson, R. Rosenswig, and M. Smith, "Origins and Development of Mesoamerican Civilization" in *The Legacy of Mesoamerica: History and Culture of a Native American Civilization*, ed. R. Carmack, J. Gasco, and G. Gossen (Upper Saddle River, NJ: Prentice Hall, 1996); R. Sharer and L. Traxler, *The Ancient Maya*, 6th ed. (Stanford, CA: Stanford University Press, 2006); and L. Shaw, "The Elusive Maya Marketplace," *Journal of Archaeological Research* 20 (2012):117–155.

16 *Tzolk'in* is the Yucatec Mayan name for this calendar system. Each Mayan language today has its own name for this calendar; for example, in Kaqchikel, it is called the *Cholq'ij*.

17 D. Stuart, *The Order of Days: The Maya World and the Truth About 2012* (New York: Harmony Books, 2011). Coe, *The Maya*. Sharer and Traxler, *The Ancient Maya*.

18 The Maya calendar and Maya writings do not prophesize the end of the world on December 21, 2012; see Stuart, *The Order of Days*.

19 Coe, *The Maya*. Sharer and Traxler, *The Ancient Maya*.

20 Sharer and Traxler, *The Ancient Maya*.

21 Ibid.

22 Ibid.

23 R. Herrera, *Natives, Europeans, and Africans in Sixteenth-Century Santiago de Guatemala* (Austin, TX: University of Texas Press, 2003).

24 Herrera, *Natives, Europeans, and Africans in Sixteenth-Century Santiago de Guatemala*; and R. L. Woodward Jr., *Central America: A Nation Divided*, 3rd ed. (Oxford: Oxford University Press, 1999). C. Lutz, *Santiago de Guatemala, 1541–1773: City, Caste, and the Colonial Experience* (Norman, OK: University of Oklahoma Press, 1994).

25 UNESCO, World Heritage Conservation, Antigua, Guatemala.

26 Herrera, *Natives, Europeans, and Africans in Sixteenth-Century Santiago de Guatemala*. W. L. Sherman, "Some Aspects of Change in Guatemalan Society, 1470–1620" in *Spaniards and Indians in Southeastern Mesoamerica: Essays on the History of Ethnic Relations*, ed. M. J. MacLeod and R. Wasserstrom, Latin American Studies Series (Lincoln, NE: University of Nebraska Press, 1983). R. Carmack, "Spanish-Indian Relations in Highland Guatemala, 1800–1944" in *Spaniards and Indians in Southeastern Mesoamerica*, ed. MacLeod and Wasserstrom. Woodward, *Central America*. E. Wolf, *Sons of the Shaking Earth* (Chicago: University of Chicago Press, 1962).

27 Woodward, *Central America*. Wolf, *Sons of the Shaking Earth*. Lutz, *Santiago de Guatemala, 1541–1773*.

28 Herrera, *Natives, Europeans, and Africans in Sixteenth-Century Santiago de Guatemala*. Woodward, *Central America*. Wolf, *Sons of the Shaking Earth*. M. J. MacLeod, "Ethnic Relations and Indian Society in the Province of Guatemala 1620–1800" in *Spaniards and Indians in Southeastern Mesoamerica*, ed. MacLeod and Wasserstrom. P. Foxen, *In Search of Providence: Transnational Mayan Identities* (Nashville, TN: Vanderbilt University Press, 2008).

29 C. Lutz and G. Lovell, "Core and Periphery in Colonial Guatemala" in *Guatemalan Indians and the State: 1540 to 1988*, ed. C. Smith (Austin, TX: University of Texas Press, 1990), 35–51.

30 Lutz and Lovell, "Core and Periphery in Colonial Guatemala."

31 Woodward, *Central America*. Stephen Schlesinger and Stephen Kinzer, *Bitter Fruit: The Untold Story of the American Coup in Guatemala* (Garden City, NY: Doubleday, 1982); and S. Striffler and M. Moberg, eds., *Banana Wars: Power, Production, and History in the Americas* (Durham, NC: Duke University Press, 2003).

32 S. M. Streeter, *Managing the Counterrevolution: The United States and Guatemala, 1954–1961* (Ohio University Center for International Studies, 2000).

33 Ibid.

34 V. Sanford, *Buried Secrets: Truth and Human Rights in Guatemala* (New York: Palgrave Macmillan, 2003); and Garrard-Burnett, *Terror in the Land of the Holy Spirit*.

35 G. Lovell, *A Beauty That Hurts: Life and Death in Guatemala*, 2nd rev. ed. (Austin, TX: University of Texas Press, 2010); see also Sanford, *Buried Secrets*; and Garrard-Burnett, *Terror in the Land of the Holy Spirit*.

36 "Ligan a proceso a Ríos Montt por genocidio durante conflicto armado," *Prensa Libre* (Jan. 26, 2012), available from www.prensalibre.com; see also E. Malkin, "Accused of Atrocities, Guatemala's Ex-Dictator Chooses Silence," *New York Times* (Jan. 27, 2012), available from www.nytimes.com.

37 "Jueza liga a Ríos Montt a un segundo proceso por genocidio," *El Periódico* (May 21, 2012), available from www.elperiodico.com.gt; see also "Guatemala Ex-leader Ríos Montt Faces Massacre Trial," *BBC* (May 22, 2012), available from www.bbc.co.uk.

38 Informe del Proyecto Interdiocesano de Recuperación de la Memoria Histórica, "Guatemala: Nunca Más," Oficina de Derechos Humanos del Arzobispado de Guatemala; see also F. Goldman, *The Art of Political Murder: Who Killed the Bishop?* (New York: Grove Press, 2008.

39 Guatemalan Commission of Historical Clarification, "Guatemala: Memory of Silence" (report, 1999).

40 Guatemalan Commission of Historical Clarification, "Guatemala: Memory of Silence." Sanford, *Buried Secrets*.

41 C. Chase-Dunn, "Guatemala in the Global System," *Journal of Interamerican Studies and World Affairs* 42 (2000):109–126.

42 See CEPAL, Impacto del Tratado de Libre Comercio de Centroamérica en la agricultura y el sector rural en cinco países centroamericanos.

43 S. Gauster and P. Sigüenza, "El Impacto de los altos precios de los commodities: Guatemala" (CONGCOOP/Instituto de Estudios Agrarios y Rurales, Guatemala: 2008).

44 Ibid.

45 Guatemalan Human Rights Commission (2010).

46 U. Gamarro and A. Ortiz, "Costo de vida llega a 7.63%," *Prense Libre* (Sept. 8, 2011), 28. INE.

47 Guatemala 2011 Acuerdo Gubernativo No. 388–2010 Salario Minimo.

48 L. Diaz Zecena. "Canasta básica vital se sitúa en Q3 mil 712.77," *Prensa Libre* (Aug. 11, 2010), available from www.prensalibre.com. INE.

49 M. Barillias, "Guatemala Verges on Status as Failed State," (Apr. 8, 2010), accessed May 28, 2011, available from www.energypublisher.com. See also S. Kinzer, "Guatemala's Challenge," *The Guardian* (Jan. 14, 2008), accessed May 28, 2011, available from www.guardian.co.uk.

50 Barillias, "Guatemala Verges on Status as Failed State," accessed May 28, 2011, available from www.speroforum.com. See also S. Kinzer, "Guatemala's Challenge."

51 S. M. Streeter, "Nation-Building in the Land of Eternal Counter-Insurgency: Guatemala and the Contradictions of the Alliance for Progress," *Third World Quarterly* 27 (2006):57–68.

52 Streeter, "Nation-Building in the Land of Eternal Counter-Insurgency." E. Beck, "Las ONG y las Mujeres: Los Pros y Contras de las ONG en Guatemala. Más que Desarrollo: Memorias de la Primera Conferencia Bienal sobre Desarrollo y Acción Comunitaria." (Bethel, VT: Wuqu' Kawoq, 2011).

53 D. Levenson, "Reaction to Trauma: The 1976 Earthquake in Guatemala," *International Labor and Working-Class History* 62 (2002):60–68. S. Kurtenbach, "Guatemala's Post-War Development: The Structural Failure of Low Intensity Peace; Project Working Paper No. 3: Social and Political Fractures after Wars" (Duisburg, Germany: Institute for Development and Peace, 2008).

54 Beck, "Las ONG y las Mujeres." Ceidec, "Guatemala ONG's y Desarrollo: El Caso del Altiplano Central" (Mexico: Ceidec, 1993).

55 Chase-Dunn, "Guatemala in the Global System."

56 A. Sridhar, "Tax Reform and Promoting a Culture of Philanthropy: Guatemala's 'Third Sector' in an Era of Peace," *Fordham International Law Journal* 31 (2007):186–229. Beck, "Las ONG y las Mujeres."

57 Ministerio de Salud Pública y Asistencia Social (MSPAS), Instituto Nacional de Estadística, Universidad del Valle de Guatemala, USAID, Agencia Sueca de Cooperación para el Desarollo Internacional, CDC, UNICEF, UNFPA, PAHO, USAID/Calidad

en Salud, "V Encuesta Nacional de Salud Materno Infantil 2008–2009" (Guatemala City: MSPAS et al., 2009).

58 INE, "Encuesta Nacional de Ingresos y Gastos Familiares 1998" (Guatemala City: INE, 1999).

59 It is well documented that far more people identify as ethnically Maya than those who report fluency in a Mayan language; see, for example, B. M. French, *Maya Ethnolinguistic Identity: Violence, Cultural Rights, and Modernity in Highland Guatemala* (Tucson, AZ: University of Arizona Press, 2010). Similarly, according to one expert estimate, perhaps only one-half of self-identifying Maya routinely speak a Mayan language (N. England, "Mayan Language Revival and Revitalization Politics: Linguists and Linguistic Ideologies" *American Anthropologist* 105 [2003]:733–743). Based on our own experience, however, we suspect that language use is greatly underestimated, because our collaborators often relate how they withhold their ability to speak a Mayan language, fearing that this disclosure may negatively impact their employment or other advancement prospects. Further, the targeting of Mayan language speakers during the decades-long civil war is still a recent memory for many communities.

60 D. Cojti, "El desarrollo socioeconomico contra el desarrollo de los idiomas indigenas," Proceedings of the Symposium on Teaching and Learning Indigenous Languages of Latin America 2011. (Notre Dame, IN: forthcoming).

61 J. M. Maxwell, "Revitalización de los Idiomas Mayas de Guatemala" in *Más que Desarrollo: Memorias de la Primera Conferencia Bienal sobre Desarrollo y Acción Comunitaria*, P. Rohloff, A. Kraemer Díaz, and J. Ajsivinac Sian (Bethel, VT: Wuqu' Kawoq, 2011).

62 M. Richards, *Atlas Lingüístico de Guatemala*. (Guatemala City: Editorial Serviprensa, 2003). Inst. de Lingüístico y Educación de la Universidad Rafael Landívar.

63 D. Greebon, "Educación Primaria Bilingüe desde el Aula" in *Más que Desarrollo*, Rohloff, Kraemer Díaz, and Ajsivinac Sian.

64 Greebon, "Educación Primaria Bilingüe desde el Aula." See also Maxwell, "Revitalización de los Idiomas Mayas de Guatemala."

65 Maxwell, "Revitalización de los Idiomas Mayas de Guatemala." Three field-school opportunities that currently exist include the Oxlajuj Aj Kaqchikel field school (Tulane University), the Kablajuj Ey Kaqchikel field school (Wuqu' Kawoq), and the Summer K'ichee' field school (University of Chicago).

66 M. Gragnolati and A. Marini, *Health and Poverty in Guatemala*. (Washington: World Bank, 2003).

67 MSPAS et al., "V Encuesta Nacional de Salud Materno Infantil 2008–2009."

68 B. Schieber and C. Stanton, "Estimación de Mortalidad Materna en Guatemala Período 1996–1998" (Guatemala: GSD Consultores Asociados/Measure/Evaluation Macro International, 2000).

69 T. Rosada and L. Bruni, "Crisis y pobreza rural en América Latina: el caso de Guatemala" (Santiago: Rimisp 2009).

70 For more discussion of this phenomena, see P. Rohloff, A. Kraemer Díaz, and S. Dasgupta, "'Beyond Development': A Critical Appraisal of the Emergence of Small Health Care Non-Governmental Organizations in Rural Guatemala," *Human*

Organization 70.4 (2011):427–437. It is common for nonindigenous professionals to refer to Mayan languages as *lengua/tongue* or *dialecto/dialect*; only Spanish is awarded the semantic status of *idioma/language*.

71 N. S. Berry, "Who's Judging the Quality of Care? Indigenous Maya and the Problem of 'Not Neing Attended.'" *Medical Anthropology Quarterly* 27 (2008):164–189.

72 Others have also convincingly shown that the fact that indigenous people are less likely to access healthcare services is not a problem of physical distance from a healthcare facility. See, for example, S. Annis, "Physical Access and Utilization of Health Services in Rural Guatemala," *Social Science and Medicine* 15 (1981):515–523. See also D. A. Glei and N. Goldman, "Understanding Ethnic Variation in Pregnancy-Related Care in Rural Guatemala, *Ethnic Health* 5 (2000):5–22.

73 An auxiliary nurse has approximately the same level of training as a licensed practical nurse (LPN) in the United States.

74 For example, it is not uncommon for family members of a hospitalized patient to be asked to purchase antibiotics for intravenous administration at a private pharmacy. For further discussion, see Berry, "Who's Judging the Quality of Care?"

75 J. Maupin, "Fruits of the Accords: Health Care Reform, Decentralization, and Community Participation in Highland Guatemala" (PhD dissertation, SUNY–Albany, 2006).

76 G. M. La Forgia, P. Mintz, and C. Cerezo. "Is the Perfect the Enemy of the Good? A Case Study on Large-scale Contracting for Basic Health Services in Rural Guatemala" in *Health System Innovations in Central America: Lesson and Impact of New Approaches*, ed. G. M. La Forgia (Washington: World Bank, 2005), 9–48.

77 Maupin, "Fruits of the Accords." See also Gragnolati and Marini, *Health and Poverty in Guatemala.*

78 J. Maupin, "Divergent Models of Community Health Workers in Highland Guatemala," *Human Organization* 70 (2011):44–53. See also Rohloff, Kraemer Díaz, and Dasgupta "'Beyond Development.'"

79 Aldo Castañeda is one of the preeminent cardiovascular surgeons in the world, formerly surgeon-in-chief at Boston Children's Hospital.

80 Personal communication, Guillermo Gaitan, director of pediatric cardiology, UNICAR.

81 Maupin, "Fruits of the Accords."

82 K. Newell, "Health by the People" in *Health by the People*, ed. K. Newell (Geneva: WHO, 1975), 191–203.

83 See www.asecsaguate.org.

84 A. Hernandez, "Auxiliares de enfermería en areas rurales de Guatemala" (presentation at 2nd Futuros Colectivos Conference, Patzun, Guatemala, Oct. 2011).

85 A. Chary et al., "The Changing Role of Indigenous Lay Midwives in Guatemala: New Frameworks for Analysis" (in submission to *Midwifery*, 2012).

86 World Bank, "Improving Health and Nutrition of Mothers and Young Children in Guatemala" (New York: World Bank, 2010), available from http://web.worldbank.org.

87 See MSPAS et al., "V Encuesta Nacional de Salud Materno Infantil 2008–2009."

88 World Bank, "International Bank for Reconstruction and Development and International Finance Corporation Country Partnership Strategy for the Republic of Guatemala," report no. 44772-GT (New York: World Bank, 2008).

89 N. Scrimshaw, "History and Early Development of INCAP," *Journal of Nutrition* 140 (2010):394–396.

90 R. Martorell, J.-P. Habicht, and J. Rivera, "History and Design of the INCAP Longitudinal Study (1969–77) and Its Follow-up (1988–89)," *Journal of Nutrition* 125 (1995):1027S–1041S.

91 A. Stein, P. Melgar, J. Hoddinott, and R. Martorell, "Cohort Profile: The Institute of Nutrition of Central America and Panama (INCAP) Nutrition Trial Cohort Study," *International Journal of Epidemiology* 37 (2008): 716–720.

92 Ibid.

93 M. Ruel, J. Rivera, and J.-P. Habicht, "Length Screens Better than Weight in Stunted Populations," *Journal of Nutrition* 125 (1995):1222–1228.

94 R. Martorell, "Physical Growth and Development of the Malnourished Child: Contributions from 50 Years of Research at INCAP," *Food and Nutrition Bulletin* 31.1 (2010): 68–82.

95 See Martorell et al., "History and Design of the INCAP Longitudinal Study."

96 N. Scrimshaw, C. Taylor, and J. Gordon, "Interactions of Nutrition and Infection" (Geneva: WHO, 1968); N. L. Solien de Gonzalez, "Health Behavior in Cross-Cultural Perspective: A Guatemalan Example," *Human Organization* 25 (1966):122–125; and J. Salomon, L. Mata, and J. Gordon, "Malnutrition and the Communicable Diseases of Childhood in Rural Guatemala," *American Journal of Public Health* 58 (1968):505–516. See also Scrimshaw, "History and Early Development of INCAP."

97 J. Rivera and M. Ruel, "The Timing of Growth Retardation in Rural Guatemalan Children with Adequate Birth Weight," *FASEB Journal* 7 (1993):A282.

98 Nutrinet, "Historia de la alimentación escolar en Guatemala" (Nutrinet: 2009), available from http://guatemala.nutrinet.org.

99 G. Gunderson, "The National School Lunch Program: Background and Development. (USDA Food and Nutrition Service, 2009), available from www.fns.usda.gov.

100 See Nutrinet, "Historia de la alimentación escolar en Guatemala."

101 L. De Leon, "La galleta escolar nutricionalmente mejorada," *INCAP Notas Tecnicas* 5 (1995):1–2. See also Scrimshaw, "History and Early Development of INCAP."

102 Personal communication, Margaret Blood, director, Mil Milagros. Mil Milagros is an NGO that develops parent-teacher associations around Lake Atitlán to improve school outcomes.

103 Food and Nutritional Technical Assistance 2, "Preventing Malnutrition In Children Under 2 Approach (PM2A): A Food-Assisted Approach" (Washington: FANTA, 2010).

104 C. Gamazo, "La Ventana de los Mil Días" *El Periodico* (Nov. 28, 2011), avaliable from www.elperiodico.com.gt.

105 Secretaría de Planificación y Programación de la Presidencia, "Pacto Hambre Cero: Retos para Guatemala" (2012), available from www.unicef.org.gt.

106 J. Rah, S. dePee, K. Kraemer, G. Steiger, M. Bloem, P. Spiegel et al., "Program Experience with Micronutrient Powders and Current Evidence," *Journal of Nutrition* 142 (2012):191S–196S.

107 P. Rohloff, N. Henretty, S. Messmer, E. Sorenson, F. Cali, J. Federico Cali et al., "Feasibility of Chispitas as a Treatment for Iron Deficiency Anemia in Rural Guatemala: Report of a Pilot Study" (Santiago Sacatepéquez: Wuqu' Kawoq, 2011).

108 J. Phuka, K. Maleta, C. Thakwalakwa, Y. Cheung, A. Briend, M. Manary et al., "Complementary Feeding with Fortified Spread and Incidence of Severe Stunting in 6- to 18-month-old Rural Malawians," *Archives of Pediatrics and Adolescent Medicine*, 162 (2008):619–626.

109 Nutributter® and Plumpy'Doz™ that make it into Guatemala are currently manufactured by Edesia, LLC, an NGO based in Providence, Rhode Island. One programmatic focus for Edesia is the development of nutrition capacity, including production, in Central America. A coalition of health and development researchers from Vanderbilt University is also advancing a well-developed concept for local manufacturing under the name Mani-Plus (personal communication, Edward Fischer, Vanderbilt University).

110 K. Dewey, "Nutrition, Growth, and Complementary Feeding of the Breastfed Infant," *Pediatric Clinics of North America* 48.1 (2001):87–104.

111 A. Chary, S. Dasgupta, S. Messmer, and P. Rohloff, "Breastfeeding, Subjugation, and Empowerment in Rural Guatemala" in *An Anthropology of Mothering*, ed. M. Walks and N. McPherson (Toronto: Demeter Press, 2011). A. Chary, S. Messmer, and P. Rohoff, "Male Influence on Infant Feeding in Rural Guatemala and Implications for Child Nutrition Interventions," *Breastfeeding Medicine* 6 (2011):227–231.

112 WHO, "Epidemiological Fact Sheet on HIV and AIDS: Guatemala" (2008). Although this number is no doubt influenced by significant underreporting, it is still quite low.

113 WHO, *Global Tuberculosis Control 2011*.

114 WHO, *World Malaria Report 2010*.

115 WHO, *Global Status Report on Noncommunicable Diseases 2010*.

116 Ibid.

117 MSPAS, "Enfermedades Crónicas No Transmisibles" (n.d.).

118 MSPAS, "Diabetes Mellitus" (2010).

119 G. Danaei, M. Finucane, Y. Lu, G. Singh, M. Cowan, C. Paciorek et al., "National, Regional, and Global Trends in Fasting Plasma Glucose and Diabetes Prevalence since 1980: Systematic Analysis of Health Examination Surveys and Epidemiological Studies with 370 Country-Years and 2.7 Million Participants," *Lancet* 378.9785 (2011):31–40.

120 WHO Diabetes Action Now; and Danaei et al., "National, Regional, and Global Trends in Fasting Plasma Glucose and Diabetes Prevalence since 1980."

121 PAHO, "Survey of Diabetes, Hypertension and Chronic Disease Risk Factors: Villa Nueva, Guatemala, 2007."

122 PAHO "Survey of Diabetes, Hypertension, and Chronic Disease Risk Factors"; and C. Gregory, J. Dai, M. Ramirez-Zea, and A. Stein, "Occupation Is More Important than Rural or Urban Residence in Explaining the Prevalence of Metabolic and Cardiovascular Disease Risk in Guatemalan Adults," *Journal of Nutrition* 137 (2007):1314–1319.

123 A. Sawaya, P. Martins, V. Baccin Martins, T. Florêncio, D. Hoffman, P. do Carmo et al., "Malnutrition, Long-term Health and the Effect of Nutritional Recovery," Nestlé Nutrition Workshop Series: Pediatric Program 63 (2009):95. L. Grillo, A. Siqueira, A. Silva, P. Martins, I. Verreschi, A. Sawaya, "Lower Resting Meta-

bolic Rate and Higher Velocity of Weight Gain in a Prospective Study of Stunted vs Nonstunted Girls Living in the Shantytowns of Säo Paulo, Brazil," *European Journal of Clinical Nutrition* 59 (2005):835. W. Leonard, M. Sorensen, M. Mosher, V. Spitsyn, A. Comuzzie, "Reduced Fat Oxidation and Obesity Risks among the Buryat of Southern Siberia," *American Journal of Human Biology* 21 (2009):664. A. El Taguri, F. Besmar, A. Abdel Monem, I. Betilmal, C. Ricour, M. Rolland-Cachera, "Stunting is a Major Risk Factor for Overweight: Results from National Surveys in 5 Arab Countries," *Eastern Mediterranean Health Journal* 15 (2009):549.

124 M. Greiner et al., "Determining Type 2 Diabetes-Related Health Care Needs in an Indigenous Population from Rural Guatemala: A Mixed Methods Preliminary Study" (in submission, 2012).

125 WHO, "Use of Glycated Haemoglobin (HbA1c) in the Diagnosis of Diabetes Mellitus" (2011).

126 Examples include Link for Health (www.linkforhealth.org), Guatemala NGO Network (La Antigua Guatemala Network, www.laantiguaguatemala.net), and Habla Guate (http://hablaguate.com).

127 See www.futuroscolectivos.com.

128 Rohloff et al., "'Beyond Development.'"

129 See the relevant organization websites for Proyecto Lingüístico Francisco Marroquín (www.plfm.org), Tulane University's Oxlajuj Aj Kaqchikel field school (www.tulane.edu), Wuqu' Kawoq's Kablajuj Ey Kaqchikel field school (www.wuqukawoq.org), and the University of Chicago's Summer K'ichee' Maya Institute (http://clas.uchicago.edu).

Suggested Websites

Guatemalan Academy of Mayan Languages: www.almg.org
INCAP: www.incap.org
Wuqu' Kawoq—Maya Health Alliance: www.wuqukawoq.org
Edesia: www.edesiallc.org
National Security Archive Guatemala Project: www.gwu.edu/~nsarchiv/guatemala
CIRMA: www.ama.edu.gt/cirma

Suggested Reading

Metz, Brent. *'Ch'orti'-Maya Survival in Eastern Guatemala: Indigenity in Transition* (Albuquerque, NM: University of New Mexico Press, 2006).

Wilkinson, Daniel. *Silence on the Mountain: Stories of Terror, Betrayal, and Forgetting in Guatemala* (Durham, NC: Duke University Press, 2004).

Coe, Michael D. *The Maya*. 8th ed. (London: Thames and Hudson, 2011).

Garrard-Burnett, Virginia. *Terror in the Land of the Holy Spirit: Guatemala under General Efraín Ríos Montt* (New York: Oxford University Press, 2011).

3 El Salvador

Jennifer Kasper and Clyde Lanford Smith

Contributors: Denise Zwahlen, Isabel Quintero, Elizabeth Rogers, Alex Lugar, Sara Doorley, Brenda Hubbard, Chico Montes, and many more people from Santa Marta, El Salvador

The health and well-being of every person in the world is greatly influenced by social, economic, political, and cultural forces. Although biomedicine (for example, anatomy, physiology, pharmacology, and biology) is important, this model falls short of explaining the diversity of health and disease inequalities. There is clear evidence that access to healthcare plays only a minor role in a person's overall risk of being ill and dying; behavior and a multitude of social factors hold much greater importance. Social medicine involves how we define health and disease, how we diagnose and treat, how we finance healthcare, and who has access to what health services.[1] Rudolf Virchow, a pioneer in medicine and advocacy, said that the health of the population is a matter of social concern.[2]

The World Health Organization's definition of health highlights the importance of people living to their fullest potential: "health is a state of complete physical, mental, and social well-being and not merely the absence of disease or infirmity."[3] The Declaration of Alma Ata stresses the critical role of many societal sectors, not just healthcare: "health is a fundamental human right, and attainment of the highest possible level of health is a most-important world-wide social goal whose realization requires the action of many other social and economic sectors in addition to the health sector."[4]

The fact that 1.2 billion people live in extreme poverty (defined by the World Bank as having income lower than $1.25 US per day[5]) is not a result of biology. Disparities in wealth and poverty translate into health inequalities. The poor consume the least in terms of material wealth, but are consumed the most by preventable illnesses and, increasingly, by non-communicable diseases such as hypertension and cancer. A keen, critical examination of this reality is necessary. And one of the ways to examine this is with the help of the poor. They should be invited to and included in the discussion. Unfortunately, in many instances, their voices are not heard, or worse yet, are silenced. In this chapter we will share the story of Santa Marta, El Salvador, a community that is working hard to have its voice heard. And we will share how Doctors for Global Health works to amplify the voices of the people of Santa Marta.

Brief History

To gain a deeper understanding of the health and well-being of the people of El Salvador today, and in particular Santa Marta, one must understand and reflect on an important aspect of social medicine: past centuries. The impoverished, indigenous people of El Salvador, primarily of Maya or perhaps Pipil descent, were once a vibrant population before the Spanish conquest. However, centuries of oppression and structural violence have drastically reduced their number. Since the time of the Spanish conquistadors in the early sixteenth century, wealth has been consolidated and controlled by a few people, while land and resources have been denied to the poor. These disparities in resources and wealth intermittently have led to revolt to redress inequities. One well-known uprising was the 1932 peasant fight for human rights and land redistribution. In response, the Salvadoran government systematically massacred between 35,000 and 50,000 indigenous people (the massacre is known as *La Matanza* in Spanish). After La Matanza, indigenous people were forced to give up their traditions and worked in earnest to assimilate into the dominant Latino culture to avoid being singled out, discriminated against, and killed; they accelerated this process of assimilation during the civil conflict of 1980–1992. Today, the primary indigenous groups of Nahua-Pipiles, Lencas, and Cacaoperas account for approximately four to ten percent of the general Salvadoran population, and they struggle to maintain their identity.[6]

By the twentieth century, 2 percent of El Salvador's population controlled 95 percent of the country's income. During the 1970s, El Salvador's people suffered from increased levels of landlessness, poverty, and unemployment. At the onset of the civil war in 1980, most farms (90 percent) were insufficient even for subsistence farming; 60 percent of rural farmers did not earn enough to purchase the most basic foodstuffs. Six families held more land than 133,000 small farmers.[7] Increased repression against the poor and organized labor, as well as assassinations of leaders of social and political movements, led to a twelve-year armed civil conflict. Salvadoran military leaders employed scorched-earth and *sacar el pez del agua* ("remove the fish from the water") policies. Serious human rights abuses ensued; one of the most well known was the El Mozote massacre, in which approximately 1,000 people—mostly women and children—were killed, and there was only one survivor. Other military tactics included the hammer-and-anvil operation: one military troop would force inhabitants to flee into the hands of another military troop. During the Río Lempa massacre, people fleeing Salvadoran forces by crossing the

Río Lempa were killed by Honduran military on the other side. People living in "free-fire zones" were subjected to aerial bombardment with napalm incendiary bombs, resulting in loss of human life and environmental degradation.

During the civil war, an estimated 75,000 were killed; innumerable people were tortured and disappeared; 1 million fled the country, and 500,000 were internally displaced. This had a devastating effect on the country's population of 6 million. The war consumed 36 percent of the national budget in 1986.[8] From 1976 to 1986, per capita spending by the Ministry of Health fell by one-third, and clinics were either destroyed or abandoned.[9]

The Chapultepec Peace Accords were signed in January 1992, ended the civil war, and mandated the creation of a Truth Commission. The commission asserted that the Salvadoran government had a systemic policy supporting violence against unarmed civilians; it was responsible for 85 percent of the human rights atrocities, while the guerilla forces were responsible for 5 percent (10 percent of abuses had undetermined perpetrators).[10] Evidence confirms that the US government's nearly $6 billion US in aid and its military school in Fort Benning, Georgia (then called the School of the Americas, or SOA, and in 2001 renamed the Western Hemisphere Institute for Security Cooperation), supported the Salvadoran government and its military in committing human rights abuses and atrocities.[11]

International NGO presence in El Salvador, including health-related initiatives from groups such as Doctors Without Borders (Médecins Sans Frontières, MSF), the International Committee of the Red Cross (ICRC) and Médecins du Monde (MDM), was greatly increased during the armed civil conflict from 1980 to 1992. However, after the signing of the peace accords, the ICRC and MSF left. Thereafter, international NGO presence has fluctuated depending on perceptions of disaster management, with increased presence during Hurricane Mitch in 1998 and the earthquake of 2001.[12]

Politics

Social medicine is also steeped in politics, and the politics of health. The right-wing Nationalist Republican Alliance (ARENA) was founded by Roberto D'Abuisson, a death squad leader trained at SOA who was responsible for many of the massacres during the civil conflict of 1980–1992. ARENA had been the dominant political party since the 1992 peace accords. The Salvadoran government practiced neoliberal policies that included privatization of social services (for example, healthcare and education). The government also proposed the Plan Contra la Pobreza (Plan to Confront Poverty), designed to provide cash assistance to 100,000 poor families, allocate hundreds of millions USD for microenterprise, and invest $200 million US to restart 100

Ministry of Health clinics. But no money was allocated for any of this, and rural, isolated communities were even more neglected in the ensuing years.

In 2009 the left-wing political party, Farabundo Martí National Liberation Front (FMLN), won the presidential elections. President Mauricio Funes inaugurated the first Economic and Social Council (this had been a part of the peace accords, but no president had put it into practice). His government instituted an ambitious platform that included job creation; improving basic infrastructure and housing; opening diplomatic ties with Cuba; strengthening nutrition and education for children; and improving access to healthcare via a more comprehensive hospital and subspecialty network. This was a tall order, as the country was $1 billion US in debt.[13] The government doubled investment in health services and removed "voluntary payments" for hospitalized patients. It created 410 community-based healthcare teams (doctor, nurse, nurse assistant, logistician, and three community health workers for every 600 families) based in approximately one-half of the municipalities. The government now provides free meals, uniforms, shoes, and supplies for every schoolchild. Small family farmers and cooperatives have received free seeds, fertilizer, technical assistance, and low-cost credit. Land titles have been granted to nearly 1,000 families.[14]

Though there are no active civil conflicts, tensions are high in Latin America. Through an agreement between the Salvadoran and US governments, an International Law Enforcement Academy (ILEA) was established in El Salvador in 2005. Although its purpose includes confronting human rights violations as well as human and drug trafficking, many are concerned that it allows for increased US intervention, militarization, and promotion of US interests in the region, and guarantees immunity to foreigners who participate in ILEA.[15] In June 2009, Honduras experienced a military coup when President Manuel Zelaya, an open critic of US foreign policy, was forced from the country and his supporters subjected to terror. Despite initial condemnation by President Obama, there was strong support of the coup leaders by some members of the US Congress, and the US government in essence supported the interim government with military aid. This set a precedent that some believe may be used for dealing with similar governments and leaders who defy US foreign policy, and sent a strong message to the new FMLN government of El Salvador.[16]

Economics

As mentioned earlier, one of the most important social factors affecting health is absolute wealth and inequalities in wealth. With 6 million people, El Salvador is the most densely populated country in Central America.[17] It also has one of the highest income disparities in the world.[18] Historically a coffee oligarchy, the economy of El Salvador is controlled by a banking oligarchy, with the combined wealth of the top five banks five times greater than the Salvadoran government's budget. More than one-third of the population lives below the poverty line.[19] The wealthiest 20 percent have 58 percent of total income, and the poorest 20 percent have 3.3 percent; two-thirds work in the informal sector, and the average monthly salary is $154 US. Salvadorans suffer from deprivations in multiple dimensions, including lack of income, poor school attendance, illiteracy, and lack of access to safe sanitation and water, or to housing that meets minimum-quality standards. There is a clear disparity between urban and rural Salvadorans: 44 percent of Salvadorans in urban settings suffer deprivations in at least two of these dimensions; this jumps to 93 percent of Salvadorans in rural settings.[20] According to the UN Development Program, El Salvador's Human Development Index (HDI) ranks it in the lowest third.[21]

Rather than tackle this problem, the ARENA government changed the country's currency to the US dollar on January 1, 2001, reportedly to stabilize the economy.[22] ARENA also led the passage of the Central American Free Trade Agreement (CAFTA-DR) during a late-night vote in December 2004. The terms of CAFTA-DR require that El Salvador change its economic and trade policies (for example, remove import and export taxes for transnational corporations, and allow weak labor laws and environmental standards) to secure foreign direct investment. CAFTA-DR exacerbated income disparity and increased poverty.[23] After CAFTA-DR's passage, food prices rose, and subsistence farmers could not compete with agribusinesses. The World Food Program stated that the sharp increase in global food prices means that average rural Salvadorans now eat 60 percent of what they used to eat.[24] Many farmers gave up their livelihoods and migrated to the capital, San Salvador, to work in *maquilas* (sweatshops). This internal migration has led to increased poverty rates. More than 25 percent of the country's population (1.5 million) lives in makeshift homes of plastic and rusty sheet metal in ad hoc urban settlements around San Salvador, accounting for 58 percent of Salvadorans living in poverty. The country relies on 13 percent sales tax, which again disproportionately affects the poor. Since CAFTA-DR was instituted, El Salvador has experienced a trade deficit.

During the civil conflict, many people fled to other countries to seek political asylum; many now flee to seek economic asylum. Since the twelve-year civil war, a steady stream of Salvadorans have risked their lives crossing into California, the desert in Arizona, or rivers in Texas to attempt to make a better life in the United States and support family in El Salvador; the country's number-one export is people. As of this writing, approximately 2.5 million Salvadorans live and work in the United States, and in 2011, their remittances accounted for $3.6 billion US, or 16 percent of GDP, according to the Banco Central de Reserva de El Salvador.[25] Even though 30 percent of households receive remittances, 20 percent of Salvadorans still live in extreme poverty (that is, less than $1.25 US per day). Without remittances, this figure would be nearly doubled.[26] The ever-growing number of hybrid, transnational families has resulted in 40 percent of Salvadoran children growing up without one or both parents.[27] The psychological, educational, and economic consequences of this situation are yet to be fully elucidated.

Finally, El Salvador is still paying off loans received from the International Monetary Fund in the 1970s and 1980s.[28] It spends nearly twice its GDP on debt relief (6 percent) as compared to health (3.8 percent).[29]

Health

The effects of war, poverty, disparities, political processes, and environmental degradation are writ large on the bodies of impoverished men, women, and children. The maternal mortality ratio is 170 per 100,000 births (the US ratio is 13 per 100,000); infant mortality is 16 per 1,000 (the US ratio is 7 per 1000); and under-five mortality is 19 per 1,000 (the US ratio is 5 per 1,000).[30] With disaggregation of the data, infants and children in the lowest income quintile have four and five times the mortality risk when compared to those in the highest quintile.[31] The major causes of death are neonatal (40 percent), pneumonia (13 percent), and diarrhea (12 percent). Malnutrition is still prevalent and plays a prominent role in these deaths: of children under age 5 years, 8.6 percent are underweight, and 20 percent are stunted.[32] A network of government health programs, including rural clinics and CHWs, has achieved a childhood immunization rate of 85 percent.

Environmental Factors

El Salvador faces many environmental burdens, which also impact health. It is the most heavily deforested country in Latin America, and 95 percent of its rivers are polluted. Most wastewater is not treated; instead, it is dumped directly into rivers and coastal waters. Analysis of river water reveals high concentrations of bacteria, metals, pesticides, and toxic gases (for example, ammonia).[33] Many people obtain their water from these polluted sources. Nationally, only 44.5 percent of people in the lowest income quintile have access to safe water, and 8 percent have access to a toilet.[34] For rural people, the situation is worse: only 33 percent have access to piped water, while 20 percent must collect water from a water hole or river; the majority use latrines, and 20 percent still have no access to sanitation. The lack of appropriate, safe water and sanitation creates a complex interplay among parasitic and diarrheal infections, malnutrition, anemia, and academic attainment in children, and this also has ramifications for their future economic success as adults.

Healthcare System

Even as infectious, communicable diseases continue to plague the poor, the country is undergoing an epidemiologic transition; the prevalence of chronic diseases such as hypertension, cancer, diabetes, asthma, and HIV is growing. El Salvador is experiencing a double jeopardy; it has a high burden of communicable and noncommunicable illnesses and an insufficient number of healthcare workers to care for the sick.

In terms of healthcare infrastructure, El Salvador is one of fifty-seven countries worldwide with a severe lack and inequitable distribution of human resources;[35] this is defined by WHO as fewer than 23 health workers (doctors, nurses, midwives, and ancillary providers) per 10,000 people to provide adequate primary care. Such care includes deliveries by skilled birth attendants and immunization, two interventions that can have a significant impact on maternal and child mortality.[36] El Salvador has historically had a highly centralized, fragmented, privatized healthcare system, with major public hospitals, including the only children's hospital in the entire country, concentrated in the capital of San Salvador. The current government has named health a human right and a public good, and is striving for greater participation of the general populace in defining health priorities, strengthening primary care, and improving access to subspecialty care, while enhancing preventive strategies, water and sanitation, reproductive health, and nutrition.[37] The government also needs to confront the fact that El Salvador pays the highest prices for medications of any country in Central America.

Even though a variety of public insurances exist—Bienestar Magísterial (Teachers' Welfare), Sanidad Militar (Military Health Services), Instituto Salvadoreno del Seguro Social (Salvadoran Social Security Institute), FOSALUD (a fund created from the taxes collected on tobacco and alcoholic drinks), and the Ministry of Health—as well as private insurance and health clinics and hospitals, they are insufficient to meet the need; nearly one-half of all Salvadorans do not have access.[38] The challenge is to create a seamless system.[39]

Regarding the MDGs, El Salvador's progress is a mixed picture, depending on the indicator and reporting source.[40] The country has reduced its extreme poverty, increased access to primary education, increased access to water and sanitation, and reduced child and maternal mortality. Yet El Salvador needs to redouble its efforts not only to achieve these goals, but also to greatly reduce hunger (which remains stagnant at 10 percent, while the percentage of people not receiving the minimum dietary energy consumption has increased from 7 to 9 percent since 2002), increase HIV prevention and treatment, and increase vaccine coverage. And the country needs to reduce, if not eliminate, the disparity between rural and urban populations.

Doctors for Global Health and Its Partnership with Santa Marta

Santa Marta is in the Department of Cabañas, northeast of the capital San Salvador, and shares its northern border with Honduras. The community suffered during the civil conflict; many were massacred by Salvadoran and Honduran armed forces as they tried to cross the Río Lempa to live as refugees in Honduras. In 1987, while armed civil conflict was still in full force, the people of Santa Marta returned to reestablish and recreate their community.

Doctors for Global Health

The mission of DGH is "to improve health and foster other human rights with those most in need by accompanying communities, while educating and inspiring others to action."[41] We do this by practicing *accompaniment*, a concept adopted from other grassroots organizations that expresses how to work with marginalized populations. Our partner communities know and approve of us, and they invite us to work with them. We engage in a participatory process *with* the community rather than imposing our way of thinking or doing things. Local partners define their priorities; we help them implement these at their rhythm.

Another defining aspect of DGH is *liberation medicine*, or "the conscious, conscientious use of health to promote social justice and human dignity."[42] Inspiration for this concept came from Ignacio Martín-Baró's *Writings for a Liberation Psychology*. Liberation medicine emphasizes using practical tools (notably the UN Universal Declaration of Human Rights and related documents, the social medicine tradition, art such as street theater, and community-oriented primary care) to plan and effect practical, palpable action.[43] Former El Salvador Archbishop Oscar Romero declared that we should be a "voice for those without voice"; DGH interprets this as a mandate to amplify the voices of the silenced. One of the most important functions of DGH is to create a space where observation, reflection, action, and evaluation toward optimal health and social justice can find respect and affirmation.

DGH fully endorses the WHO definition of health and the charge from the Declaration of Alma Ata that to obtain optimal health, we must involve many different sectors in society.[44] While striving for equity, DGH also recognizes the opportunity and responsibility to celebrate life through art, music, and theater, and to provide a "vaccination of hope" with others in the struggle. DGH puts this spirit into practice during its annual general assemblies (meetings that bring together people from our partner communities and from all walks of life in the United States who are interested in health and human rights, equity and social justice). Principles of Action guide the vision and everyday work of DGH.

Doctors for Global Health Invitation to Work in Santa Marta

In 1998, DGH was initially invited to work with rehabilitation health promoters in Santa Marta. This came about because of a remarkable woman, Brenda Hubbard. Brenda is a US physical therapist who arrived in San Salvador in August 1989 to accompany the women of a Salvadoran organization called Co-Madres. Her experience was life-changing, as she saw how US tax dollars were being spent to torture, slaughter, and disappear Salvadoran youth and adults, and to destroy the infrastructure of the country. Brenda helped establish a rehabilitation program for people injured in the conflict, and trained local people to be rehabilitation health promoters in Santa Marta. When Brenda learned of DGH's work, she asked DGH to collaborate.

The original invitation for DGH coordination centered on asthma management, including solicitation of medications, and DGH responded positively. Asthma is a serious problem worldwide, affecting an estimated 235 million people; it is the most common pediatric chronic disease. More than 80 percent of deaths due to asthma occur in low- and middle-income countries, including El Salvador.[45] Since our initial invitation, the rehabilitation health promoter program has greatly expanded to include services to promote early infant development and activities for the elderly.

The Santa Marta Rehabilitation Center

The mission of the Santa Marta Rehabilitation Center is to improve the overall physical, mental, and emotional health of the community by providing a holistic approach to the management of congenital disabilities, developmental delays, overuse syndromes, physical and emotional war- and poverty-related trauma, and environmentally induced disease. The two health promoters from the community who staff the center have received training from Brenda and a series of DGH volunteers. Lola is a mother of two children, and Ana is a young therapist who also works with youth groups in the community. Ana and Lola are in charge of community outreach; they make home visits and organize numerous weekly workshops to educate community members on health promotion issues, which serve to complement individual patient treatments:

- *Vamos a Jugar* (Let's Play) is a workshop that seeks to encourage interaction and play between parents and children, in order to promote early stimulation and learning in all areas of child development, while forging the establishment of nurturing family bonds. A special Vamos a Jugar workshop is held separately for disabled children and their parents.
- *Masaje para Bebés* (Massage for Babies) is a workshop for mothers and

babies, who are invited to learn how to stimulate young babies using soothing and relaxing massage techniques.

- *Mayores en Movimiento* (Elderly on the Move) is an initiative to include the elder members of the community via programs of exercise and massage, in order to improve their overall well-being.

Among the individual patient treatments, the most successful initiative has been Espacio Mujer (Women's Space), a program of massage exclusively for women. Massage is used to address the physical pains of hard manual labor (for example, carrying large loads of wood on the head), the emotional stress of poverty, and as yet unaddressed post-traumatic stress from the civil war and oppression. Many suffer from back problems, headache, and insomnia. It has been a long struggle to convince these women to abandon their daily chores from time to time, and to treat themselves to an uplifting massage. There is a great need for this kind of attention.

One of the women who has benefitted from these treatments is Lita, a sixty-seven-year-old woman suffering from fibromyalgia. The lack of adequate health services during the civil war caused Lita to have an emergency cesarean section in a makeshift clinic. A gauze from the surgery remained in her abdomen for years, and she suffered from terrible pains. Lita is particularly fond of the head and leg massages (she is always on her feet), and throughout the treatment she often talks of her hardships. Through massage, she has learned to live with the pain of her illness, the recurring memories of the war, and the hard conditions she has overcome. Lita also attends the Mayores en Movimiento workshop: in the first five minutes, people share comments about this-and-that aching limb, and then the music starts and smiles appear as Ana and Lola demonstrate gentle movements with their arms.

In recent years, the rehabilitation center's scope of activity has expanded, and a series of exchanges has taken place between health promoters in Santa Marta and those at another DGH partner site in Estancia, Morazán. DGH volunteers and psychologists from Italy accompanied the health promoters during these first exchanges, in which Ana and Lola enjoyed sharing their experience and knowledge with other Salvadoran communities.

DGH volunteers have played an important role in providing technical assistance and training for the health promoters in occupational, physical, and speech therapy, and in bodywork and psychology. A DGH board member–physical therapist provides ongoing mentorship. Additionally, DGH provides economic support for Ana and Lola in the form of a monthly stipend.

Another effort has focused on addressing the mental health needs of the community. Italian psychologists from the organization Psicologi per I Popoli

(Psychologists for the People, PPP) teamed up with DGH and began the Bien-estar en El Salvador (Well-Being in El Salvador) project for Santa Marta and Estancia in 2008. This program sends volunteers to provide biannual training and support for the rehabilitation health promoters and school teachers. PPP is also helping community members approach and preserve their historical memories with the creation of Comité 16 de Enero (the January 16th Commit-tee) and provides mental health support to community members under threat because of their anti-mining advocacy.

The health promoters in the rehabilitation center value their unique op-portunity to work hands-on for the mental and physical well-being of their community. As Ana notes,

> As a therapist I feel I still have a lot to learn, but I hope in the future I will have the opportunity to do so thanks to the volunteers that come. I like this profession because I can help people with muscular problems, backaches, etc., and because it's very important to help people with [mental] trauma, whether it's from the war or due to abuse, etc. I chose to participate in the rehab center to learn more about how to treat these people, and at the same time for the opportunity to be able to help people from my own community, who need it a lot.

A Vibrant Youth Group Tackles Sex, Gender, and AIDS (and a whole lot more)

The Comité Contra SIDA (Committee Against Aids, COCOSI) is one of a kind in El Salvador. It is the only grassroots organization working and edu-cating in HIV prevention and gender-based violence in isolated rural com-munities in Cabañas. COCOSI is a community-based nonprofit organization founded in 1999 by young people who were born in the Mesa Grande refugee camp during the civil war. People in Cabañas and elsewhere were frightened that people could be living with HIV or AIDS in their community; and the Ministries of Health and Education did not take a leadership role in HIV pre-vention to address the fear and to separate myth from reality. In 1999, the Sal-vadoran foundation Contrasida visited Cabañas and brought an HIV-infected woman and her daughter. They gave their testimony, and inspired the young impoverished Salvadoran youth to found COCOSI. The COCOSI youth realized that in order to have an impact in HIV prevention, it was imperative that gen-der inequality, sexual orientation, masculinity, sexuality, and human rights be addressed; in short, both women and men needed to learn how to take care of their bodies. COCOSI youth receive training, and they teach via popular educa-tion techniques (by the people, for the people) that make it possible to educate and sensitize people who cannot read or write. This participatory teaching method makes learning not only fun, but also visceral. It creates bonds and friendships, and develops trust and self-confidence that are not promoted in public school.

COCOSI operates three programs: (1) HIV prevention, (2) accompaniment and mitigation, and (3) social and political advocacy. The prevention program, through its Womyn's Space and Men in the Gender Process projects, provides HIV education in schools and prisons. Two theater groups—Reality on Stage (adolescents) and CoCoLocos (children and preadolescent clowning and theater)—make the educational experience come alive. In the Sensuntepéque Prison, COCOSI implemented Drama Therapy and Freedom Writers in the women's sector, and Men in the Gender Process in the men's sector. The accompaniment program works with people with HIV/AIDS, homosexuals, and sex workers. Activities include assisting patients with their appointments and medications, fighting discrimination and stigma, and coordinating with the Ministry of Health and the central penal system. Due in part to COCOSI's advocacy, Sensuntepéque Hospital now has a weekly HIV clinic, which provides privacy and antiretroviral drug access to people with HIV. The social and political advocacy program promotes human rights and educates through the weekly radio program *Life and Reality*, which reaches five departments in El Salvador and one in Honduras, and the COCOSI web page. It is responsible for denouncing human rights abuses, and for communication, coordination, and follow-up with governmental and nongovernmental organizations.

The Economic and Social Development Association Santa Marta (Asociación de Desarrollo Económico Social [ADES]), an NGO formed by Salvadorans, was instrumental in securing funds during those first years. ADES and COCOSI participants coordinate to this day in leadership training and gender workshops. Much has changed for the better as a result of COCOSI's work. During the early years, COCOSI members were accosted while walking through their communities, to and from school and work. People yelled things like "contaminated creep" and "AIDS loser." In 1999, adolescents, many only age thirteen or fourteen, comprised about 85 percent of pregnancies. Today, teen pregnancy is rare. People are much less afraid of HIV-infected people; discrimination and hatred are declining. Women are beginning to denounce violence perpetrated by their male partners or husbands. In recognition of its work, COCOSI received the 2010 UNAIDS Red Ribbon Award. COCOSI is now a legally recognized NGO and is a member of the national network PrevenSida.

COCOSI recognizes that education about HIV prevention and about gender-based violence are linked, and the organization wants to provide safe alternatives for at-risk women. There are no legal avenues for Salvadoran women who denounce domestic violence. A victim and her children are at risk for retribution by her partner. The only shelter for battered women is in the capital San Salvador, which is not accessible to rural women. If a woman who has experienced violence leaves her home and is forced to live on the streets, she is more likely to become infected with HIV if she has to resort to risky behaviors in order to support her family.

DGH Advocacy and Accompaniment Role in Santa Marta

Ever since the first DGH volunteers worked in Santa Marta in 2001, DGH has had a strong connection with young people, who have played a key role in many of the community initiatives. One area that high school youth wanted to study was the effect of pesticide use on health and potential alternative agricultural practices. A DGH volunteer taught them how to use community-based participatory research methods to interview subjects, collect and analyze data, and present the results in an easy-to-understand way to the community. In 2004, the youth of Santa Marta successfully advocated for a full-time high school. Two years later, the same young people graduated from the high school they helped establish. Since then, they have secured funding to attend the National University in San Salvador while continuing to serve the community.

Radio Victoria and Gold Mining in El Salvador

Radio Victoria is another critically important organization led by the Santa Marta youth. Located in Victoria, the regional capital, this station has been transmitting since 1994. It is not affiliated with any political party or religious organization and makes its airwaves available to diverse groups and individuals. Programs include twice-daily news (local, national, and international), music, and weekly programs presented by different local groups to publicize events and services. The station broadcasts in five departments in El Salvador and one in Honduras. Radio Victoria is one of the founding members of the Salvadoran Association of Participative Radios and Programs (ARPAS), which is a member of the Latin American Radio Education Association and the World Association of Community Radios.

The radio staff is committed to defending human rights and denouncing electoral fraud. As of this writing, they are fighting against gold mining in Cabañas. In 2002, Pacific Rim Mining Corp., a Canadian gold-mining company with subsidiaries in the United States, obtained a permit and began exploring in Cabañas because preliminary reports revealed promising veins of gold. The mining process uses large volumes of cyanide-laced water to extract gold from subterranean rock. People in the communities became concerned when wells and rivers started to dry up and water became contaminated.[46]

Members of the Cabañas Environmental Committee traveled to other mining communities in Central America to gain a better understanding of the potential environmental impact. They learned how in other sites, the water and the soil had been contaminated by cyanide and other toxic chemicals used in the mining process. They were also concerned because El Salvador is prone to earthquakes, and a natural disaster such as this could crack open cyanide containers and cause devastation on a massive scale.

Pacific Rim conducted an environmental impact assessment (EIA), but did not release it to the general public; an independent expert said that the EIA would never have met the necessary criteria to pursue exploration in another country. Even though Pacific Rim declared that its mining practice was "green" and that the communities would be able to detoxify the water and make it potable, the people of Cabañas still had concerns, which were confirmed by experts. Not only were the local communities at risk—the country at large was at risk. Local rivers are tributaries of the Lempa, the major aquifer in El Salvador that provides water to more than one-half of the country's people.[47]

The National Round Table against Metal Mining in El Salvador (known as Mesa) coordinated local protests, and the local Catholic Church hierarchy took a stand against gold mining in El Salvador. They and the people of Cabañas convinced the Salvadoran government to deny the gold extraction permits to Pacific Rim.

In the face of increasing resistance to gold mining, violent intimidation arose. Marcelo Rivera, an active community leader, led the opposition to mining in his community. He was found dead in a well in July 2009. His autopsy showed signs of torture.

Throughout this period, Radio Victoria used its airwaves to educate the local people about the negative health and environmental effects of mining. It denounced Marcelo's torture and assassination. As a consequence, the station's reporters have received repeated death threats. Other messages have targeted community activists for their work in defense of human rights and denouncing electoral fraud. Three more anti-mining activists have been murdered; the most recent assassination was in June 2011.[48]

Despite the local environmental organizations' insistence that the National Civilian Police and the Attorney General's Office conduct an investigation into the "intellectual authors" of the murders and provide adequate police protection for those threatened, these demands have not been met. The only people arrested and jailed for short-term sentences were the gang members found guilty of the killings. But they were recently released, and upon release, some of them were assassinated. Perpetrators are acting with impunity.[49]

In 2008, Pacific Rim stopped exploratory mining, and has since sued the

Salvadoran government under CAFTA-DR for violating the rights of its investors to make a profit.[50] With the price of gold skyrocketing, the company has much at stake. Meanwhile, environmental groups under the leadership of Mesa are working to pass a law that would ban all metal mining in El Salvador.[51]

What is the role of an organization like DGH in this situation that threatens members of its partner community? This is where DGH accompaniment comes into play, a role it takes very seriously. DGH's partner organization, PPP, the Italian NGO of psychologists and educators with expertise in treating people experiencing trauma, happened to be in Santa Marta in the wake of Marcelo's murder. PPP has provided ongoing psychological support to those threatened.

DGH posted an action alert on its website asking its members to send letters to El Salvador's Attorney General's Office and National Civilian Police, and to US legislative representatives to support an investigation of the crimes committed. DGH alerted human rights organizations and asked them to get involved. As US citizens, DGH members have sought to repeal provisions in free trade agreements such as CAFTA-DR that prioritize foreign investment rights over government interests in preventing environmental degradation or activities that jeopardize public safety. DGH remains vigilant because attacks continue to this day.[52]

Oscar Beltran, reporter from Radio Victoria, describes the role of the radio:

> One of our primary goals is the defense of the environment. We have to provide information about threats to its integrity. There is no other institution out there that provides this information. Not only do we have to educate people, but we also have to take a position, to show what can be done about the situation. Thanks to the radio, communities like San Isidro, which has been at the center of the resistance against gold mining in the country, have learned about the experience of Santa Marta in their own struggle. This knowledge has given them inspiration and tools to organize in their own community. Even though Santa Marta has not been directly implicated in the gold-mining issue (there is not gold in Santa Marta), we know that we are in this together.[53]

The Long Road to Education Access
From the Refugee Camps of Honduras to University Degrees

During the civil conflict, more than 600 schools were closed across the country, 60 percent in the five departments most involved in the conflict with the government (including Sensuntepéque, where Santa Marta is located). ADES was created in 1993 to address the needs and problems of returnees to rural communities in the Department of Cabañas.[54] Against great odds, ADES and Santa

Marta have made significant accomplishments in education. The road began in the Mesa Grande refugee camp in Honduras, where the people of Santa Marta lived from 1981 to 1987. Members with some education but no formal training as teachers took it upon themselves to teach others using liberation teaching methods in the tradition of Paolo Freire. This form of popular education responds to the realities of the most marginalized and excluded people; rather than using a hierarchical teacher-learner model, it is more egalitarian and participatory. NGOs in the refugee camps gave the teachers support and guidance.[55]

When they returned to Santa Marta in 1987, these newly trained teachers faced daunting tasks: to resume classes in the community school, while also receiving their own formal education training at the university. And they also needed to support their families. By 2003, forty-three teachers had graduated with university degrees in elementary education and passed the Salvadoran competency exam. This was a huge milestone. But Santa Marta still lacked a building for high school classes; only a small number of students had the financial means to study in a high school outside Santa Marta.

In 2001, the Ministry of Education provided resources for a part-time high school education. This meant that two teachers gave classes on the weekends in their homes, and during the week the students studied on their own. Self-study was challenging, but it paid off. Parents, students, and ADES advocated for a full-time high school program on-site. Eventually, the Ministry of Education provided more teacher positions. Most children in Santa Marta now graduate from high school every year.

It became clear that for the new graduates to obtain jobs, they would have to continue their studies at the university level. ADES took a leadership role in seeking funding. A major supporter was COCODA (Companion Community Development Alternatives), a US-based NGO that made a ten-year commitment to support this education initiative. The first class enrolled in 2006 and graduated in 2011, another significant accomplishment for a community that built its education program from the ground up. These various initiatives operate under several guiding principles:

- The initiatives were created with the active participation of all concerned—parents, students, teachers.
- An emphasis was placed on bringing into the classroom the local, national, and international realities in which the students lived.
- High school and university student involvement was prioritized in community initiatives.
- Many different individuals and groups, who knew the community and were committed to help, were asked to participate: people from abroad

who had spent time in the community, DGH volunteers, emigrants from Santa Marta who now live in Virginia, and other NGOs.

Many DGH volunteers have collaborated on various aspects of the educational program. They have taught classes, tutored students, mentored teachers, and raised money to support the program.

Conclusion

The work of Liberation medicine and accompaniment continues to this day. The people of Santa Marta and their commitment to the struggle for human rights, equity, and social justice are an inspiration to DGH. DGH Santa Marta volunteer Elizabeth says, "Learning from the people of Santa Marta has been nothing short of life-changing, their resiliency and community-mindedness humbling. I count myself lucky to participate in my own small way through DGH." And DGH Santa Marta volunteer Alex notes, "It seems to me that at the foundation of Santa Marta's health projects is a cohesive community struggle for the flourishing of human potential."

The Santa Marta community knows no boundaries. In Reston, Virginia, there is a vibrant community of people who migrated from Santa Marta during the armed conflict and afterwards. They all have their own stories of survival, of how they made and continue to make a dignified life for themselves and their families in the United States and back home in Santa Marta. They have faced numerous challenges, including confrontations with the Minutemen (an outspoken, anti-immigrant group in the United States). They have participated in DGH General Assemblies. They continue to support their community of origin in El Salvador. They are an inspiring example of cross-border solidarity; interconnectedness; and "globalization from below," a process that illustrates and elevates the importance and priority of individual and community-level communication and interaction instead of corporate-driven policies and priorities.

With the Salvadorans in Virginia, the members and volunteers of DGH and the people of Santa Marta, the work of understanding the social determinants of health, amplifying the voices of the silenced, accompaniment, and liberation medicine continues until all in Santa Marta are able to live a life of dignity and optimal health and well-being.

The Comments of Isidra Garcia Villalobos, Santa Marta High School Teacher

We could never rely on the government to provide our community with the kind of education we wanted. Our priority has always been to work for the community. We use a popular education method. My first experience with teaching was in the refuge camps in Honduras. I was a teacher for one year. When we came back to Santa Marta, we knew right away we could not expect the government to rebuild our school and hire teachers. We took matters in our own hands. With the support of the international community and some local organizations, we somehow gathered the financial resources to build our school and to start teaching. We decided we needed to get formal training. But at the same time, we continued to teach. So it took many years to complete our training part-time from Friday to Sunday while teaching Monday through Thursday.

It took years until the Department of Education started to pay us. We graduated with a degree to teach elementary school. But later on, when the high school was open, we started teaching these grades as well. Now we are in school again on the weekends to complete our training to teach those grades. We keep learning, not just to get a degree or just for our own gain, but to provide the best teaching possible. We are not alone. We work together with the health clinic, with cocosi. We also have had the help of volunteers. They taught English, sciences, and reproductive health. Now many of the youth we taught at the high school are completing their college education in several different institutions. That will provide them with a door to a career and will mean that fewer will need to go north to find employment that will give them the means to support their families. We can already observe this change. Fewer young people are leaving the community.

Notes

1 M. Anderson, C. Smith, and V. Sidel, "What Is Social Medicine?" *Monthly Review* 56.8 (2005), accessed Feb. 1, 2012, available from http://monthlyreview.org.
2 L. Eisenberg, "Rudolf Karl Virchow, Where Are You Now That We Need You?" *American Journal of Medicine* 77 (1984):524–532.
3 World Health Organization, accessed Feb. 4, 2012, available from www.who.int.
4 *Declaration of Alma Ata: International Conference on Primary Health Care, Alma-Ata, USSR, 6–12 September, 1978*, accessed Feb. 4, 2012, available from www.who.int.
5 World Bank, accessed Feb. 4, 2012, available from http://web.worldbank.org.
6 "Assessment for Indigenous Peoples in El Salvador," 6, accessed Feb. 1, 2012, available from www.cidcm.umd.edu; and Minority Rights Group International, "World Directory of Minorities and Indigenous Peoples," accessed Feb. 1, 2012, available from http://www.minorityrights.org.
7 L. R. Simon, J. C. Stephens, and M. Diskin, *El Salvador Land Reform 1980–1981*, Impact Audit Series (Boston: Oxfam America, 1982).

8   Instituto de Derechos Humans de la Universidad de Centroamerica, "La salud en tiempos de guera," *Estudios Centroamericans* 46 (1991):653–671.

9   J. L. Fiedler, "Recurrent Cost and Public Health Care Delivery: The Other War in El Salvador," *Social Science and Medicine* 25 (1987):867–874.

10 UN Security Council, "Annex, From Madness to Hope: The 12-Year War in El Salvador: Report of the Commission on the Truth for El Salvador" (S/25500, 1993), 5–8, available from www.usip.org; R. White, "The Problem That Won't Go Away," *New York Times Magazine* (July 18, 1982); and J. L. Thomsen, J. Gruschow, and E. Stover, "Medicolegal Investigation of Political Killings in El Salvador," *Lancet* 333.8651 (1989):1377–1379.

11 C. Krauss, "U.S., Aware of Killings, Worked with Salvador's Rightist, Papers Suggest," *New York Times* (Nov. 9, 1993); B. Levy and V. Sidel, eds., *War and Public Health* (New York: Oxford University Press, 1997). 16: 238–253; SOA Watch, "What Is the SOA?" accessed Jan. 11, 2011, available from http://soaw.org; M. Danner, *The Massacre at El Mozote* (New York: Vintage, 1994), and "The Truth of El Mozote," *New Yorker* (Dec. 6, 1993), 50–133; and Amnesty International, *El Salvador "Death Squads": A Government Strategy* (London: Amnesty International, 1988).

12 F. A. Solís and P. Martin, "The Role of Salvadoran NGOs in Post-War Reconstruction," *Development in Practice* 2.2 (1992):103–113, available from www.jstor.org; and L. J. Bowman, "Community Perceptions of an NGO's Impact on Disaster Preparedness in Los Planes de La Laguna, Santa Ana Volcano, El Salvador" (MS thesis in geology, Michigan Technological Institute, 2009), accessed Jan. 25, 2012, available from www.geo.mtu.edu.

13 North American Congress on Latin America, "A New Day in El Salvador: The FMLN Victory and the Road Ahead," *NACLA Report on the Americas* 6 (Nov./Dec. 2009); and T. Hayden, "El Salvador Rising," *The Nation* (June 15, 2009).

14 E. Achtenburg, "El Salvador: Social Programs Bolster Support for Funes Government," NACLA blog (July 22, 2011), available from https://nacla.org.

15 Federal Law Enforcement Training Center, "International Law Enforcement Academies," available from www.fletc.gov, and ILEA San Salvador, available from www.ileass.org.sv; accessed Feb. 2, 2012; and "Rice Announces Plan to Build International Law Enforcement Academy in El Salvador," *SALVANET* (Spring/Summer 2005), 4.

16 Committee in Solidarity with the People of El Salvador, "ILEA Background Information" (June 12, 2006), accessed Feb. 2, 2012, available from www.cispes.org.

17 Democracy NOW! "What's Behind the Honduran Coup? Tracing Zelaya's Trajectory" (July 1, 2009), available from www.democracynow.org.

18 See www.cia.gov, accessed Nov. 15, 2011.

19 See http://hdrstats.undp.org, accessed Nov. 15, 2011; and see www.cia.gov, accessed Nov. 15, 2011.

20 See www.cia.gov, accessed Nov. 15, 2011.

21 United Nations Development Program, *Regional Human Development Report for Latin America and the Caribbean 2010: Acting on the Future: Breaking the Intergenerational Transmission of Inequality* (New York: UNDP, 2010), accessed Jan. 25, 2012, available from www.beta.undp.org.

22 See http://hdr.undp.org. accessed Nov. 15, 2011; and see http://hdrstats.undp.org, accessed Nov. 15, 2011.

23 CNN, "El Salvador to Launch U.S. Dollar as Official Currency," (Dec. 29, 2000).

24 SHARE Foundation, "CAFTA Educational Packet," accessed Feb. 4, 2012, available from http://share-elsalvador.org.

25 World Food Program, "Skyrocketing Food Prices Threaten Nutritional Crisis for Poor Central Americans" (Feb. 26, 2008), available from www.wfp.org.

26 Banco Central de Reserva de El Salvador, "Comunicado de Prensa No. 46/2011," accessed Jan. 25, 2012, available from www.bcr.gob.sv.

27 Central Intelligence Agency, "El Salvador" in *The World Factbook* (Washington, DC: CIA), accessed Nov. 20, 2011, available from www.cia.gov.

28 L. J. Abrego, "Rethinking El Salvador's Transnational Families," *NACLA Report on the Americas* 6 (Nov./Dec. 2009).

29 International Monetary Fund, accessed Nov. 20, 2011, available from www.imf.org.

30 I. Ortiz, J. Chai, and M. Cummins, "Identifying Fiscal Space: Options for Social and Economic Development for Children and Poor Households in 182 Countries," UNICEF (Oct. 2011), accessed Feb. 4, 2012, available from www.unicef.org.

31 Health Resources and Service Administration, "Women's Health USA 2010: Maternal Mortality," accessed Jan. 11, 2012, available from http://mchb.hrsa.gov; and Measure DHS, "El Salvador," accessed Jan. 25, 2012, available from www.measuredhs.com.

32 USAID, CDC, Ministry of Health, San Salvador, El Salvador, FESAL, "Encuesta Nacional de Salud Familiar" (Feb. 2009).

33 USAID Country Health Statistical Report. El Salvador, November 2008, see https://dec.usaid.gov; and WHO Global Health Observatory Data Repository, El Salvador, 2008, available from http://apps.who.int/gho/data. Current data states that 20.6 percent of children under five in El Salvador are stunted and 6.6 percent are underweight.

34 M. Heiber, "Between a Growing Economy and an Alarming Water Situation," *International Ecological Engineering Society* (Apr. 24, 2009), accessed Feb. 1, 2012, available from www.iees.ch.

35 UNDP, *Regional Human Development Report for Latin America and the Caribbean 2010*; and Facultad Latinoamericana de Ciencias Sociales, www.flacso.org.sv.

36 Pan American Health Organization, "El Salvador: Iniciativa de Indicadores Básicos Regionales de Salud" (May 2010), available from http://new.paho.org.

37 *Spotlight on Health Workforce Statistics* 6 (WHO, Nov. 2008), accessed Aug. 11, 2010, available from www.who.int.

38 Sistema Nacional de Salud, "Política Nacional Participación Social en Salud," San Salvador, El Salvador (Apr. 2009). M. I. Rodriguez, "Construyendo la Esperanza, Estrategias y Recomendaciones en Salud, 2009–2014" (Oct. 2009), available from www.mspas.gob.sv. Declaration of the National Health Forum: "Building Social Participation in Health" (San Salvador, May 2010).

39 PAHO, "Health Systems Profile: El Salvador" (Oct. 2007), accessed Feb. 2, 2012, available from http://new.paho.org.

40 E. Espinoza and F. Barten, "Health Reform in El Salvador: A Lost Opportunity for

Reducing Health Inequity and Social Exclusion?" *Journal of Epidemiology and Community Health* 62.5 (2008):380–81.

41 "Millennial Development Goals Indicators: El Salvador," accessed Feb. 1, 2012, available from http://mdgs.un.org. PAHO, "Millennium Development Goals: El Salvador," accessed Feb. 1, 2012, available from www.paho.org. International Bank for Reconstruction and Development/World Bank, *Improving the Odds of Achieving the* MDG, Global Monitoring Report 2011, accessed Feb. 1, 2012, available from http://siteresources.worldbank.org.www.dghonline.org

42 See www.dghonline.org.

43 See www.dghonline.org.

44 C. L. Smith, "Building Health Where the Peace is New in Near-Postwar El Salvador," *Development* 50.2 (2007):127–133.

45 J. Kasper and C. L. Smith, "Liberation Medicine and Accompaniment in El Salvador: The Experience of Doctors for Global Health" in *Rights-Based Approaches to Public Health*, ed. E. Beracochea, C. Weinstein, and D. Evans (New York: Springer, 2010); and C. L. Smith, T. H. Holtz, J. Kasper, "Doctors for Global Health: Applying Liberation Medicine and Accompanying Communities' Struggles toward Health and Social Justice" in *Comrades in Health: U.S. Health Internationalists, Abroad and at Home*, ed. A. E. Birn and T. M. Brown (forthcomimg)

46 WHO, "Chronic Respiratory Diseases: Scope: Asthma," accessed Jan. 25, 2012, available from www.who.int. Nation Master, "Mortality Statistics: Asthma by Country," accessed Jan. 25, 2012, available from www.nationmaster.com.

47 C. Starr, "Radio Victoria Chronology of Death Threats and Action" (May 2011), available from www.radiovictoria.org.

48 M. Busch, "El Salvador's Gold Fight," *Foreign Policy in Focus* (July 16, 2009), available from www.fpif.org; J. Freeston, "Shredding Social Fabric: Company Promoters 'Contaminate' Communities in El Salvador," *The Dominion* (Nov. 11, 2008), available from www.dominionpaper.ca; and P. Broad and J. Cavanaugh, "Like Water for Gold in El Salvador," *The Nation* (Aug. 8, 2011), available from www.thenation.com.

49 J. Wallach, "Another Anti-Mining Activist Shot in Cabanas, El Salvador, Hit Man Tied to Pacific Rim is Detained," *Voices on the Border in El Salvador* (Aug. 13, 2009), available from www.votb.org.

50 Amnesty International, "Urgent Action: Journalists Threatened and at Risk" (May 10, 2011) http://www.amnesty.org.

51 M. Busch, "CAFTA's Casualties: El Salvador Battles a Multinational Corporation Over Mining Rights," *Dissent* (July 22, 2009).

52 E. Achtenberg, "A Mining Ban in El Salvador?" *NACLA Report on the Americas*, (Sept./Oct. 2011), available from www.nacla.org.

53 Oscar Beltran, personal communication with the author.

54 Voices on the Border, "A New Attack Against Cabañas Anti-Mining Activists" (Jan. 25, 2012), available from http://voiceselsalvador.wordpress.com.

55 S. Loose with J. A. Argueta, R. A. Veliz, and I. G. Villalobos, "Una Sistematización de la Educación Popular en el Cantón Santa Marta, Cabañas, El Salvador, 1978–2001," (San Salvador: ADES Santa Marta, 2003)

Suggested Reading

Benitez, Sandra. *Bitter Grounds: A Novel*. New York, NY: Picador, 1997.

Benitez, Sandra. *The Weight of All Things*. New York, NY: Hyperion, 2001.

Clements, Charlie. *Witness to War*. New York, NY: Bantam, 1984.

Danner, Mark. *The Massacre at El Mozote*. New York, NY: Vintage, 1994.

Dilling, Yvonne. *In Search of Refuge*. Scottsdale, PA: Herald Press, 1984.

Famer, Paul. *Pathologies of Power: Health, Human Rights, and the New War on the Poor*. Berkeley, CA: University of California Press, 2003.

Galeano, Eduardo. *Open Veins of Latin America*. New York: Monthly Review Press, 1997.

Gorkin, Michael, Marta Pineda, and Gloria Leal. *From Grandmother to Granddaughter: Salvadoran Women's Stories*. Berkeley, CA: University of California Press, 2000.

Kim, Jim Yong, Joyce Millen, Alec Irwin, and John Gershman, eds. *Dying for Growth: Global Inequality and the Health of the Poor*. Monroe, ME: Common Courage Press, 2000.

LaFeber, Walter. *Inevitable Revolutions: The United States in Central America*. New York, NY: W.W. Norton and Company, 1984.

MacDonald, Mandy, and Mike Gatehouse. *In the Mountains of Morazán: Portrait of a Returned Refugee Community in El Salvador*. New York: Monthly Review Press, 1995.

Maiz, Equipo. *Historia de El Salvador*. 6th ed. San Salvador, El Salvador: Equipo Maiz, 2005.

Mann, Jonathan M., Michael A. Grodin, Sofia Gruskin, and George J. Annas, eds. *Health and Human Rights: A Reader*. New York, NY: Routledge, 1999.

Montgomery, Tommie Sue. *Revolution in El Salvador*. 2nd ed. Boulder, CO: Westview Press, 1994.

Tula, Maria Teresa. *Hear My Testimony: Maria Teresa Tula Human Rights Activist of El Salvador*. Edited and translated by Lynn Stephen. Cambridge, MA: South End Press, 1999.

Werner, David, with Carol Thuman and Jane Maxwell. *Where There Is No Doctor: A Village Health Care Handbook*. 2nd rev. ed. Berkeley, CA: Hesperian Foundation, 1992 (12th rev. printing: 2011).

Werner, David, and Bill Bower. *Helping Health Care Workers Learn: A Book of Methods, Aids, and Ideas for Instructors at the Village Level*. Berkeley, CA: Hesperian Health Guides, 2012.

Suggested Websites

Doctors for Global Health: www.dghonline.org

Association of Socioeconomic Development (Asociación de Desarrollo Económico Social, ADES): www.adessm.org

Committee Against Aids (Comité Contra el SIDA, COCOSI): www.cocosi.org

4 Honduras

Ryan Alaniz and Peter J. Daly

In his Fulbright field notes from December 2009,
Ryan Alaniz writes,

Take the chicken bus north from Tegucigalpa, Honduras for about 35 minutes and soon you will descend into a beautiful area called the Valle de Amarateca. You will notice thousands of pine trees, green scrub brush and pockets of identical houses scattered about the valley. Billows of smoke rise from the Café Indo coffee processing plant on the right and the Café Maya plant on the left. The smell is inviting on a calm day. Soon you are in the lowest part of the valley where streaks of brown reveal the dirt roads that wind their way up into the mountains well worn by foot, tire, and hoof. You will turn left on the last dirt road—the one before you head up the mountain on the other side. Remember to hold onto the seat in front of you to avoid hitting your head on the roof due to the dips and bumps. Climb around the cow pastures and follow the sign up the hill. There, workers cutting grass will stop and wave or nod, wondering who is entering their community. If they know you they will shout with a raised hand "compa" or "hermano," endearing names that remind you of the friendship you maintain. Notice the skinny dogs and roaming cattle on the road and as you enter the community you will see a microcosm of the glory and sadness that is Honduras. People laughing alongside burning trash, kids playing barefoot with a flat soccer ball, abandoned cars alongside beautiful gardens, and gentle smiles that turn into growls when talking about politics. In this country, the third poorest in the Western Hemisphere by most standards, life is both simpler and more complicated than in the United States.

Indeed, volunteering in a health-related capacity in Honduras can be both a simple and a complex experience. This chapter offers a broad perspective of the people, national challenges, history, and culture of this warm and beautiful country. It also highlights some important issues concerning the logistics of becoming a health volunteer, and asks some questions to help readers think critically about their role and relationship with the Honduran people they will serve.

Brief History

According to legend, the name *Honduras* was born in the harsh Atlantic Ocean. As the story goes, Christopher Columbus, on his last trip to the New World in 1502, encountered rough seas off the northeastern coast of an "unnamed" land. That early August hurricane season was treacherous, and it took the fleet twenty-eight days of negotiating the length of the tropical coastline to finally find calmer waters off the east coast of what was later called Nicaragua. After arriving safely, Columbus is cited as saying, "Gracias a Dios que hemos dejado estas honduras" ("Thank God we have left these depths"). The far eastern state of Honduras received the name *Gracias a Dios* (Thank God) and the country as a whole was called Honduras.

Because of its position at the center of the Americas, Honduras was a crossroads for indigenous cultures. Among these, the Maya settled in the valley of Copán and developed a city known for its achievements in science, astronomy, and the arts. Impressive hieroglyphs have been discovered there. Copán fell into ruin around 800 AD. At the time of the conquest, the Lenca were the dominant tribe and there were no major cities in the region. Since it gained independence from Spain in 1821, Honduras has had a long history of political challenges. Wealthy Spanish-descendant elite were able to maintain control over land and property throughout the nineteenth and twentieth centuries, finding economic prosperity in land use for natural resource expropriation (minerals, fruits, coffee, fish, and so on).

Land control by a few did not encourage broad economic growth or a strong middle class, and this resulted in a two-tier society with a small elite and a largely poor, self-subsistent citizenry. A system of patronage and corruption, political infighting, an inefficient bureaucracy, dependency on raw materials, isolation from the broader world market, and ties with international corporations contributed to the poor, underdeveloped economy.[1] With such an inauspicious beginning, Honduras as a nation had little opportunity to jumpstart the economic progress necessary for long-term sustainable growth. In 2007, 60 percent of Honduran households lived below the poverty level. The inequitable distribution of income within the country determines who is poor, and there is significant underemployment with low-productivity jobs. Most jobs are in agriculture (35 percent), trade (21 percent), and manufacturing (15 percent).

Poverty has also been perpetuated by two international influences: corporations and the US government. Economically, Honduras became known as the quintessential "Banana Republic" after international corporations such as Standard Fruit Company turned much of the north coast into banana plantations, keeping the majority of the resulting wealth. Politically, the Honduran government has maintained close ties with the United States, first to protect the corporations working in the country, and later as a geopolitically key location. As social movements and later revolutions began to form during the 1960s through 1990s in Guatemala, Nicaragua, and El Salvador, the US used Honduras as a staging ground to intervene in the civil wars of these countries. An example of this was the construction of Palmerola (or Soto Cano),[2] the largest air force base in the region, built by the United States in 1981. Palmerola was a base of operation for the counter-revolution against Nicaragua in the 1980s but now is used for the war on drugs as well as humanitarian missions throughout Central America.

Geography

Honduras is in the heart of Central America. Bordered by three countries—Guatemala to the west and north, El Salvador to the southwest, and Nicaragua to the east and south—the nation also touches the Pacific and Atlantic Oceans. Honduras may be divided into four geographic quadrants: (1) the western mountains, (2) the central hills and plains, (3) the tropical north coast, and (4) the eastern rainforest. From the southwest corner, where the country touches the Pacific at the Gulf of Fonseca, plains rise to hills in the central country, and slowly slope and widen to the broad north coast. There is a particular beauty in each of the major areas: dry and arid in the south, and progressively more wet when heading north. Six islands dot the Caribbean coast. The two largest, Roatan and Utila, are the country's chief tourist attraction as excellent diving locales. The interior highlands comprise 80 percent of the country; this is where the majority of Hondurans live. The soil is poor because Honduras lacks rich volcanic ash that, over time, leads to the creation of fertile soil of the type found in other Central American countries. The rugged terrain of Honduras has also made the land difficult to cultivate and traverse.[3] Additionally, the country has a long history of hurricanes, floods, and landslides; and 20 percent of Hondurans live in a disaster-prone area.

The People

Honduras is often described as demographically homogenous, but there are many small and important subgroups scattered throughout the country. Of the nearly 8 million residents, 90 percent consider themselves mestizo, or of mixed blood. There are nine culturally distinct ethnic groups numbering approximately 500,000 people. The largest minority (7 percent) is composed of various indigenous tribes and communities, located mostly in the western highlands and the northeast forests. Finally, a small but culturally important group of Garifuna (descendants of African slaves) lives mostly on the north coast and Bay Islands. These indigenous groups suffer more effects of poverty, as well as limited access to basic services.

The nation is similar to many others in Latin America. The estimated median age of Hondurans, according to the Central Intelligence Agency's (CIA) *World Factbook*, is twenty-one years.[4] A historically higher birth rate, cultural acceptance of adolescent pregnancy, religious values, machismo culture,[5] and the difficult living conditions created by poverty create this youthful population. Following a global trend, however, the birth rate has been slowly declining at least since the 1970s, dropping from 47 births per 1,000 women to 38 per 1,000 in 1990 and 27 per 1,000 in 2008.[6] The 2011 age estimates show that 37 percent of Hondurans are under age fourteen, about 60 percent are between ages fifteen and sixty-four, and fewer than 4 percent are sixty-five or older. Additionally, most Hondurans have only an eleventh-grade education, live on $4,200 US per year,[7] and consider themselves Roman Catholic or Evangelical Christian.[8]

Hurricane Mitch

Perhaps the most important nonpolitical event in recent Honduran memory is the Hurricane Mitch disaster of 1998. The Category 5 hurricane devastated the small Central American nation. Tied for the fourth strongest Atlantic hurricane on record, surpassing even Katrina, Hurricane Mitch topped out at a central pressure of 905 millibars with winds averaging 155 knots (180 mph). Not only the wind but the rain ravaged the country. As the hurricane slowed and later stalled, becoming a tropical storm over central Honduras, it deposited approximately twenty-five inches in thirty-six hours, and ten inches in six hours, between October 29 and 31, according to 2011 information from the Met Office, the United Kingdom's national weather service. Affecting more than one-half of the population, the hurricane killed 5,657 people, injured over 12,000, and displaced 2.1 million people. According to some agencies, the country was set back fifty years in its development. About 70 percent of the vital national infrastructure was damaged. Highways were washed away or layered with sediment, 170 bridges were badly damaged or completely destroyed, and seventy-five dams broke, flooding whole communities. Many health centers were damaged or destroyed as well as the nation's water distribution system. The normally quiet Choluteca River that snakes through the downtown of Tegucigalpa, the capital city, had record-level flooding, leaving eighteen feet of mud and a massive amount of destruction in its wake.[9]

As is often said, there is no such thing as a natural disaster. A natural hazard becomes a disaster only in relationship to a vulnerable human population. According to disaster scholar Greg Bankoff and coauthors, "The concept of vulnerability expresses the multidimensionality of disasters by focusing attention on the totality of relationships in a given social situation which constitute a condition that, in combination with environmental forces, produces a disaster."[10] Over the past sixty years, Honduras, like many Global South countries, has witnessed a signification population shift from rural to urban areas due to changes in the economy and growing poverty. This exponential growth of the urban population, increasing city density, and the inability to cope with more people made Honduras particularly vulnerable, and redefined Mitch from a natural meteorological occurrence into a disaster. Since Mitch, numerous torrential rains and smaller hurricanes have left thousands homeless each year.

The Reconstruction

The global community coalesced to serve the Honduran people. The international call to rebuild Honduras was that reconstruction must not be at the expense of transformation. Money, development workers, NGOs, and experts filed into the country to make the nation a model of post-disaster recovery. It was considered the most significant reconstruction plan of its time. Thirteen years later, evidence of this effort can be seen throughout the country. Large signs are posted in multiple languages on bridges, highways, and other infrastructure thanking various countries for their donations. Rows of identical houses built for survivors can also be found near the major cities. The question more recently is, *Was the reconstruction a success?* The answer depends on what is being measured.

There have been gains in the social, infrastructural, and economic arenas. Socially, citizens and NGOs saw major improvements in their ability to make government listen and respond. Although initially marginalized by the Honduran government, international donors demanded the inclusion of civil society. INTERFOROS, a grassroots organization of more than 500 community groups, gained a prominent voice and political leverage in the reconstruction process.[11] Gender issues were also addressed as never before, providing women with greater economic opportunity and safeguarding against domestic violence. Infrastructure in many places has been greatly improved to withstand future disasters, and new communities have been built to relocate disaster survivors away from high-risk housing on hillsides and along riverbanks.

Economic and Political Challenges

The dream of transformation has yet to be fulfilled in many ways.[12] More specifically, looking at national statistics from 1997 to 2010, the Honduran government has had a steadily declining record of financial transparency (except for a blip immediately after Mitch, due to international oversight) and ranks significantly lower than its neighbors, Guatemala and El Salvador.[13] Transparency International measures the perceived levels of public sector corruption in 183 countries worldwide.[14] In 2011, the organization's Corruption Perceptions Index ranked Honduras at 129, illustrating how public officials abuse their entrusted power to benefit privately at the expense of their citizens. The wealth gap has also continued to climb between the rich and the poor. According to the United Nations, 60 percent of the national earnings are in the highest income quintile, while 40 percent of the poorest Hondurans receive less than 10 percent of earnings. The World Bank has also found that the gap in wealth increased slightly from 1997 to 2009, with the richest 10 percent of Hondurans receiving approximately a 2 percent wealth increase, while the poorest 10 percent saw a decrease of nearly 25 percent.[15]

Honduras has been a democracy since 1981, following ten years of a military dictatorship. Politically, as recently as June 2009, Congress and the Supreme Court mandated the removal of President Manuel Zelaya from the country in what was considered by most nations as a coup d'état. The 2010 election of Porfirio Lobo Sosa, known as Pepe Lobo, was a peaceful process, but the country still has a long way to go. Deposed president Zelaya returned to Honduras on May 28, 2011, but the same politicians who engineered the coup are still in power as of this writing, and have not been prosecuted. Internationally, Honduras, which had lost its position after the coup, was only recently permitted to rejoin the Organization of American States.

As of November 2011, the nation holds the rank of highest murder rate per capita outside of a warring country, with particularly high rates of homicide in drug-related areas. Contributing factors include increased drug trafficking, youth gang activity, and failure of police to apprehend the criminals. Honduran government response to the increased violence has included using the military in high conflict areas.[16]

Healthcare System

The Honduran health system consists of three parts: (1) the Ministry of Health, (2) the Honduran Social Security Institute (IHSS), and (3) the private sector. First, the Ministry of Health oversees eighteen Departmental Health Regions in the country, with two Metropolitan Health Regions, one centered in the capital city Tegucigalpa and the other in the more industrial San Pedro Sula. The Ministry of Health regulates outpatient facilities, rural health centers, and hospitals. It also provides partial funding for services in public hospitals. It is responsible for organizing and implementing national and local health initiatives, including reducing infant mortality rates, malnutrition, and communicable disease rates (for example, malaria, TB, and Chagas disease).

In June 2010, an outbreak of dengue fever occurred, prompting the Honduran Ministry of Health to declare a Dengue Fever Red Alert. In 2004 and 2005, Honduras reported 19,000 dengue fever cases per year.[17] However, from June 2010 to December 2010 alone, over 66,000 cases were reported and eighty-three deaths.

The second portion of the Honduran health system is the IHSS, which provides health benefits to formal contributing wage earners; but this amounts to only 11 percent of the Honduran population. Most working Hondurans earn their living in the informal sector. IHSS delivers healthcare through a network of private and public providers at community clinics and outpatient facilities, IHSS hospitals, and referrals to the specialty hospitals in Tegucigalpa and San Pedro Sula. Lastly, the private sector is available on a fee-for-service basis, and via private health insurance.[18]

Despite the theoretical strategy and order in the Honduran health system, it unfortunately is fragmented and inadequately funded by the government. The lack of resources to properly coordinate the health system has resulted in significant adverse effects on public health. In a 2006 country report,[19] the World Health Organization noted that political instability and frequent changes in authority negatively impacts the health system, which is already uncoordinated and disjointed. More concretely, the national health providers (Ministry of Health and IHSS) have little coordination with the private sector, thereby duplicating some responsibilities while leaving other areas unprotected. Additionally, the frequent changes in authority (political nepotism is rampant, and with the change of government, jobs are often handed over to party supporters) contribute to work inefficiencies. Those who do stay in their positions often do not have the economic or technological resources to implement educational or medical initiatives, conduct investigations about health concerns, or check on the quality of care received by patients at clinics or hospitals.

All of these factors result in significant healthcare inequality. The wealthiest 5 percent of the population has private sector insurance, and they commonly obtain their care at private sector hospitals and facilities. These facilities are competing for this small number of insured patients and for those able to pay without insurance. There is little financial incentive to help the rural, indigent majority of the population. An additional 11 percent, such as teachers' unions, have health insurance via IHSS. Because 44 percent of Hondurans live on $2 US per day, and 66 percent live below the poverty line, the remaining 84 percent of the population is uninsured and tries to access the government-run public hospitals and primary care clinics. Although the actual hospital bed may be seen as "free" by the patient, surgical implants and other items often cost extra, making care unavailable for many. These public hospital facilities are overwhelmed with trauma and emergencies, so that electively treated conditions such as hernias, prostate enlargement, gynecologic conditions, nasal obstructions, torn tendons, and joint abnormalities—all disabling conditions—are the losers in the triage scheme, which consequently keeps people out of work and out of hope.

Nongovernmental Public Health Organizations

To supplement the low coverage resulting from difficulties within the healthcare system, NGOs have found ways of addressing the multiple needs of the Honduran people. A significant organization serving in the country is Doctors Without Borders (Médecins Sans Frontières, MSF), which has worked in Honduras since 1974. The organization's projects have included services for youth overcoming addiction to glue sniffing, young girls involved in commercial sex activities, victims of violence, and flood relief.[20] Like Doctors without Borders, the organization Global Brigades also addresses issues of preventive healthcare, and provides mobile clinics, all staffed by thousands of college-aged volunteers each year.

Numerous smaller organizations provide specialized health services to citizens: these include ENLACE Foundation, which maintains a clinic in Taulabe; numerous medical schools; and church missions, which provide everything from general services in rural areas to serious dental and eye surgeries. Another NGO, Shoulder to Shoulder, has connected short-term medical volunteers and sustainable development by partnering US medical schools' family medicine trainees with community health boards in Honduras communities. Since 1990, these interventions have established cancer screening, pregnancy care, and community-based water filtration programs.[21] Honduras also had one of the largest contingents of Peace Corps volunteers in the world. More than 5,750 volunteers have served from 1962 until the Peace Corps ended the program in 2012 because of safety concerns.

Honduran Culture

Honduras has confronted major structural barriers to economic growth, and has experienced political upheaval and devastating disasters. Yet with all of this strife and conflict, there is resilience in the face of significant challenges. The Honduran culture is as warm, generous, and inviting as one could find anywhere. Indeed, it is why we keep returning to the country. *Bienvenidos* (welcome) captures this sentiment, as many *catratchos* (Hondurans) are quick to offer a foreigner a place to stay, a cup of coffee, or a friendly game of soccer. This can be found throughout the country, whether visiting the Bay Islands, traveling through the cities, seeing the beautiful Copán ruins, or walking the beaches of Amapala—Hondurans are often kind and gracious.

Over the years, volunteers have shared stories about their time in Honduras. Of course, there are stories of stolen wallets, forgotten bags, and concern for safety when walking in the city late at night. But far more common are the stories of volunteers who received *un jalón* (a ride hitchhiking) across the country, were invited to someone's home when they didn't have a place to stay, and were treated like family rather than a stranger. There is a feeling among many foreigners that if they needed assistance, they would rather be in need in Honduras than in their own country.[22]

Additionally, medical volunteers commonly encounter restaurant owners who open their patio for groups to enjoy an authentic Honduran meal. This scene usually includes the establishment's family members serving the food and joining the group for coffee and a pastry at meal's end. The Honduran people are particularly grateful to volunteers who bring their skills and resources to the battle for health and wellness in impoverished conditions.

Nuestros Pequeños Hermanos
An Inspiration

Thirty-six kilometers northeast of Tegucigalpa sits a large orphanage with nearly 550 children. Nuestros Pequeños Hermanos (NPH) was started in 1986 by a long-term German volunteer Reinhart Koehler, who had previously worked at the sister house in Cuernavaca, Mexico. The philosophy of the orphanage is simple: NPH is a Christian mission that strives to provide a permanent family and home for orphaned, abandoned, and other at-risk children who live in conditions of extreme poverty. NPH programs provide quality education, healthcare, and spiritual formation with the goal of raising good Christians and productive members of their respective societies.

NPH is unique in that unlike most people's concept of an orphanage, the children are not available for adoption. NPH's founder, Father William Wasson, believed that these children needed to be relieved of the emotional instability of moving from one institution to another, and he did not want siblings to be separated. So he created a permanent home that provides a stable, loving family life complete with food, clothing, chores, educational opportunity, faith, and of course, love. It was at an NPH fundraising event where the authors of this chapter met; it was the place that inspired them both, and it continues to be an anchor for their efforts—like the mission of NPH—to meet the needs of Hondurans.

Children arrive at NPH from all over the country and for dozens of reasons. Some have lost parents to AIDS, others come from poverty-stricken families that can no longer care for their children, and some are abandoned because of physical or mental disabilities or have been abused. What they all have in common is that the entering child has no family members willing to provide care, and if there is more than one child in the family, all the children must come as a unit. These rules prevent future issues involving relatives who suddenly want to be the caretaker, or a family selecting one or some of the children but not others. Also, keeping brothers and sisters together provides children with consistency in their lives during the difficult transition of moving to a new home.

This work with underprivileged children is only the first of many roles that NPH plays in rural Honduras. Over the years, and with generous donations from organizations and individuals, NPH has been able to expand its work to increasingly support the needs of the local community, especially in the field of medicine. Medical brigades have been using NPH as a staging point to serve surrounding areas since the late 1990s. The organization has maintained living facilities for volunteers who can work internally serving the kids, at the external clinic to serve the local population, or by traveling to nearby communities to provide services, including dental, optometry, and basic first aid.

Case Study: Angela's Journey

On one of those volunteer trips, Dr. Peter Daly, an orthopedic surgeon, and his wife LuLu, a pediatric nurse, met a nine-year-old girl named Angela. Before Angela arrived at the NPH orphanage, she had suffered the loss first of her father and then, four years later, of her mother—both to HIV/AIDS. (Honduras has an HIV rate of 0.8 percent and accounts for 60 percent of the HIV/AIDS cases in Central America.[23]) The family had always lived in extreme poverty. The mother worked hard washing and ironing clothing, which barely provided enough to pay the rent for a small room in which the entire family lived, and for a little food each day. On her deathbed, the mother beseeched a neighbor to take care of the older sister, Cynthia. She left Angela and her little brother Christian with her eighteen-year-old brother. The mother's brother made a living selling trash, requiring him to be on the move constantly. In the end, neither the neighbor nor the brother could provide for the children, and they sought assistance from the local authorities. Finding the children in squalid conditions, the authorities immediately moved the children to a government home for temporary shelter, and later informed NPH about Cynthia, Angela, and Christian. Along with devastating poverty, Angela also suffered from a severe bone growth plate condition that caused her knees to bend inwards ("knock-knee") 65 degrees on each knee (normal being 0 degrees). She had to scissor one leg in front of the other to stand or walk. She used a wheelchair for longer distances, and she couldn't participate in physical activities such as soccer or dancing. The local medical community lacked a diagnosis or any resources to treat her condition. When Dr. Daly evaluated Angela, he recognized that her severe deformity could not be fixed with one operation in the local facility, so he and his wife brought her to their US home for a year, during which Angela received several surgical procedures and months of rehabilitation. She can now run and dance like her peers.

Holy Family Surgery Center

Like Angela, many patients arrive at the NPH community clinic needing surgery. But these patients either can't afford the surgery or can't get the services in the few public hospitals of Honduras because the hospitals are consistently overloaded with emergencies. The hospitals regularly lack supplies and have other shortages, also resulting in a lack of services.

NPH envisioned the ability to provide quality surgeries to the poor of Honduras who otherwise would not have access. In 2003, with the support of the Dalys, fundraising began. By 2004, $500,000 US was raised, and building began on what was to be called the Holy Family Surgery Center (HFSC), or Centro Quirúrgico Sagrada Familia.

Beyond providing surgery to the poor, NPH Honduras aimed to establish a permanent link between local surgeons and surgeons on medical missions from the United States, in a collaborative effort to work together and learn from each other. This partnership provides many types of surgery, as well as attentive post-operative care to avoid the negative consequence that can result when medical and surgical brigades come and go without an ongoing follow-up program.

Along with the primary care clinic facilities located on the property of NPH Honduras's Rancho Sante Fe, HFSC provides a rich educational opportunity for the NPH children. In addition to the standard curriculum of primary and secondary school, the children currently can receive vocational training in auto repair, metalworking, electricity, sewing, cosmetology, and shoe making. Healthcare career development is a natural extra vocational option made available by the presence of the surgery center.

My Path from the NPH Orphanage to Become an Orthopedic Surgeon

A testament to the success of NPH's educational system is Dr. Merlin Antunez, who grew up at the NPH orphanage and will complete orthopedic surgical residency training in December 2013. What follows are his reflections on observing and receiving healthcare as a Honduran, and then pursuing a medical career.

My life does not differ much compared to many other Hondurans. I find my life very fortunate in every single way. My family lived in a small village, where the fact of having food on the table for the next meal depends on the work the man of the house is able to do. My parents had just a few years of education and had to struggle with my father's progressing Parkinson's disease. Those were really bad times for my two brothers and me. We were just three, five, and six years old. I consider that period of time the beginning of a twisted, but blessed path in my life. My parents divorced on May 16, 1985. We did not see our mother for many years after that day. After several weeks our father took the three of us to the road and someone gave us a fourteen-hour ride to Tegucigalpa city. We lived for nine months in a government orphanage and attended public school. We then were taken to a new place. There are a few memories that still live clearly in my mind—a warm bed, pancakes, honey and butter (my favorite breakfast ever since), and smiles and hugs from strangers who were very happy to see us. From that day on I called that place "home." My two brothers, a friend and I were the very first to join what now is the family of Nuestros Pequeños Hermanos (NPH, meaning "Our Little Brothers and Sisters").

Every once in a while I took a look around myself and could tell that my parents were gone, but somehow I understood I had other issues to worry about, like dreaming and planning my life. The best part was that I had the support I needed 24/7. I planned the next thirty-five years of my life when I was seven years old, even before I could spell my name. My biggest goal: to become a doctor.

Twenty-five years have passed and I have walked through most of that path fearless. If I could go back in time, I would make sure my life would be exactly the same and that not even a period was changed.

The early death of two of my other brothers, and the illness in my early childhood, all must have been strong and unconscious reasons regarding my decision to become a doctor. However, the fact that my father's Parkinson's disease was getting worse was definitely my real inspiration. I always thought that if I were not able to heal my Dad, I could help others with their medical issues along the way. Maybe I was aiming to the moon, but a step forward every day got me closer all the time. Just now I have had the chance to realize it was harder than what I thought, especially when no one of my family members had more than six years of school.

In 1999, I had the chance to work at the NPH Honduras clinic as a nurse assistant. Before getting to go to the university, we usually work three years at our NPH home, doing different activities to compensate for all the help we have received in our early years. It allows us to share our experience and knowledge with our younger brothers at the NPH home. They consider us their example, and during that time I became more mature. During that year, I discovered something really special—the relationship between a patient and a doctor. And I had no doubt I had made the best decision ever in my life.

I would love to say the public health system in Honduras offers everybody the same opportunities, but I cannot. I would not say it is the worst system, either. Maybe the better description is that there is too much politics in between patients and doctors, and it is too centralized. Many people must travel long distances to have medical care, and once they get to the hospital, they realize that it is not "It," not the end of their journey. It is just part of the odyssey. There is a lot of trauma, and the government does not pay for the surgical implants. Elective surgeries are often canceled. Patients with chronic illnesses do not always receive their outpatient medication.

Nevertheless, beyond [those] lines, we see huge amounts of outpatients and emergency patients, and help those that we can. As a traumatology and orthopedic surgical resident, I can tell that many of my colleagues love taking care of patients. Like me, many times they will fall asleep on a chair to get a couple hours of rest after working more than thirty hours in a row.

Many other patients have the chance to get medical attention with private health insurance, and a small percentage can afford private clinics, which are very expensive. Many of the patients I see in the public hospitals will have to work for years in order to afford an elective private surgery.

Since the beginning of NPH in Honduras (1985), I had the chance to see nurses and doctors from different countries. Some stayed for days, weeks, months and years. There are some that are still here. Healthcare is expensive everywhere, and many families have to pay an onerous price at all costs. I see that reflected in the footprints of disease in my family saga. I have this great admiration for the medical groups that come to my country to share their knowledge to heal my people.

Foreign medical brigades come down to Honduras leaving behind the comfort and security they have at home, working hard hours in the service of patients who desperately are looking for a medical solution to their complaints. Some of these doctors have been my inspiration all these years. A smile on the face of these patients and the joy in their eyes would explain it better than my words, and can be considered more than enough in a priceless world. Perhaps the best ingredient to understand it would be to stand in their shoes for a few seconds. Maybe the hardest part will be the follow-up of some of the patients and seeing that not too many of them found the help they sought, because of time and logistic limitations.

Every once in a while, when I look back upon my life, my eyes betray me and shed some tears. Part of that realization is the fact that currently, more than 3,000 NPH children have had the same opportunity I was given, with no conditions attached.

Merlin Antunez, MD
December 2012

The Fútbol Project

Ryan Alaniz was also inspired to start a 501(c)3 NGO at NPH. After a year of volunteering, Ryan found himself returning annually to visit the kids. Before one of his trips around Christmas, he wanted to provide all 550 children with a gift they would enjoy and would also encourage healthy habits. Remembering that the children often played soccer with plastic bottles because they didn't have real soccer balls, Ryan went to local soccer leagues in California to raise money. After he had surpassed his goal of $400 US by fivefold, and with the support of the local community, Ryan founded a 501(c)3 nonprofit called The Fútbol Project to provide orphaned and underprivileged children with soccer equipment. Yet, to avoid creating future dependency, before receiving any equipment or tournament sponsorship, the young people were asked to do a service project for their local community. This philosophy of "pay it forward" promotes numerous social benefits for the kids (such as empowerment, trust, and connection among youth and residents) and for the community (betterment of the neighborhood, a connection to the local youth, and the encouragement of resident participation). Since 2006, the organization has supported children in twelve countries to implement projects such as planting trees (Honduras), picking up trash (South Africa), painting a school (Brazil), and cleaning up the neighborhood (Costa Rica).

Together, HFSC and The Fútbol Project highlight how health issues can be addressed on different levels and in different ways while maintaining a goal of sustainability. On one hand, HFSC has created a bricks-and-mortar locale that will be of service to Hondurans as long as there is need. With the capacity and medical instruments to conduct complex surgery, this facility will have a life-changing impact on the lives of thousands. But life-changing impact is not restricted to those receiving medical treatment. HFSC has been a vehicle for career development for the older children, or *pequeños*, growing up at the orphanage. Several pequeños have progressed through medical school and nursing programs, and assist with the care given at HFSC. Medical volunteers there serve as mentors to these young people—a key component of fighting poverty—one child at a time.

On the other hand, The Fútbol Project also aims for sustainability, not as much in terms of physical change as social and emotional change. By looking to instill the value of service in youth, along with a feeling of empowerment and agency to create positive change, the Fútbol Project views its sustainability in terms of affecting underlying culture. Both organizations hope to give participants the ability to pay it forward by using the benefits they received in the service of others.

Challenges for Global Health Workers

Healthcare in Honduras faces significant challenges in providing citizens with necessary and lifesaving treatment. Some of these challenges are structural and come with working in an impoverished nation—for example, lack of adequate infrastructure and inefficient bureaucracy. In what follows, we will convey some of the contemporary issues that the Honduran state and people face, and that medical volunteers should understand.

In the developing world, there are many practical issues in healthcare delivery, including the lack of previously taken-for-granted infrastructure. Electricity is a simple example. Power outages, voltage surges (abrupt excess amounts), and brownouts (weak voltage) are all too frequent, and cause severe damage to expensive medical equipment. Voltage-regulating transformers and surge suppressors are necessities for equipment longevity. Diesel-fueled backup generators are also needed, and must have an automatic transfer-switch capacity to guarantee that power is established within seconds in emergency and operating room settings. In addition, water quality for human consumption and operating room sterilizers is essential. To create the distilled water needed by smaller sterilizers, larger sterilizers must first be used to avoid the ubiquitous, machine-killing sediment contained in the water sources of many developing nations. Power supply, water quality, and equipment maintenance and service are all difficult and expensive, and they remain some of the most basic hurdles to be addressed before care can be delivered.

Guidelines for Collaborative Health Services

Medical volunteers often do not realize that they are entering an existing medical and political arena when they visit a developing country. When Dr. Daly first began volunteering in Honduras, he introduced himself to the local university orthopedic surgeons, made rounds with them, and discussed his plans to participate in surgical brigades at an outreach site where a new surgical facility was being constructed. Although the local surgeons were grateful for the help, their reception was tempered by a legacy of untoward complications following prior visiting brigades. When Dr. Daly visited the local hospital wards he saw many examples of well-intentioned procedures gone wrong. Infection, inadequate surgical follow-up, poor social conditions to which the patients had returned, and a lack of communication between patient and doctor sometimes reversed the hard work of medical brigades. These patients then showed up on the local medical provider's doorstep, occasionally with devastating results, including amputation. Meanwhile, the original treating medical-volunteer was unaware of this situation, having left after the surgery. In contrast, volunteering with an organization that provides the structure and collaboration with the local medical community is an important ethical consideration in order to ensure continuity of care for these patients.

A common misconception of the medical volunteer, which undermines collegiality and impairs communication with the local medical community, is the assumption that the severe cases of disease and disability are the result of poor-quality care given by local physicians and workers. Dr. Daly believes that the opposite is the reality: Honduran physicians and medical workers are very determined to provide the best care for their patients, and in this digital information age, they know the best practices for clinical conditions. The difficulty is that the treatments they have available do not usually constitute best practice. Often, these medical professionals must choose less than best-practice treatments while following the dictum "First, do no harm." Because medical volunteers are not privy to the information and resources that the previous provider had available, they must refrain from judging the previous treating clinicians. Often, inadequate treatment may be more harmful than no treatment, and hence, patients in developing countries can justifiably present with advanced disease due to the limited local resources and economics.

Impact of Volunteers

Opportunities for volunteers in Honduras are vast and visible. As US citizens, we are privileged to have the time, talent, and treasure to give back through volunteering. Even small, conscious efforts can have a big impact.

At NPH each child has multiple "godparents" in the United States or Europe who sponsor the child for $30 US per month. The sponsors occasionally send pictures or letters to their godchild. A child, feeling so loved by a sponsor for the support and connection, often will keep the sponsor's picture under his or her pillow, and pray for the godparent every night. When Ryan visited a poor family in a post-Mitch community, he observed that among the multiple framed photos of family and friends was a framed high-school graduation photo of an American girl. The family explained that the girl had come with a youth group to volunteer for only one week, and they had maintained contact over the years. These Hondurans were so touched by the foreigners in their lives that they had put their pictures in places of honor. In these two examples above, the change that these US citizens made, knowingly or not, has had a long-term positive impact via their transnational connection.

Yet broad and visible change has been much more elusive when volunteers fail to link their efforts to programs that foster sustainable change. The following example describes a project where a lack of coordination actually made the situation worse. As noted earlier, in 1998 Hurricane Mitch caused massive devastation throughout the country, necessitating an equally large rebuilding effort for residents who lived in high-risk areas. One efficient international organization that had connections already in Honduras quickly built houses in a disaster-safe area, La Colina. But once the houses were finished, the organization left and moved on to another housing project. Unfortunately, three factors—the lack of a continued NGO presence, a highly traumatized population, and a large gang problem—combined in La Colina. A gang took control of the area and forced the 355 families to pay a monthly "war tax" to keep their donated homes and the invitation to continue living in the community. Crime, drug trafficking, and murders became so common in the area that not even the police would enter. Although the organization had intended something positive by building houses for disaster survivors, its plan was short-sighted and had long-term negative consequences that could have been avoided.

In summary, there are broad possibilities to accomplish positive social change in Honduras and in oneself, but they will ideally be vetted through a self-critical process. Whether a volunteer is spending a week doing health checkups or a lifetime teaching at a home for street children, how the work is being done is as important as what is being done.

Bringing the Experience Home

During the significant experience of volunteering abroad, many youth and adults have a "mountaintop experience." They feel good about what they have done and look forward to doing it again. But after being back at home for a few weeks, when humdrum "normal" life returns, ex-volunteers are often lulled into the same routines and habits of their previous lives. This is not to say that they have not changed, but rather that they re-acculturate to their old ways, and the change they had hoped for becomes almost imperceptible. So how do we maintain a fire for service once we return home?

Over the years, we have seen a spectrum of post-experience responses. On one end of the spectrum are those who valued the opportunity to serve, but did very little to change the way they lived, or never again participated in a similar project. On the other end, there are people who capitalize on their life-altering experience to start nonprofits or to become active in justice issues as part of their new personas. Most people are somewhere in the middle.

We make no judgment about falling on either end of the spectrum. Each person is called to serve in a different way. However, for those interested in bringing the experience home, the following suggestions may help. First, some people have found it worthwhile to keep a journal, blog, or other written record of what they are experiencing and learning. Using concrete language and anecdotes to anchor specific moments, ideas, and feelings will make it easier to remember them later. Second, volunteers often find value in giving back to those who supported them in their choice to go abroad. Most people have a network of friends and family who encouraged their decision to go. A great way to extend the experience and give back to those who were supportive is through a presentation of pictures and stories about the experience and broader issues. Third, many people make a point of continuing to learn. Having lived in another country, albeit briefly, people often have fun delving deeper to learn why things are the way they are: What was the history of Tegucigalpa? Why is there a large Christ statue above the city? Who built the ancient temples in Copán? Why is the country so poor? Finally, some volunteers have found ways to continue relationships with people they met. These long-distance relationships can be very fulfilling, and with current technologies such as inexpensive calling plans, email, social media (Facebook, for example), and free video calling (Skype), it's easier than ever.

Conclusion

Honduras, as its legendary name and geography implies, is a land of mountaintops and valleys. This is also an apt metaphor for the country's contemporary social situation. Among the mountaintops are cultural values and a beautiful countryside. Values such as hospitality, family, resiliency, and faith are tangible. Hondurans are amazingly generous people, especially to those from the United States because they often have relatives or friends living in the States. The country is as beautiful as it is diverse. From cascading waterfalls to well-preserved Mayan ruins, white-sand beaches to dense tropical forest, and long mountain ranges to Technicolor coral, the nation offers a lifetime's worth of venues to see and explore.

Even so, there are also deep valleys in the small isthmus nation. Politics continue to divide the nation, especially after the 2009 coup. Economic inequality between the wealthy and the growing number of poor has continued to expand, as has crime. For example, in Tegucigalpa 3 percent of the population owns more than 40 percent of the land, and those living under the national poverty line rose from 51 percent of the population in 2009 to 65 percent in 2011.[24] In this nation of contrasts, global health volunteers have the opportunity to reflect upon not only what they have to offer Hondurans, but also about what they have to gain.

Notes

1 Tim Merrill, ed., *Honduras: A Country Study* (Washington: Government Printing Office for the Library of Congress, 1995).

2 Global Security, "Soto Cano Air Base, Honduras," accessed Nov. 25, 2011, available from www.globalsecurity.org.

3 Merrill, *Honduras.*

4 Central Intelligence Agency, "Honduras" in *The World Factbook* (Washington: CIA), accessed May 18, 2011, available from www.cia.gov.

5 See Patricia M. Hernandez, "Myth of Machismo: An Everyday Reality for Latin American Women," *St. Thomas Law Review* 15 (2002):859–882. There, Hernandez explains *machismo* as "the cult of virility. The chief characteristics of this cult are exaggerated aggressiveness and intransigence in male-to-male interpersonal relationships and arrogance and sexual aggression in male-to-female relationships" (p. 862).

6 United Nations Data (UNDATA), "Crude Birth Rates," accessed May 13, 2011, available from www.data.un.org.

7 CIA, "Honduras."

8 Ibid. The CIA claims that 98 percent of Hondurans are Catholic. My own study finds that the number is significantly lower.

9 Plutarco Castellanos, "Transformacion Del Sector Salud: A Presentation by the Former Secretary of Health," Tegucigalpa, Honduras (Mar. 2011).

10 Greg Bankoff, George Frerks, and Dorothea Hilhorst, *Mapping Vulnerability* (Sterling: Earthscan, 2004), 11.

11 Sarah Bradshaw, Brian Linneker, and Rebeca Zúniga, "Social Roles and Spatial Relations of NGOs and Civil Society: Participation and Effectiveness in Central America Post Hurricane 'Mitch,'" *Nicaraguan Academic Journal* 2.1 (2001):73–113.

12 Sally O'Neill, "Central America 15 Months On: Reconstruction But No Transformation," *Humanitarian Exchange Magazine* 16 (Mar. 2000), accessed Apr. 28 2011, available from www.odihpn.org. Paul Jeffrey, "Rhetoric and Reconstruction in Post-Mitch Honduras," *NACLA Report on the Americas* 33.2 (1999):28–37. Bradley E. Ensor and Marisa Olivo Ensor, "Hurricane Mitch: Root Causes and Responses to

the Disaster" in *The Legacy of Hurricane Mitch: Lessons from Post-Disaster Reconstruction in Honduras,* ed. Marisa O. Ensor (Tucson, AZ: University of Arizona Press, 2010).

13 Transparency International, "Corruption Perception Index," accessed Oct. 10, 2010, available from www.transparency.org.

14 Ibid.

15 World Bank, "Honduras," accessed May 24, 2011, available from www.data.world bank.org.

16 Palash R. Ghosh, "Honduras Has World's Highest Murder Rate: UN," *International Business Times,* accessed Nov. 25, 2011, available from www.ibtimes.com.

17 Pan American Health Organization, "Honduras" in *Health in the Americas, 2007 Volume II–Countries,* accessed Jan. 13, 2012, available from www.paho.int.

18 Ibid.

19 World Health Organization, "Country Cooperation Strategy at a Glance: Honduras," accessed Nov. 2, 2011, available from www.who.int.

20 Doctors Without Borders, "MSF in Honduras," accessed Nov. 2, 2011, available from www.doctorswithoutborders.org.

21 Jeffrey E. Heck, Andrew Bazemore, and Phil Diller, "The Shoulder to Shoulder Model–Channeling Medical Volunteerism Toward Sustainable Health Change." *Family Medicine* 39.9 (2007):644–650.

22 In generalizing about a country, there is the risk of essentializing a people, culture, or place. As in every country, not all citizens, subcultures, or areas share the same values.

23 UNAIDS, "UNAIDS Report on the Global Aids Epidemic 2010," accessed Nov. 2, 2011, available from www.unaids.org.

24 United States Agency for International Development (USAID), "Land Tenure and Property Rights Portal, Country Profile: Honduras," accessed May 13, 2011, available from www.usaidlandtenure.net.

5 Nicaragua I

James Saunders, Margo J. Krasnoff, and Benjamin Jastrzembski

Nicaragua is a land of amazing natural beauty with a rich cultural heritage. It is also the second poorest country in the Western Hemisphere, behind Haiti. Nicaragua's history of political unrest, foreign interventions, revolution, and natural disasters has resulted in extreme poverty. Healthcare delivery in rural areas of the country is further hampered by geographical isolation caused by mountains, rivers, and poorly maintained roads. These factors have had a profound impact on the health of the population, and on a healthcare system that struggles to meet their needs.

The poverty and struggling healthcare system set the stage for a large volume of foreign healthcare volunteers. Highly committed and resourceful Nicaraguan health professionals are eager to partner with visiting physicians, nurses, and allied healthcare workers. Despite a troubled history with the United States, Nicaraguans are interested in and feel connected to US culture, with no animosity toward visitors from the States. Medical volunteering in Nicaragua can be an extraordinarily rewarding experience and can lead to substantial improvements in the health of the Nicaraguan people.

To explore the context within which healthcare volunteers work, this chapter reviews Nicaraguan history and society with an emphasis on how these features influence health issues. We describe the Nicaraguan healthcare system and major public health concerns. We then review our experiences with two volunteer medical programs. The first focuses on students collaborating in development projects. The second program integrates surgical and specialty care such as otolaryngology and audiology into existing Nicaraguan health systems, and includes extending the care of children with hearing loss from the operating room into the classroom. We conclude with strategies to improve the effectiveness of volunteer surgical missions. The authors of chapter 6, "Nicaragua II," focus on the Caribbean Coast region of Nicaragua, with an emphasis on dental medicine and indigenous populations.

History

The Spanish arrival to western Nicaragua in 1522 precipitated a demographic implosion among the indigenous people who had lived in a well-developed agrarian society. By 1555, the population had plummeted from one-half million to less than 50,000.[1] Deaths from diseases brought by the Spanish dwarfed the number of deaths from direct conflict with the conquistadors. The Spanish caused further devastation by shipping survivors to Peru to work as slaves in the gold mines.[2] Subsistence agriculture and cattle ranching became the primary economic activities.[3] During the colonial era, two major cities emerged: Granada, a center of trade and connection to Spain, and León, the intellectual and artistic center. The pro-business Conservative Party aligned with Granada, and the Liberal Party with León. Feuds between these two competing political parties have shaped much of Nicaragua's history.

William Walker and Postcolonial Nicaragua

Nicaragua gained independence from Spain in 1821, but this only heralded a new era of foreign domination as the United States and the British competed for influence.[4] Nicaragua attracted the attention of foreign powers because it was the site of a potential transoceanic canal via Lake Nicaragua and the San Juan River.[5] With the 1848 discovery of gold in California, the importance of Nicaragua's potential transoceanic link grew.[6]

Soon after, members of the Liberal Party approached a San Francisco mercenary, William Walker, for support in defeating their Conservative Party rivals.[7] Walker and his band of mercenaries successfully wrestled control of Nicaragua from the Conservatives, but Walker soon overshadowed his Liberal allies and proclaimed himself president of Nicaragua in a sham election.[8] In 1856, both the Conservatives and Liberals united to oust Walker and were helped by a broad coalition of Central American armies. A famous battle in the campaign against Walker occurred at the San Jacinto ranch. Even though the Nicaraguans lacked ammunition and were reduced to throwing stones against the well-armed mercenaries, the Nicaraguans proved victorious. As Walker retreated, he burned the city of Granada to the ground. In 1860, Honduran authorities executed William Walker after he attempted a second Central American invasion.[9]

The so-called Walker Affair represents the beginning of US political and military influence on Nicaragua that continues to this day. After the disgrace of the Liberals' collusion with Walker, the Conservative Party took control of Nicaragua's government.[10] The relative peace during the subsequent Conservative rule from 1857 to 1893 was in part due to diminished US interest in Nicaragua. The completion of the US transcontinental railroad and the trans-Panama railroad reduced the importance of Nicaragua as a transportation link to the western United States.[11] During this period of relative peace, one of Nicaragua's national heroes, the poet Rubén Darío, rose to fame. Considered one of the greatest poets of Castilian Spanish, Darío remains an iconic hero in Nicaragua, with his image present in nearly every school and governmental office.

In the 1870s, the coffee industry emerged, bringing economic and social transformation.[12] Coffee plantations required significant capital and large pools of labor. Although the coffee boom provided economic benefit for a small group of elites, it did not improve the welfare of most Nicaraguans.[13] Peasants were coerced into working indefinitely on the plantations to pay their debts to the wealthy landowners.[14] The government also passed laws prohibiting the communal system of land ownership previously used by the indigenous farmers, and this facilitated the violent takeover of land by coffee planters.[15]

In 1902, the United States chose Panama rather than Nicaragua as the site of the future transoceanic canal. In light of this, the United States perceived Nicaraguan president José Santos Zelaya's ambition to reunite Central America as threatening to US dominance in the region. In response, US companies and members of the Nicaraguan Conservative Party organized a rebellion to defeat Zelaya. A powerful figure inside the US government also had reason to want Zelaya out: US Secretary of State Philander Knox, who had connections to a gold-mining outfit in Nicaragua, publicly called for Zelaya's overthrow, and Zelaya was forced to resign as president.[16] The toppling of Zelaya is significant in the history of American foreign policy because it represents the "first real American coup."[17] Adolfo Díaz, the financial secretary of the gold-mining company that Secretary of State Knox was associated with, became president of Nicaragua in 1911.[18] Díaz continued to receive a salary from the US gold-mining company while president.[19] His government also arranged loans from US banks that gave the United States control over Nicaragua's finances and infrastructure.[20]

Anger over the threat to Nicaraguan sovereignty and growing American economic control sparked an uprising against President Díaz. Only with an American military intervention did Díaz manage to stay in power. To protect American investments, and because of Nicaragua's strategic importance, the United States had a continual military presence in Nicaragua until 1933. Later in the occupation, the United States trained the Nicaraguan National Guard, which it hoped would replace the US Marines.

Sandino and the Somoza Family Dictatorship

One general, Augosto César Sandino, refused to accept the presence of US troops in Nicaragua. From 1927 to 1933, Sandino led a guerrilla war against the US troops and the new US-trained Nicaraguan National Guard. Sandino was a nationalist whose principal grievance was that American occupation violated Nicaraguan sovereignty. With fewer than 1,000 fighters, Sandino cultivated a support base of rural peasants and effectively harassed the enemy through targeted raids. The US and Nicaraguan National Guard responded with indiscriminate force, using airplanes to bomb villages suspected of supporting the Sandinistas.

Under pressure from Sandino, the United States finally withdrew the marines from Nicaragua and transferred control of the National Guard to Anastasio Somoza García, a young, charismatic, US-educated military officer.[21] With the departure of the US military, the politically ambitious Somoza began to align the Nicaragua National Guard as a partisan force loyal to him personally, rather than as an apolitical stabilizing institution.[22] After the US withdrawal, Sandino promptly signed a peace agreement.[23] However, in 1934 General Somoza invited Sandino to a dinner meeting where Sandino was captured and executed.[24] Two years later, Somoza overthrew President Juan Bautista Sacasa, and consolidated his own power by declaring himself president of Nicaragua.[25] The legacy of Sandino's movement would reemerge decades later when a reborn Sandinista movement, named in his honor, would eventually lead the effort to overthrow the Somoza family dictatorship.

The Somoza family dictatorship ruled Nicaragua for the next forty-two years. Anastasio Somoza García ("Tacho") ruled from his ascension in 1936 until he was assassinated in 1956. His eldest son, Luis, succeeded him and ruled until he died from a heart attack in 1967. Luis's younger brother Anastasio Somoza Debayle ("Tachito") was "elected" president in 1967 and became the most brutal of the three rulers.[26]

The key to Anastasio Somoza's success was his control of the powerful and loyal National Guard, which infiltrated every aspect of Nicaraguan life.[27] The systematic extortion of businessmen through bribes, smuggling, and kickbacks secured the loyalty of the guardsmen and led Somoza to amass a great fortune.[28] Betrayal was punished with prison, torture, and execution.[29] Somoza pronounced his political strategy as "bucks for my friends, bullets for my enemies."[30]

In addition to the National Guard, Somoza also secured his power by maintaining a close relationship with the United States. He demonstrated his loyalty by supporting the United States' staunch anticommunist foreign policy during the Cold War.[31] Somoza offered one of his private plantations as a training base for the overthrow of the left-leaning Guatemalan president in 1954.[32] In return for his support, Somoza received extensive military assistance for the National Guard,[33] as well as economic aid from the United States. Although these initiatives provided opportunities for Somoza and the upper class, they did little to lift the majority of Nicaraguans out of poverty.[34] Increased military aid facilitated the National Guard's operations against an emerging guerrilla movement, the Frente Sandinista de Liberación Nacional (FSLN), named in honor of the martyred Sandino.[35] Sandinista leaders included Edén Pastora, Tomás Borge, Daniel Ortega, Dora María Téllez, and Carlos Fonseca, among others.

Managua Earthquake and the Revolution

On December 23, 1972, a magnitude 6.3 earthquake struck the Nicaraguan capital Managua.[36] The disaster killed at least 10,000 Nicaraguans, destroyed the capital, and left most residents homeless.[37] In the wake of the tragedy, Somoza channeled relief funds to himself and his allies while downtown Managua remained in ruins.[38] The corrupt response of the regime to the earthquake fueled opposition to Somoza, including successful operations by FSLN in 1974.

Somoza's response to the Sandinista rebels was ferocious. In a counterinsurgency campaign intended to destroy FSLN, the National Guard attacked Nicaraguan civilians, especially in the Matagalpa and Caribbean regions. Catholic clergy and missionaries from these areas publicized cases of torture, rape, and murder of civilians.[39] These human rights abuses threatened support from the United States, especially because President Jimmy Carter had made human rights promotion a centerpiece of his foreign policy.[40] The newspaper *La Prensa* published daily exposés, and a group of respected and famous Nicaraguan leaders formed The Twelve, which called for Somoza's resignation.

In January 1978, gunmen linked to the Somoza regime assassinated the award-winning *La Prensa* editor Pedro Joaquín Chamorro as he drove to work. The murder was the beginning of the end for the Somoza dictatorship. Thousands of mourners and protesters took to the streets of Managua, many elites denounced the regime, and the United States canceled a military aid loan.[41] The Nicaraguan National Guard needed air strikes and heavy ordnance to suppress uprisings in the coming months.[42] One of the turning points in the insurgency came when a band of nineteen FSLN guerillas, led by Edén Pastora, stormed the National Palace and successfully held 2,000 hostages, including some members of the legislature.

The success of the Sandinista operation immediately galvanized the opposition, but the National Guard again suppressed the resistance with the use of overwhelming force and human rights abuses. As 1978 drew to a close, the economic situation in Nicaragua became dire. After months of preparation, the FSLN rebel radio station called on all Nicaraguans to support a final military and political push to finish the Somozas. The guerrillas captured National Guard barricades across the country as volunteers joined their ranks.

The National Guard inflicted heavy casualties on civilians during the combat, including the bombing of Sandinista-controlled neighborhoods in Managua. The Carter Administration attempted unsuccessfully to arrange a negotiated settlement; the Sandinistas refused to include members of Somoza's party and the National Guard in the government. On July 17, 1979, Somoza and his top aides fled to Miami and then into exile, as the Nicaraguan Revolution reached its dramatic triumph and the National Guard disintegrated.[43]

After the Revolution

After the revolution, the Sandinistas governed through a Council of State until national elections were held in 1984 when Daniel Ortega was elected president. Although many in Washington and upper-class Nicaraguans feared that the revolution heralded the coming of a Soviet-style state, Sandinista policy proved to be moderate.[44] The Sandinistas were influenced by socialism, but they were also pragmatic and sought to maintain broad diplomatic relations.[45] After negotiations with international creditors, the Sandinistas agreed to honor outstanding debt inherited from the Somoza regime. The Sandinistas did nationalize Somoza properties as well as some industries, such as mining, banking, and insurance, but advocated for an economy with both public (state-owned) and private sectors.[46] The executive political body and legislature included upper-class elites as well as Sandinistas.[47]

The most spectacular successes of the Sandinistas were social programs, such as the literacy campaign and health reforms. In 1980, the Sandinistas organized 85,000 volunteer teachers to teach basic reading and writing in the "second war of liberation." The Sandinistas also recruited thousands of the volunteers to be trained as auxiliary nurses in the government's new health system. The Sandinistas sought to provide free medical care to the population through a new system of local and regional health centers and national hospitals.[48] Healthcare became the second-largest government expenditure, behind education.[49] The Ministry of Health (MINSA) dedicated resources to primary care, and focused on the most vulnerable people living in urban slums and rural areas. Although US funding for several new hospitals in Nicaragua was cancelled, hundreds of new primary care health posts were built, including some in former mansions of Somoza supporters.[50] Vaccination campaigns on People's Health Days dramatically reduced the incidence of polio, measles, and pertussis.[51] An effort to eradicate malaria counted on 240,000 volunteers to distribute anti-malarial medications to 70 percent of the Nicaraguan population. Although unsuccessful in malaria eradication, the effort did significantly reduce malaria cases and increased public awareness about the illness.[52]

The Contra War

Despite the promising beginning to the decade, conditions in Nicaragua during the 1980s soon degenerated as the United States adopted a policy designed to topple the Sandinistas. US President Ronald Reagan pursued a coordinated policy across Central America to support right-wing anticommunist governments and movements. In the case of Nicaragua, the Reagan Administration sponsored a group of contra-revolutionaries (referred to as the "Contras") who attacked the Sandinista government. They consisted of former Nicaraguan National Guardsmen and former Sandinistas who were disillusioned with the direction Daniel Ortega had taken.

Beginning in 1981, the Reagan Administration terminated all economic aid to Nicaragua and allocated $20 million US for the CIA to support the contra-revolutionary guerrillas. The Contras, and later the CIA directly, began attacking bridges, oil refineries, health centers, and other infrastructure targets as well as mining Nicaraguan harbors. In response to the threat posed by the Contras, the Sandinista government was forced to cut social programs and to increase military spending, including distributing automatic weapons to civilians.[53] In addition, 10,000 Miskito indigenous people were forced to evacuate their homeland along the Río Coco, and some Miskitos joined a Contra organization out of frustration with the regional Sandinista leadership.[54]

Despite the challenges posed by the Contra War, the Sandinistas forged ahead with elections in November 1984. US diplomats discouraged opposition candidates from participating in an attempt to delegitimize the election, but international observers and the US-based Latin American Studies Association concluded that the election was fair. The Sandinista party won a resounding victory, and the guerrilla leader Daniel Ortega became president for a five-year term.[55]

Following Ortega's election, the Reagan Administration enacted a complete embargo on trade with Nicaragua, which ultimately was as devastating as the Contra War. Nicaragua's GDP, which had grown immediately following the revolution, fell precipitously in the late 1980s. Soon, the Sandinistas began to pay for the growing demands on their government by printing money, which led to a skyrocketing inflation rate. Inflation eventually became so uncontrolled that the government resorted to stamping new, higher denominations on paper bills rather than actually printing new bills with the higher values. Opposition to funding the Contras led to the US Congress prohibiting such support. Nonetheless, Reagan remained determined to sustain the Contras by whatever means possible.

In November 1986, news reports revealed what became known as the Iran-Contra Affair, an illegal funding scheme for the Contras. Reagan Administration officials secretly organized the sale of more than 1,500 missiles to the Iranian government of Ayatollah Khomeini. In exchange, the Iranian government facilitated the release of American hostages held by Iranian terrorists in Lebanon. The $2 million US of profits from the covert arms sales to Iran were then funneled to the Nicaraguan Contras.

Once it was publicized, the Iran-Contra Affair put future US support of the Contras into doubt, and gave the United States' right-wing allies across Central America incentive to begin peace negotiations. In 1987, Sandinista amnesty laws prompted thousands of Contras to disarm, Nicaragua enacted a new constitution, and a new law granted the people of the Caribbean more autonomy. Still, by the time of the 1990 elections, Nicaragua was exhausted. The Contra War alone had resulted in 31,000 casualties, and the economy had failed to improve despite austerity measures and the introduction of a new currency. The remaining Contra forces intensified their attacks prior to the election in an effort to weaken the Sandinista position.

Contemporary Politics

In the 1990 election, the National Opposition Union (UNO) a coalition of more than a dozen parties, opposed the Sandinistas. The UNO Candidate, Violeta Barrios de Chamorro, widow of the martyred *La Prensa* editor, unseated Ortega, and there was a peaceful transfer of power. President Chamorro moved quickly to end the Contra War and significantly reduced the size of the army. She expanded the economic austerity programs initiated in the final years of the Sandinista government. In order to qualify for international loans, Nicaragua agreed to neoliberal structural adjustment reforms involving government downsizing, deregulation of private enterprise, and the reduction of tariffs on imports and exports. Government spending dropped by one-half as government properties were sold, state-owned businesses were privatized, agriculture cooperatives were disbanded, and teachers, health workers, police officers, and soldiers were laid off. The effect of reduced government spending was disastrous for Nicaragua's poor. Free services were curtailed, and many impoverished Nicaraguans found it impossible to pay for healthcare and education. These economic adjustments led to stabilization of the currency as well as economic growth, but the growth was concentrated in goods that catered to the wealthy minority. In 1995, unemployment in Managua remained high, at 32 percent.

The old Liberal Party, mentioned earlier in the chapter, was transformed in the mid 1990s to become the Liberal Alliance (Alianza Liberal [AL]). In the 1996 election, President Chamorro did not run and Arnoldo Alemán, mayor of Managua and leader of the AL, won the presidency over FLSN candidate

Daniel Ortega. President Alemán continued the cost-cutting measures of the Chamorro administration. In addition, Alemán diverted public funds for his personal enrichment and that of his closest allies. In 1998, Hurricane Mitch devastated Nicaragua, killing 2,400, destroying crops, and leaving 20 percent of Nicaraguans homeless. After years of downsizing, the Nicaraguan government did not have the resources to adequately respond to the disaster. Alemán worsened the situation by funneling relief funds to municipalities under the control of his party.

In 2000, in order to consolidate their political power, Alemán and Ortega negotiated a "pact" between themselves and their parties; they united in order to appoint loyal party members to some of the most important government institutions. This agreement saved both Alemán and Ortega from investigation of accused crimes, and changed the election law to make it more difficult for third parties to compete.

In the 2001 elections, the Liberal Alliance nominated Alemán's vice president, Enrique Bolaños Geyer. Bolaños, who promised to fight corruption, won the election. Bolaños then surprised many by opening investigations against Alemán, who was accused of stealing more than $100 million US from Nicaragua. In 2004, Alemán was convicted of corruption but was allowed to serve his sentence under house arrest. The Nicaraguan Supreme Court later overturned the conviction.

In 2006, Bolaños succeeded in achieving some debt reduction for Nicaragua and signed a free-trade agreement, CAFTA-DR. The free-trade-zone assembly plants in Nicaragua (*maquilas*) have grown since then, and by 2012, they employed approximately 103,000 people, primarily in clothing assembly and tobacco.[56] Wages in the assembly plants are low, and concerns have been raised about environmental and labor protections.

Prior to the 2006 presidential elections, the allies of FSLN and PLC enacted changes in the election laws in a manner that favored Daniel Ortega, who was reelected to the presidency in 2006 and 2011. One important success of the second Ortega Administration has been to reform the practice of school fees, policies of prior administrations that had reduced primary school access for Nicaragua's poor. Ortega forged a close alliance with President Hugo Chávez of Venezuela, who provided Nicaragua with extensive aid. Money was invested in health and education programs, as well as in new auxiliary power generators, which reduced electricity shortages in the country.

Geography

Nicaragua is the largest country in Central America and is slightly smaller than New York State. It has a population of roughly 6 million, similar to its neighbors Honduras and Costa Rica, but because of its larger geographic size, Nicaragua has the lowest population density in Central America.[57] The majority of the population lives in the major urban centers of the Pacific lowland region. Overcrowding is a significant problem in the urban areas, yet the vast Central Highlands and Caribbean Coast are sparsely inhabited. The geography of the Caribbean Coast is discussed in chapter 6.

Pacific Lowlands

Nicaragua is referred to as the Land of Volcanoes and Lakes because of the geography of the country's western region.[58] The Pacific Lowlands extend 75 kilometers inland from the Pacific Ocean, and are relatively flat except for a line of volcanoes. Two major tectonic plates collide here, and many of these volcanoes are active, including the Masaya Volcano near Managua, which is now a national park. Its last major eruption was in 1772, but numerous minor eruptions have occurred, including one in 2003. Just east of this line of volcanoes is a rift valley, with farmlands made fertile from the volcanic ash, punctuated by Lake Managua and Lake Nicaragua, the largest freshwater lakes in Central America. Lake Nicaragua is the only lake in the world with freshwater sharks.[59] These lakes drain into the Caribbean Sea via the San Juan River, which forms the southern national border with Costa Rica.

The Pacific Lowlands are home to the major urban centers. The city of Granada is located on the shores of Lake Nicaragua near the Mombacho Volcano. The island of Ometepe was formed by two volcanoes that arise directly out of Lake Nicaragua: the Concepción and Maderas Volcanoes. Further north, the colonial city of León lies in the shadow of the Momotombo Volcano. The capital city of Managua is located on the southwestern shore of Lake Managua, almost halfway between the rival colonial cities.

Managua

With a population of nearly 2 million, Managua is home to one-third of the people of Nicaragua and is the second-largest city in Central America. It has all of the attributes of a bustling urban center except for the conspicuous absence of high-rise buildings. The downtown area was never rebuilt after the massive earthquake of 1972. The original streets, the abandoned buildings, and the partially destroyed cathedral remain as an eerie reminder of this destructive period in Nicaragua's history.

As the country's foremost industrial, cultural, and commercial center, Managua's economy is based primarily on trade. Its principal products include beer, coffee, textiles, matches, auto parts, jewelry, and shoes. Most travelers enter Nicaragua via the Augusto Sandino Airport in the northeast border of

Managua, far from the cultural or commercial center of town, but conveniently located on the Pan-American Highway.

Near the downtown is the crater lake of Tiscapa, with the iconic statue of Sandino looking out over the capital city. The industrial center of Managua is along the southeastern side of town, but most of the recent retail commercial development is along the corridor that eventually leads to the town of Masaya, the Carretera de Masaya. Nowhere in Nicaragua are the stark economical disparities more palpable than in Managua, where in less than five minutes one can travel from a neighborhood of families huddled under makeshift shacks to a galleria shopping mall.

Central Highlands

Rising up out of the center of the country, the Central Highland region borders Honduras and is dominated by the Segovia Mountains. The eastern section is known for its gold-mining communities of Bonanza, Siuna, and Rosita. Due to the rugged terrain, the Central Highland region is sparsely populated outside of its three principal municipalities: Estelí, Matagalpa, and Jinotega. The Pan-American Highway runs through the town of Estelí, making it a major commercial center and the third-largest city in Nicaragua. The climate in Estelí is ideal for cigar tobacco, and the city has attracted many Cuban cigar manufacturers. Matagalpa and Jinotega are both major coffee-producing centers. Matagalpa was originally founded as an indigenous village by the Matagalpa Indians. Jinotega is situated in a high valley of the Segovias, accessible only by a steep and winding road that isolates it geographically from the rest of the country. The Central Highlands are also the homeland of Augusto Sandino, and were the site of intense fighting during the Sandinista revolution.

Roads and Transportation

Because of the mountainous terrain, the major highways in Nicaragua run north and south along the coast and along the Pan-American Highway through the Segovia Mountains. Rental vehicles are available at the airport, and there is a public bus system but no rail system. Light aircraft service provides access to the Caribbean Lowlands and to the mining district of the eastern mountains. But, very poorly maintained rural roads limit land travel to these areas, as well as land travel from east to west in the mountains.

An interesting and unique feature of Nicaraguan life is that most streets do not have names, and there is no numeric address system.[60] Addresses throughout the country, including those in urban areas, are designated by the number of blocks from well-known landmarks or businesses. For example, a typical address in Nicaragua might be "two blocks south and one block east of the Texaco." To complicate things further, in Managua, *down* or *abajo* means west, and *up* or *arriba* means east. To the amazement of visitors, landmarks are still used to designate an address even if they no longer exist. For instance, an address might refer to "where the Texaco used to be." This situation makes postal service (especially international parcel service) to Nicaragua difficult. As international trade becomes more common in Nicaragua, there is an effort to establish an address system, but change has been slow, and the reality is that most Nicaraguans know how to get where they are going.

Public Health Priorities

According to 2011 statistics, life expectancy at birth is 69.6 years for men and 74 years for women.[61] The infant mortality rate has declined significantly since 2001, but is still one of the highest in Latin America at 29 per 1,000 live births.[62] Nicaragua's population is relatively young, with 36 percent of the population younger than fifteen years, and the majority of the population is of reproductive age. The fertility rate has declined somewhat, but remains relatively high at 2.7 children per woman. Maternal mortality is 170 deaths per 100,000 live births.[63] As might be expected, both the fertility rate and the infant mortality rate vary between the rural and urban populations, with significantly higher rates for rural Nicaraguans.[64] These health conditions and the fact that a large portion of the Nicaraguan population is of reproductive age are important factors in defining the national health agenda.

A ten-year National Health Plan was approved in 1994 and revised to cover the period 2004–2015.[65] Health promotion priorities include legislating environmental protection; establishing community-based programs for health, personal hygiene, and nutrition; promotion of physical activity (especially in children); coordinating activities to promote occupational safety and hygiene; and providing educational programs to prevent traffic accidents and violence (especially family violence). Disease prevention priorities include strengthening surveillance systems and controlling both communicable and noncommunicable disease; preventing maternal and child mortality; implementing a comprehensive reproductive health plan, with promotion of prenatal and postnatal care; encouraging breast-feeding programs; strengthening the national vaccination program; promoting policies on food and water safety; developing counseling services for mental illness and violence reduction; and promoting gender equity. In 2007, the government adopted a family- and community-centered healthcare model (MOSAFC) with the goals of building effective health services, generating higher levels of user satisfaction, and improving financial protection in health. This healthcare model promotes further decentralization of healthcare and the provision of more comprehensive services at the local level (see SILAIS, in "Healthcare System" section that follows).[66]

The implementation of these health priorities is limited by budgetary constraints, given that public health expenditures in 2010 were only 4.8 percent of GDP with a per capita health expenditure of $54 US per year for each Nicaraguan.[67] Although these figures are low, they have gradually increased since 2000, reflecting a greater national commitment to health.

Economy

With a GDP of $16.62 billion US (adjusted for purchasing power parity), Nicaragua is a lower-middle-income country with an average per capita income slightly over $1,000 US.[68] But there is tremendous economic disparity between the classes, and roughly 48 percent of Nicaraguans live below the international poverty line of $1 US per day.[69] The Nicaraguan economy is based primarily on agriculture. Mining, fishing, and light industry are also important.[70] Coffee is cultivated in the volcanic ash–enriched soil of the Western Highlands,[71] and has been Nicaragua's most important export since the nineteenth century; the price of coffee strongly influences the national economy.[72] Tobacco, particularly cigar tobacco and cigars from the Estelí region, and rum from Chinandega are well-known exports. Other exports include bananas, sugar, and beef. In addition to those who grow these commercial crops, many Nicaraguans live on small subsistence farms. Nicaraguans living abroad also contribute significant economic support through remittances.

Language and Literacy

Central American Spanish is spoken by 90 percent of the population, and many indigenous Nahuatl words have been preserved in the national dialect. On the Caribbean Coast, many people speak Creole or English as well as Spanish. Because of a National Literacy Crusade of the Sandinista governments in 1980, the illiteracy rate was cut in half; but the illiteracy rate has climbed in recent years to 32.5 percent.[73]

Educational System

Primary. Six years of primary education is compulsory and free in
Nicaragua. Most children attend school for a half-day, either morning
or afternoon. Enrollment and attendance have improved with the
educational initiatives over the past thirty years, but enrollment is
still only 94 percent at the primary level. Of those enrolled in primary
school, 76 percent complete primary education.[74] As expected, there

are dramatic regional and geographic variations in school enrollment and completion across the country, with lower rates in the eastern autonomous regions and rural areas.

Secondary. The enrollment and attendance for secondary education is much worse than for primary, with only 40 percent of males and 46 percent of females enrolled in secondary school.[75] Secondary education is free aside from the cost of uniforms and supplies, but it is not compulsory.

Universities. León is the original home of the state university of Nicaragua, the Universidad Nacional Autónoma de Nicaragua (UNAN, National Autonomous University of Nicaragua), founded in 1812. A second UNAN campus was founded in Managua in 1982. In addition, there are multiple small universities, colleges, and technical institutes in Nicaragua. The two most prominent institutions are the University of Central America (UCA, Universidad Centroamericana), a private Catholic university originally founded in El Salvador with campuses all over Central America, and the Universidad Americana in Managua. Despite the strong educational and literacy campaign in the post-Somoza era, in 2005 only 7 percent of Nicaraguans held a university degree.[76]

Medical Schools. There are four accredited medical schools in Nicaragua: two at the private institutions of the Universidad Americana and the Universidad Católica Redemptoris Mater (UNICA) in Managua, and two campuses of UNAN. One medical campus of UNAN is in the university's original home in León, and the other is in Managua. Medical education in Nicaragua is a six-year course of study, and a prior university degree is not a requirement for admission. All graduating doctors are required to work for one year as primary care providers in government clinics before they can enter a residency position.

Healthcare System

In general, there is a relative scarcity of healthcare providers to meet the needs of Nicaraguans; and like the people, these providers are distributed unevenly across the country. In 2007, there were 2,404 doctors in the country, or a ratio of 1 doctor for every 2,500 inhabitants. Roughly one-quarter of these physicians work in Managua. In that same year, there were 2,440 professional nurses, or a ratio of 1 nurse for 909 inhabitants.[77] MINSA controls all aspects of healthcare delivery, including the network of public clinics and hospitals, medical specialty training, research, and humanitarian medical aid. Since the 1990s, the public hospitals and community clinics within each of the seventeen departments in Nicaragua have been managed by the regional entities called SILAIS (System of Locally Integrated Health Service). These public hospitals and clinics from the United Health System (Sistema Nacional Único de Salud, or SNUS). Though all SILAIS providers and administrators are employees of MINSA and subject to the same bureaucratic challenges, this decentralization of services does allow local authorities some autonomy. From a practical standpoint, any significant event, such as creating a new position for a Nicaraguan provider or requesting a visiting medical brigade to work in the government hospital, must be requested by the local SILAIS and then approved by MINSA.

The MINSA strategy of healthcare delivery places a strong emphasis on primary healthcare. Through SILAIS, MINSA has 877 primary healthcare units that provide primary care for approximately 3 million people (that is, slightly less than one-half of the nation's population has direct access to these facilities). Each of these primary care units is supported by 177 health centers that feed into 33 hospitals, many of which are regional hospitals within each department.[78] These regional SNUS hospitals provide emergency services, surgical care, high-risk obstetric care, and some other specialty services. In 2008, MINSA began a national program that focuses more on community-based care with expanded basic healthcare delivery (EBA, Equipo Básico de Atención). Each unit is given the task of providing basic health benefits as defined by the Conjuntos de Prestaciones de Salud (CPS, Joint Health Benefits).[79]

Provision of surgical subspecialty care is particularly sparse, with many other subspecialties that are lacking at the regional level, including otolaryngology, ophthalmology, neurosurgery, cardiothoracic surgery, urology, and the pediatric specialties. For example, only six of seventeen departmental hospitals provide regional otolaryngology services. MINSA provides these services at its tertiary hospitals in Managua, where the residency programs are based. These hospitals include Lenin Fonseca Hospital (for surgery and surgical subspecialties), Hospital Infantil Manuel de Jesús Rivera "La Mascota" (the national children's hospital), the Roberto Calderon Hospital (for trauma), Bertha Calderon Hospital (for women's health and neonatal care), the Fernando Vélez Páiz Hospital (for maternal and infant care), and Centro Nacional de Oftalmología (for ophthalmology). There is no residency training in the country for cardiac care, and these services are currently available only at three private hospitals.

The lack of specialized services in the rural regions creates multiple challenges for patients. The geographic isolation of many communities makes access to specialized care practically impossible. These specialty hospitals in Managua are inundated with a volume of patients that they can't possibly care for at their relatively small, poorly funded institutions. Further, there is no system of triage to coordinate the care for these patients. Those who can make it to the specialty hospitals often arrive at the hospital gate with a note from their local provider and their health record in hand.

Approximately 35 to 40 percent of the population still lacks direct access to the public health system because of geographical limitations,. and all hospitals in the SNUS healthcare system suffer from the common problems of a deteriorating infrastructure and lack of basic equipment and supplies.[80] These conditions, and the low wages for doctors, create poor morale among providers. MINSA doctors are among the lowest paid in Central America, earning between $250 and $350 US per month. Virtually all MINSA doctors must supplement their pay by working in the afternoons in private "clinics" often run out of their homes. This means that the hospital clinics are staffed by attending physicians only in the mornings, further limiting their capacity.

Approximately 20 to 25 percent of Nicaraguan healthcare is provided by Nicaraguan government-administered institutions other than the SNUS public health system.[81] Roughly 8 percent of Nicaraguans who work in government jobs (for example, Ministry of Defense) that provide their own health facilities and approximately 16 percent of the population are employed by private industries that are eligible for the social security healthcare system managed by the Nicaraguan Social Security Institute (INSS), which is also under the auspices of MINSA.[82] These systems are supported in part by contributions from employers and employees. They provide a basic package of services, and any care above this is theoretically covered by the National Health System. INSS consumes roughly 25 percent of the national healthcare budget, and its per capita cost is twice that of the public sector coverage.[83] The government and military health networks provide care to some dignitaries, military personnel, and dependents, altogether accounting for 6 to 8 percent of the population. Finally, an estimated 4 percent of the population receives care at private hospitals. There are seven such hospitals in Managua, with roughly 200 beds. Most of this private care is provided on a fee-for-service basis, with a small portion covered by various insurance entities. These hospitals, such as Hospital Metropolitano, provide high-quality services to wealthy Nicaraguans.

The poverty of Nicaragua and the unequal provision of healthcare have created a situation in which many people supplement their healthcare with that provided by NGOs. One estimate suggests that 14 percent of healthcare costs are supported by foreign NGOs.[84] This is particularly true in rural areas, where access to adequate care through the SNUS public healthcare system is most limited. This international aid includes free-standing clinics staffed by Nicaraguan physicians who are paid by foreign organizations; MINSA clinics and providers that are fully or partially supported through the donation of funds or equipment; volunteer brigades working with Nicaraguan doctors in MINSA hospitals; and ad hoc medical clinics set up by international brigades in churches, schools, or private homes. The need to mobilize services in order to address the disparities of rural healthcare has been recognized by MINSA, which has organized several internal Nicaraguan brigades. Many Cuban physicians are working within the Nicaraguan system, and many Nicaraguan physicians have trained in Cuba or elsewhere. In 2011, Cuban providers collaborated with MINSA to conduct a comprehensive national survey of people with disabilities.[85]

Regulation of Health Research

The research output for Nicaragua is limited, and publications related to the major health problems (for example, diarrhea, TB, perinatal conditions, and lower respiratory conditions) make up only 20 percent of the published work.[86] A National Policy on Science and Technology was created in 1995, but as of this writing, it has no operational budget.[87] Most research funding in Nicaragua comes from a variety of outside sources. The national health research priorities are infectious diseases (especially infant diarrhea), labor medicine, and epidemiology. MINSA requires that health research be consistent with the National Health Plan. The regulation of research is administered by the Department of Research in Health (Dirección General de Investigación en Salud) in MINSA.

The recently created Centro de Estudios Epidemiológicos y Demográficos and the Centro de Investigación de Salud, Trabajo y Ambiente at UNAN–León are conducting studies on occupational exposure to pesticides, traditional medicines, and epidemiology.[88] In addition, the Centro de Enfermedades Infecciosas at UNAN–León studies infectious diseases. UNAN–Managua houses the Centro de Investigación y Estudios en Salud (Center for Health Research and Studies).[89]

Leading Health and Environmental Issues

Deaths from noncommunicable diseases have significantly increased in recent years, with circulatory diseases, tumors, and trauma being the leading causes of death in adults.[90] Diabetes and hypertension rates are highest in Managua, reaching a prevalence of 9 percent and 25 percent respectively there. Trauma accounts for 18 percent of all emergency visits, with falls, domestic violence, assaults with weapons, and motor vehicle accidents most commonly seen. Not surprisingly, deaths from trauma are more common for males. The leading causes of infant death are intestinal infectious diseases, perinatal distress, acute respiratory infections, congenital anomalies, and malnutrition.

Child malnutrition disproportionately affects rural children and children living in the areas of the Northern Autonomous Atlantic Region (RAAN), Jinotega, Matagalpa, and Madriz. Respiratory diseases are the greatest cause of morbidity. Although the overall incidence of acute respiratory illness seems to be increasing, the mortality from respiratory disease is declining.[91]

TB remains endemic, with high rates in the Caribbean Coast.[92] The overall incidence of TB is 41.1 per 100,000 people.[93] The incidence of HIV/AIDS remains lower than 1 percent, but rates have slowly increased since 2000.[94] One triumph of the National Health Plan has been relatively high vaccination coverage rates and a subsequent reduction in measles, mumps, and rubella, as well as the eradication of polio.[95] Despite these efforts, congenital rubella syndrome accounted for 1 to 2 percent of deafness in children in Jinotega in 2005.[96] This finding underscores the fact that in spite of the broad national vaccination programs, only 22 percent of Nicaraguan communities achieve a rubella vaccination rate greater than 95 percent.[97] Malaria rates have also declined in recent years, but remain a concern in the Pacific Lowlands, the San Juan River basin, and the Caribbean Coast.[98] The mosquito-borne illness most commonly associated with Nicaragua is dengue or "break-bone" fever (see Glossary). Cases of the parasitic disease leishmaniasis have climbed dramatically in recent years, primarily in Jinotega and Matagalpa. Blood smears for the parasite that causes Chagas disease were positive in 10 percent of schoolchildren in one study, indicating exposure in these youths.[99]

Gender-based violence is a significant health problem for women, with 27 percent of women reporting physical abuse at some time in their lives, and 13 percent reporting at least one instance of sexual abuse. Although the majority of women have access to some form of contraception, this remains a somewhat controversial issue due to cultural and religious factors, and the teenage pregnancy rate is the highest in Latin America.[100] Abortion for any reason is illegal in Nicaragua. Cervical cancer is the most common fatal malignancy in women, with a prevalence of 13.9 cases per 100,000 women in 2002, far exceeding that of the United States. Cervical cancer and breast cancer together make up roughly 20 percent of all cancer deaths in Nicaragua.[101]

The major environmental risks to health result from poor air quality in Managua, secondhand smoke from poorly ventilated wood stoves, and the seemingly ubiquitous exposure to pesticides for agricultural workers; building fumigations (especially in the Pacific and Central regions) also pose a risk.[102] Active volcanoes indirectly expose the population to heavy metals, particularly arsenic and mercury, with high levels of mercury found in fish from both Lake Managua and Lake Nicaragua.[103] Some communities and populations have specific environmental issues. Industrial exposures to chemicals are poorly regulated, and mining communities in the northeastern region are exposed to high levels of lead and mercury.[104] Most rural communities and poor urban neighborhoods do not have adequate sewage management systems, and only 27 percent of rural homes have connections to potable water sources.[105]

Global Health Agencies and Initiatives

WHO has funded three major global health initiatives in Nicaragua that focus on specific conditions consistent with the MDGs. These programs include Roll Back Malaria, Stop TB, and the Global Alliance of Vaccinations and Immunizations (GAVI). Nicaragua adopted the strategies of the Roll Back Malaria initiative in 2000, and this is considered a success story in the control (but not eradication) of the disease, thanks to a strong commitment by MINSA and the Nicaraguan government.[106] Nicaragua joined the GAVI alliance in 2005.[107] Nearly $10 million US has been disbursed to Nicaragua to support health systems, immunization services, and access to new vaccines. The Stop TB initiatives have been supported by the Global Fund, and include improving supervision and monitoring activities, assuring second-line drug availability, strengthening the laboratory testing network, and providing incentives for patients to comply with treatment.[108]

USAID funds several major public health programs in Nicaragua. The FamiSalud program has enhanced family and child health through family planning, birth plans that include maternity care and deliveries by trained medical personnel, improved services to remote populations, upgrades of potable water sources, vaccination campaigns, child growth monitoring, and HIV/AIDS testing. The Health Care Improvement Project and the Maternal and Child Survival and Health Program have made significant advances in obstetric and neonatal care through health systems upgrades and hospital-based quality improvement initiatives. USAID has also provided more than 1,000 scholarships for Nicaraguan healthcare workers to study abroad in the United States.[109]

International and National Institutions

NicaSalud, a network federation composed of twenty-eight NGOs and established after Hurricane Mitch in 1998, is designed to help its member NGOs increase the attention they receive from MINSA and other institutions or donors. NicaSalud supports better alignment with MINSA policies, and allows the NGOs to play a stronger role in setting MINSA health priorities.[110] It also strengthens the involved organizations through technical and administrative assistance. NicaSalud recognizes the value of health research, both in ensuring the delivery of evidenced-based medicine and as a means of monitoring its programs.

Many universities in the United States have teamed up with academic institutions in Nicaragua. The University of North Carolina began collaborating with UNAN–León in 2002, focusing on the study of gastrointestinal diseases, renal disease, and rotovirus immunization.[111] Researchers from Duke and Johns Hopkins Universities also collaborate with UNAN–León to study febrile diseases.[112] Other collaborators with UNAN–León include Umea University, Sweden; Yale University; Universidad Autónoma de Barcelona, Spain; and the University of California–Davis, which has recently installed a state-of-the-art telemedicine center in León.[113] The University of Massachusetts has partnered with UNAN–León to improve emergency medical services (GEMINI), and there is ongoing cooperative work in other fields including otolaryngology and orthopedics.[114] UNAN–Managua and other medical institutions also have relationships with foreign academic partners.

Dartmouth Cross Cultural Education and Service Program

Dartmouth College, located in Hanover, New Hampshire, founded a Cross Cultural Education and Service Program–Nicaragua (CCESP) in 2001 under the auspices of the college's William Jewett Tucker Foundation.[115] The Tucker Foundation seeks to cultivate conscience and heart in students to complement intellectual attainment as part of a true liberal arts education. Community service is a major feature of student life at Dartmouth, where more than 60 percent of undergraduates participate in a community service program. The goals of the CCESP program are to serve targeted community health and development needs in Siuna, and to foster transformative change in the participants. Through both the pre-trip seminars and intensive in-country experiential learning, CCESP strives to prepare students to act as ethical leaders who think critically and commit themselves to service, cross-cultural exchange, and global learning.

The CCESP group consists of twenty-seven students (twenty-four undergraduate and three medical), medical professionals, and faculty. The team splits into community health and community development groups. The NGO partner is Bridges to Community, which began its work in Nicaragua in 1992. This organization emphasizes the empowerment of communities and not just the advancement of individuals. Service projects are identified by in-country Bridges staff, and are given shape by local community leaders (92 percent of those served earn less than $2 US per day). Projects are ongoing throughout the year, and include building homes and water systems, economic development, and education. Serving multiple communities in five regions of Nicaragua, Bridges expanded its work into the Dominican Republic in 2012. Bridges provides a crucial liaison to the CCESP program to ensure real community collaboration as well as efficient logistical and translator support.

Bridges engages and bolsters community leadership, solicits a diagnostic report from the community, and provides resources and support to accomplish the projects. All families are required to pay a nominal contribution, usually 15 percent of the material costs. The family later pays a portion of the project cost back into a community fund as a non-interest loan. These funds are then reinvested by those communities for future projects, creating a vehicle for long-term sustainability.

CCESP is co-led by student leaders and faculty. The cultivation of leadership skills is an important objective of this program. The annual two-week trip takes place between semesters in December, but preparations begin during the fall with a series of ten weekly two-hour seminars. To achieve the specific learning objectives, student leaders design the curriculum. This educational component is vital to the program's success in that it requires students to learn about Nicaragua before they travel there, and it also familiarizes students with the ethical dilemmas and cross-cultural issues that can result from service work. Everyone has required reading and there is skill training for the medical team. Structured reflection is emphasized through individual journal writing and group discussions.

The community health team works in a rural health post in close collaboration with Nicaraguan community health nurses and a physician, if one is present at that site. Patients travel to clinic by foot or horseback from either local or distant communities. Undergraduate students observe medical students and faculty in clinic.

The health team provides public health seminars for groups of health promoters and midwives, as well as community education programs on topics such as HIV prevention. One of the risks of short-term brigades is the risk of making a diagnosis or referral that can overwhelm the local health infrastructure. The Dartmouth team works closely with the Bridges staff and the community health nurse to help manage patients who need ongoing care after the team leaves.

The community development team collaborates with Bridges staff and local families to construct fuel-efficient cookstoves that ventilate outdoors, build gravity-fed water systems, and contribute to sustainable agricultural practices. Each year, students from the University of the Autonomous Regions of the Caribbean Coast of Nicaragua (URACCAN) work side by side with Dartmouth students on these projects, and close bonds are formed. In 2007, six URACCAN students and one professor came to Dartmouth for a two-week exchange, furthering the concept of bidirectional learning.

The Dartmouth students who visit the Siuna region are profoundly affected by witnessing poverty firsthand. The team sleeps under mosquito nets on bunk beds in rustic dwellings without electricity or plumbing. *Intercambio,* or cross-cultural exchange, is emphasized through nightly reflection sessions in which both Nicaraguans and Dartmouth students share hopes and lessons learned. Informal learning occurs by reading books with children, playing soccer and baseball, and by singing and dancing together.

After they return to campus, the students are required to write a reflection paper to analyze their experiences in Nicaragua, and to participate in a post-trip debriefing session. Often, students report that they experience compassion in the real sense—experiential compassion. They think more critically about the challenges to development, as well as how to act as ethical leaders in the global community. Many students report that the CCESP experience even leads them to rethink their academic goals and their career paths.

How Bridges to Community Fosters Change
KENIA RAMIREZ, Country Director for Bridges to Community

I am originally from Siuna, and I have been working for Bridges to Community for nine years. Bridges is a Nicaragua-based nonprofit organization focused on service learning in the context of sustainable community development. Bridges hosts over 800 volunteers from the United States and Canada each year, who come to learn, share, and experience life in Nicaragua.

When I began to work with Bridges to Community it was for two important reasons. When I asked the Bridges staff what type of projects we'd be working on in Siuna, they said that, "we needed to discover how we could be a support in Siuna." In this moment I immediately realized that Bridges was a different type of NGO. I was used to NGOs that had pre-established projects that are then offered to communities instead of NGOs that listen to community needs—something I feel is very important and necessary in ensuring sustainable change. The second reason I decided to work for Bridges was that I was told we were going to work with groups from the United States committed to working on projects, but more important, groups who would work in Nicaragua to learn about Nicaragua, the country, her people and communities. Bridges is not only focused on local change—but global change—connecting communities and strengthening communities from different countries to work toward and to ensure a more just world.

Working with Bridges has given me the privilege to learn and be empowered. I have witnessed changes in our communities when opportunities are given to people. When we started working in the community of Santa Rosa, only the men would participate in the projects, and the children could only attend school through third grade because there were insufficient teachers and teacher training. Then, with the support that Bridges offered in the area of education, more and more went to fifth grade and now some of them even go on to college.

There are many positive things for students who are hosted by families in Nicaragua. They get to experience life in Nicaragua firsthand, which is not the same as reading about poverty in a book. They learn that in Nicaragua, people are organized. We have health leaders, midwives, and community leaders who plan activities, working hard with the few resources they have and eager to take advantages of any opportunities to learn and develop their communities. Most of the time groups come to Nicaragua with the mentality that they are coming to help. For me, groups come to Nicaragua to learn, experience, share, and especially to support the work that members of communities are already doing with the few resources they have.

Specialty Care and Education—Mayflower Medical Outreach

In 1998, a volunteer mission team from Mayflower Congregational Church in Oklahoma City traveled to Nicaragua to provide general medical care as well as nonsurgical otolaryngology, ophthalmology, and gynecology care to multiple Nicaraguan communities. Initial contact with patients in Jinotega revealed that hearing loss and otolaryngology diseases were fairly common and underserved by the existing healthcare system. Mayflower Medical Outreach (MMO) was founded to address these specific health needs.[116] Collaborative efforts and funding by MMO has led to a full-service clinic for otolaryngology and audiology at La Victoria Mota Hospital in Jinotega that is staffed by a Nicaraguan otolaryngologist. Funding for this position was gradually transitioned from MMO to MINSA. An audiology technician and nurse continue to be funded by MMO. The first MMO surgical brigade to the La Victoria Mota Hospital took place in 2000. Historically, there had been virtually no training in ear surgery in Nicaragua, and the basic equipment required to do this type of surgery was nonexistent. MMO has sponsored roughly fifty outreach trips to this clinical site, where visiting physicians, nurses, and audiologists have joined with Nicaraguan providers to perform hundreds of surgeries and provide more than 500 hearing aids to Nicaraguans from all over the country. The volunteers for these trips come from throughout the United States and Canada, and include lay personnel and medical providers from a variety of religious backgrounds. From the very beginning, MMO has strived to incorporate the training and equipping of Nicaraguan physicians and allied health providers. MMO's primary focus has been on otology, audiology, and deaf education.

In 2005, providers with MMO completed a detailed study of the prevalence and causes of childhood hearing loss in this remote area of Nicaragua, the Jinotega region.[117] This study surveyed children in rural schools with no known history of hearing loss, and performed a detailed analysis of ninety-eight patients with severe hearing loss in childhood, to try to determine the underlying causes and risk factors. Approximately 18 percent of the children failed hearing screening exams. Both familial hearing loss and infections were relatively common. The more detailed study of children with severe to profound hearing loss discovered that risk factors for hearing loss were common, and that many children had multiple risk factors. Among the identified risk factors were familial hearing loss, exposure to medications that cause hearing loss, meningitis, perinatal distress, and maternal infections. Ongoing research projects include an analysis of the hearing loss effects of heavy metal toxins (for example, mercury, lead, and arsenic) and an assessment of the genetic and socioeconomic factors associated with childhood hearing loss.

A disturbing finding of this study was that approximately two-thirds of deaf children in the Jinotega region were receiving no educational services for their severe to profound hearing loss. The most common reason for this was the long distance of the children from services. It became clear that we were not able to address the needs of these children with surgery, traditional hearing aids, or the existing educational system. To address this need, MMO built the Mayflower Alberque as a residential facility for deaf children to attend a special education school during the week, and to receive after-school services. Twenty-five children live at this center and learn Nicaraguan Sign Language. This project also includes an on-site bakery and Internet café that serves as a vocational program for older students and as a source of revenue to support the residential home. To establish and maintain this program, MMO has developed close working relationships with the Casa Materna Foundation, which provides local program management; Los Pipitos, a Nicaraguan NGO that provides support to families of disabled children; Escuela Max Sengui, the special education school in Jinotega; and the local chapter of the Association of the Deaf in Nicaragua (ASNIC).

Parallel to the work in Jinotega, MMO has supported the education and training of Nicaraguan otolaryngology doctors and audiologists. MMO has helped to established otology services at Lenin Fonseca Hospital in Managua through the donation of key equipment and the training of physicians, including the mentoring of four Nicaraguan otolaryngologists at academic institutions in the United States. MMO continues to provide consult and surgical support to the Managua clinic, and has also established basic audiology services at Lenin Fonseca Hospital. As of this writing, MMO is working with the local universities to establish a certificate of training for audiometry. Audiology services are coordinated by a US-trained Nicaraguan audiologist, and all hearing aid molds are manufactured in-country. Discounted hearing aids are obtained through an international hearing aid purchasing consortium that is also managed by MMO.

Because of its close working relationship with Casa Materna Foundation, MMO also provides some gynecology support in Jinotega. Casa Materna's primary function is to provide housing in town for women with high-risk pregnancies and to support women's health programs. Some interesting concepts relating to Casa Materna include a pilot project that was completed to assess the feasibility of a "see-and-treat" screening program for cervical cancer, in contrast to the way cervical cancer screening is performed in the United States (with a Papanicolaou, or Pap, smear). This process involves a pathologist who reads the slides and a return visit for the patient. The see-and-treat method uses a solution of acetic acid (vinegar) to paint the cervix, which is then directly examined for areas that are suspicious for cancer. Suspicious lesions are removed with a hot wire cautery loop in the same setting, thus eliminating the need for pathology or a follow-up visit. In a pilot study comparing traditional Pap smear results to see-and-treat specimens in 120 patients, cervical dysplasia and inflammation were common, and no lesions were missed with the see-and-treat method. Limitations to implementing this methodology on a larger scale include the costs of the cautery equipment and training of providers, the reluctance of some providers to perform "invasive" procedures in the clinic, and the expectation of many women that a Pap smear pathology report is provided after their visit.

Big Inspiration from a Small Boy

KAREN MOJICA ALVAREZ MD, Chief of Department of Otolaryngology at Hospital Central Managua, and Nicaraguan Medical Director of Mayflower Medical Outreach

In 2002, during my first year of residency in ENT, I met a three-year-old boy. His mother told the story of how they had tried so hard to get pregnant. During her pregnancy she was healthy and so happy for the arrival of her first child. The child was healthy and grew without illness until he was nine months old, when he got sick with a high fever. After a few weeks, his parents worried because the child stopped talking and did not pay attention to sounds; their beautiful child was deaf. There began their fight. They struggled with worry and despair for over two years, until they met the doctors of MMO. I had the opportunity to participate in this boy's care, the first cochlear implant surgery in Nicaragua. This surgery brought an opportunity for this child to have a normal life without disability. MMO brought hope to this family and made the great difference in this child's life, from silence to a life full of sounds. Nine years after surgery, he speaks normally and attends a regular school. His radically changed life was, and continues to be an inspiration for me.

I first participated with the MMO team when I was a resident of otolaryngology. In 2005 MMO provided an opportunity to continue my education at the University of Oklahoma with additional training in surgery of the ear. MMO has also provided some supplies for me to evaluate patients, but my hospital does not have the necessary equipment to perform ear surgery. Even if we have training out of the country, if we don't have the money to buy the equipment, then we can't perform the surgeries we have learned. Overall, my experience has been very fruitful. Each day I try to provide medical care with high standards of quality and scientific knowledge gained through this experience.

Although Nicaraguan physicians are confronted with certain disadvantages, their willingness to serve is strong. The organizational changes of the government have made the implementation of projects to be carried out slow in some cases. However, this has not been so negative, and by continuing to work we will continue to provide better service each year.

My experience through MMO has been very important and beneficial, both to me professionally and to my people because of the healthcare we could provide. We expect to continue this laudable work and to provide better services to the poorest of my country. No matter the differences and distance between our countries, we have a bridge full of hope and the heart to help our people.

Guiding Principles of Humanitarian Surgical Service

Many of the conditions responsible for the health burden in Nicaragua and other developing countries require surgical management. As we already have seen, many of the common causes of morbidity and mortality in Nicaragua, such as trauma and malignancies, often require surgical treatment. Chronic respiratory diseases, and especially otitis media and its sequelae, may also require surgical management.

Several underlying principles of humanitarian service are particularly applicable to surgical service. By its very nature, surgery has the potential to permanently alter a patient's health through a single encounter. Even surgical missions that involve a single visit to an impoverished area may benefit patients who would otherwise not have access to surgical care. This is certainly true in Nicaragua, where there is a rural primary care network but limited access to specialists and surgical care. Such vertical or so-called parachute missions can be a tremendous resource, provided that patients are appropriately counseled, selected, and cared for after surgery. In their article on the role of surgery in global health, Paul Farmer and Jim Kim urge surgeons not to abandon the traditional vertical mission format, but they argue that these efforts can be even more effective when integrated with other strategies for building sustainable healthcare.[118]

Farmer and Kim offer some suggestions on the best way to accomplish this goal—through a careful assessment of public health in the regions served in, as well as through investment in infrastructure and building services within the public sector.[119] Surgeons must consider very carefully the needs and resources of the community. All too often, visiting physicians want to provide the specific interventions or treatments that they are most comfortable with, regardless of whether there is a need or a capacity to support this care. For example, in the United States, many deaf children might be treated with cochlear implant surgery. Although cochlear implants are quite successful in allowing deaf children to communicate orally, they are very expensive and require many hours of rehabilitation over many years to develop these language skills. Even if the implant devices were supplied free of charge, these rehabilitative resources are not available to families in Jinotega. Based on these realities, MMO has chosen to support programs that provide sign language–based education to deaf children in Jinotega. In contrast, children in Managua who have access to the rehabilitation services are offered cochlear implants as an option.

There is often a disparity between the surgical needs in developing countries and the skills of visiting surgeons. One example of this is the use of endoscopes and laparoscopes. These instruments reduce the morbidity and pain of modern surgery, and many surgeons are trained primarily in these techniques. This is especially true for younger surgeons in the United States, who may have limited exposure to more basic, open techniques. Surgeons in developing countries are often quite interested in acquiring these skills, yet the necessary equipment is often not available and, if available, is too expensive to maintain. Thus, visiting surgeons may need to move outside their comfort zone and work with local providers to optimize basic techniques that are best suited to the resources available.

The greatest potential to build sustainable surgical programs comes from the training of local providers. The experience of the MMO program is that this must occur at multiple levels. Nicaraguan physicians are involved with every surgery during MMO surgical trips. The first priority is to train local resident educators so that they may pass on these skills to their residents. In the beginning, the visiting surgeon may need to simultaneously train the residents and the faculty. A good way to jump-start faculty training is through observational rotations in US academic programs. There, the young faculty members can observe multiple surgical techniques and study the surgical anatomy in more detail. The American Academy of Otolaryngology–Head and Neck Surgery Foundation (AAO–HNSF) began an International Visiting Scholarship Grant program in 2007 to help provide this type of training experience to young otolaryngology faculty from all over the world. To make the most of this observational experience, the surgeon-in-training must have hands-on training under the direct supervision of an experienced surgeon in his or her home country. Even with two to three surgical visiting trips each year, this can be difficult. Because of the long gaps between these training opportunities, it may take years for a young surgeon to master the necessary skills.

Farmer and Kim also recommend that surgeons integrate healthcare into social projects, and they challenge surgeons to think about the broader public health issues involved in the diseases they treat.[120] From the outset, the surgeons of MMO recognized that much of the hearing loss they encountered could not be treated with surgery alone. Audiology support and educational expertise were then developed to address these needs. Similarly, the failure to provide rural deaf children with special educational services was addressed by constructing a residential center for these children. Finally, if the broader health issues related to a disease are not readily apparent, surgeons may be uniquely equipped to research the underlying etiologies. Understanding the etiology of a disease is the first and most critical step to prevention. The research studies of MMO on the genetic, socioeconomic, and toxic causes of hearing loss are good examples of this strategy.

Seven Sins of Humanitarian Medicine

In their article in the *World Journal of Surgery*, David Welling and colleagues point out these same principles of humanitarian medicine from a slightly different perspective. Rather than give surgeons recommendations for establishing a successful program, they offer a list of things to avoid, or as they call them, the "deadly sins" of humanitarian medicine. Although these principles are good advice for any medical team, they have particular significance for surgeons. According to the authors, these are the seven sins of humanitarian medicine:

1. *Leaving a mess behind.* Just as surgery offers an opportunity to alter a patient's health through a single encounter, it also has the potential to create significant morbidity that can not only harm the patient, but permanently derail the program. In the first MMO surgical trip to La Victoria Mota Hospital, the team arrived to find the hospital director suddenly much less cooperative. We later found out that a team of well-meaning and well-trained cleft palate surgeons had visited the week before, and 80 percent of their surgical wounds had opened after the team had left. Fortunately, we were able to help manage these complications and restore the faith of the administration in MMO.

2. *Failing to match technology to local needs and abilities.* One of the hardest things for a surgeon to do is to walk away from a patient in need. Nevertheless, every effort should be made to avoid performing surgeries that are either beyond the visiting surgeon's expertise or beyond the capabilities of the local providers and systems. Questions such as these must be addressed: Am I capable of performing this technique in this setting? Is an intensive care unit needed? What about blood transfusion if there is significant blood loss?

3. *Failing of NGOs to cooperate and help each other.* Often, organizations are too steeped in a particular philosophy to collaborate with other partners, both within the country and from abroad. An example of this in the work of MMO is the conflict between the philosophies of oral deaf education and sign language education. These differences can present roadblocks to much-needed collaboration, with the needs of deaf children being lost in the debate.

4. *Failing to have a follow-up plan.* It's critical that surgical patients have providers in-country that are trained in postoperative care, including the management of complications. The biggest failure of the cleft palate team just mentioned was not the surgical complications per se, but the lack of a local provider who could manage these complications after the team had left.

5. *Allowing politics, training, or other distracting goals to trump service, while representing the mission as "service."* Foreign volunteers sometimes bring with them personal attitudes that may stem from preconceived notions about what is needed that are based on the volunteers' needs

or religious agendas. Donations or resources may be conditional, or may be directed to specific areas for reasons other than the recipient's need. There is sometimes a delicate balance between maintaining a cooperative relationship with local entities and allowing the program to become a political instrument.

6. *Going where we are not wanted, or needed, and/or being poor guests.* Many Nicaraguans are polite and don't tell foreigners that they are upset or that their needs are not being met. This is particularly true if they fear that offending visitors may result in care being withdrawn. It's critical to seek out local partners who are not only capable, but confident enough to be honest with volunteers.

7. *Doing the right thing for the wrong reason.* There are lots of wrong reasons for volunteering. Some common examples might be to gain personal acclaim, to enjoy an exotic vacation, or to fulfill the desire to augment one's training with a large volume of cases in a short amount of time. When contemplating volunteering on a medical trip, ask yourself about your motivations, and try to make sure these align with the goals of the mission.[121]

Planning Global Health Work in Nicaragua

Because of the sheer volume of foreign healthcare volunteers working in Nicaragua, MINSA has specific regulations to manage these visits to ensure that healthcare volunteers are appropriately credentialed, local providers are informed of their plans, and medications do not end up being sold on the black market. Brigades must identify where they intend to work, and if they plan to work in a public clinic or hospital, they must supply a letter of invitation from that entity. All medical providers are required to supply notarized copies of their school diplomas, current licenses, curriculum vitae, and specialty certifications, if appropriate. Medications must be thoroughly indexed, including dose, quantity, cost, and expiration date. Medications that are within six months of their expiration date are not allowed into the country, and some medications are specifically prohibited. Community pharmacies are also available in Nicaragua that sell quality, low-cost generic meds to visiting teams with MINSA authorization. Donated equipment and supplies must be documented, including serial and model numbers. Equipment that will be used by the team during the visit ("temporary internment"), but not donated, must also be documented.

These documents should be presented to the MINSA Oficina de Regulación Sanitaria at least one month before the group's arrival; it's best to have a local partner who is able to hand-carry these documents to the ministry and respond to any concerns. Large groups are generally met at the airport by a MINSA representative to ensure that papers are in order and to assist with passage through customs. Items donated to MINSA hospitals are carefully inventoried by hospital administrators and may not be redistributed by the NGO once they are inventoried by the hospital.

Conclusion

Global health work in Nicaragua can be extremely rewarding. Nicaraguans are a proud and creative people with a rich cultural heritage who have persevered in spite of tremendous adversity. Our Nicaraguan colleagues are eager to work with partners from the United States and elsewhere to improve their capacity and training. In the words of one of our Nicaraguan colleagues, "Our friends from the United States provide one hand to help and we provide the other. The two hands working together do more than either can do alone." His words prove that all Nicaraguans are poets at heart.

Notes

1 Elizabeth Dore, *Myths of Modernity Peonage and Patriarchy in Nicaragua* (Durham, NC: Duke University Press, 2006), 34.
2 Walker and Wade, *Nicaragua*, 9.
3 Ibid., 10.
4 Ibid., 11.
5 Ibid.; and Karl Bermann, *Under the Big Stick: Nicaragua and the United States Since 1848* (Boston: South End Press, 1986), 15.
6 Walker and Wade, *Nicaragua*, 11.
7 Bermann, *Under the Big Stick*, 55.
8 Ibid., 64.
9 Ibid., 62–70.
10 John A. Booth, *The End and the Beginning: The Nicaraguan Revolution*, 2nd ed., Westview Special Studies on Latin America and the Caribbean (Boulder, CO: Westview Press, 1985).
11 Bermann, *Under the Big Stick*, 103.
12 Walker and Wade, *Nicaragua*, 89.
13 Ibid., 89–90.
14 Dore, *Myths of Modernity Peonage and Patriarchy in Nicaragua*, 118–119.
15 Ibid., 71–72.
16 Michael Gismondi and Jeremy Mouat, "Merchants, Mining and Concessions on Nicaragua's Mosquito Coast: Reassessing the American Presence, 1893–1912," *Journal of Latin American Studies* 34 (2002):864.
17 Stephen Kinzer, *Overthrow: America's Century of Regime Change from Hawaii to Iraq* (New York: Times Books, 2006), 70.
18 Gismondi and Mouat, "Merchants, Mining and Concessions on Nicaragua's Mosquito Coast," 869–871.

19 Ibid., 874.

20 Scott Nearing and Joseph Freeman, *Dollar Diplomacy: A Study in American Imperialism* (New York: B. W. Huebsch and Viking Press, 1925), 162–165.

21 Walker and Wade, *Nicaragua*, 22–25.

22 Booth, *The End and the Beginning*, 47–48.

23 Walker and Wade, *Nicaragua*, 22.

24 Booth, *The End and the Beginning*, 52.

25 Walker and Wade, *Nicaragua*, 22, 26.

26 Ibid., 25–30.

27 Booth, *The End and the Beginning*, 55.

28 Ibid.

29 Ibid., 56.

30 Ibid., 61.

31 Ibid.

32 Stephen C. Schlesinger and Stephen Kinzer, *Bitter Fruit: The Story of the American Coup in Guatemala*, 4th rev. ed., David Rockefeller Center Series on Latin American Studies, Harvard University (Cambridge, MA: Harvard University, David Rockefeller Center for Latin American Studies, 2005), 114.

33 Booth, *The End and the Beginning*, 60.

34 Walker and Wade. *Nicaragua*, 29, 30, 93.

35 Bermann, *Under the Big Stick*, 257–258.

36 Ibid., 253.

37 Ibid.

38 Walker and Wade, *Nicaragua*, 31–32.

39 Bermann, *Under the Big Stick*, 259.

40 Walker and Wade, *Nicaragua*, 33.

41 Booth, *The End and the Beginning*, 159–160.

42 Ibid., 160–161.

43 Ibid., 179–182.

44 Walker and Wade, *Nicaragua*, 43–44.

45 Ibid., 44–45.

46 Tani Adams, "Life Giving, Life Threatening: Gold Mining in Atlantic Nicaragua Mine Work in Siuna and the Response to Nationalization by the Sandinista Regime" (MA dissertation, Department of Anthropology, University of Chicago, 1981). Walker and Wade, *Nicaragua*, 45, 97–99.

47 Walker and Wade, *Nicaragua*, 46–47.

48 Richard Garfield and Glen Williams. *Health and Revolution: The Nicaraguan Experience* (Oxford: Oxfam, 1989), 25–29.

49 Ibid., 4.

50 Ibid., 25–32.

51 Emory M. Petrack, "Healthcare in Nicaragua: A Social and Historical Perspective," *New York State Journal of Medicine* 84.10 (Oct. 1984):523–525.

52 Garfield and Williams, *Health and Revolution*, 49–62.

53 Walker and Wade, *Nicaragua*, 50–52.

54 Charles R. Hale, *Resistance and Contradiction: Miskitu Indians and the Nicaraguan*

State, 1894–1987 (Stanford, CA: Stanford University Press, 1994), 29, 99; and Walker and Wade, *Nicaragua*, 49.

55 Ibid., 52, 53, 56.

56 Ricardo Guerrero, "Maquilas con más de 100,000 empleados," *El Nuevo Diario* (Mar. 16, 2012), available from www.elnuevodiario.com.ni.

57 Central Intelligence Agency, *The World Factbook* (Washington: CIA, 2011).

58 Hazel Plunkett, *Nicaragua in Focus: A Guide to the People, Politics and Culture* (New York: Interlink Books, 1999), 61.

59 Walker and Wade, *Nicaragua*, 2.

60 Oakland Ross, "A City of 2 Million Without a Map" (Apr. 21, 2002), *World Press Review* 49.7 (July 2002).

61 CIA, *The World Factbook* (2011).

62 Jack Reynolds and Annette Bongiovanni. "Nicaragua Health Program Evaluation," USAID Global Health Technical Assistance Project Report No. 08-001-063 (USAID, 2008), iii.

63 World Health Organization, "Country Page, Nicaragua" in WHO *Global InfoBase: Data for Saving Lives* (2010), available from https://apps.who.int.

64 National Institute of Information Development, "Encuesta Nicaragüense de Demografía y Salud 2006/07" (Nicaraguan Demographic and Health), accessed Oct. 11, 2010, available from http://www.inide.gob.ni.

65 Pan American Health Organization, "CARMEN Country Profiles: Nicaragua," available from www.paho.org, accessed Oct. 11, 2011

66 J. Muiser, R. Sáenz Mdel, and J. L. Bermúdez, "Sistema de salud de Nicaragua" (The Health System of Nicaragua), *Salúd Publica de México* 53 Suppl 2 (2011):s233–s242.

67 WHO, "Global Health Observatory Repository: Nicaragua Country Statistics," available from http://apps.who.int/ghodata, accessed Jan. 23, 2012.

68 CIA, *The World Factbook* (2011).

69 UN Statistics Division, Millennium Development Goals Indicators, available from http://mdgs.un.org, updated July 2, 2012, accessed Nov. 23, 2012.

70 CIA, *The World Factbook* (2011).

71 Walker and Wade, *Nicaragua*, 2.

72 Plunkett, *Nicaragua in Focus*, 43.

73 Juan B. Arrien, "Literacy in Nicaragua," Education for All Global Monitoring Report 2006, *Literacy for Life*, 3–6.

74 United Nations Educational, Scientific and Cultural Organization Institute for Statistics, 2010.

75 World Bank, "World Development Indicators (WDI)" database, available from http://data.worldbank.org.

76 Dirk van den Boom, Klaus-Peter Jacoby, and Stefan Silvestrini, Evaluation of Higher Education Programs in Nicaragua and South-East Europe 2005–2009 Final Report, p.19, from the Prepared Center for Evaluation, Austrian Development Agency, July 10, 2010, http://www.oecd.org, accessed Nov. 25, 2012; and Philip G. Altbach, Liz Reisberg, and Laura Rumbley, "Trends in Global Higher Education: Tracking an Academic Revolution, a report prepared for the UNESCO 2009 World Conference on Higher Education, p. 196, available at http://unesco.org, accessed Nov. 25, 2012.

77 Muiser et al., "Sistema de salud de Nicaragua."

78 Diego Angel-Urdinola, Rafael Cortez, and Kimie Tanabe, "Equity, Access to Health Care Services and Expenditures on Health in Nicaragua," in *HNP Discussion Papers* (World Bank, 2008).

79 Muiser et al., "Sistema de salud de Nicaragua."

80 Ibid.

81 PAHO, "Health System Profile Nicaragua: Monitoring and Analyzing Health Systems Change," 3rd ed. (2008), http://new.paho.org/PAHO-USAID, accessed Nov. 25, 2012.

82 Muiser et al., "Sistema de salud de Nicaragua."

83 Inke Mathauer, Eleonora Cavagnero, Gabriel Vivas, and Guy Carrin, "Health Financing Challenges and the Role of Institutional Design and Organizational Practice for Health Financing Performance in Nicaragua," discussion paper no. 2 (Geneva: World Health Organization, 2010), 4, 5, 12.

84 Proyecto Informe de Desarrollo Humano (Nicaragua), *El desarrollo humano en Nicaragua: Equidad para superar la vulnerabilidad*, 1st ed. (Managua: Programa de las Naciones Unidas para el Desarrollo, 2000).

85 "E. Todos con VOZ en Nicaragua," Ministry de Salud Sept. 13, 2011, http://www.minsa.gob.ni, accessed Nov. 24, 2012.

86 Nadia Ali and Cayce Hill, "The Global Health Research Agenda: A Case Study Approach," New York University Robert F. Wagner Graduate School of Public Service: Advanced Projects in Health Policy (2005), 41.

87 Ernesto Medina and Edumndo Torres, "Doing Research in Nicaragua" (submitted for publication in *Annual Report*, International Foundation for Science).

88 Centro de Investigación en Salud, Trabajo y Ambiente (CISTA), www.unanleon.edu.ni.

89 Centro de Investigción y Estudios en Salud (CIES), www.cies.edu.ni.

90 WHO, "Country Page, Nicaragua."

91 PAHO, "Health System Profile Nicaragua," 13–16.

92 Ibid., 13.

93 Ministry of Health, "Statistical Compendium 2006–2007," available from www.minsa.gob.ni, accessed Nov. 10, 2011.

94 Muiser et al., "Sistema de salud de Nicaragua."

95 PAHO, "Health System Profile Nicaragua," 13.

96 James E. Saunders, Sharon Vaz, John H. Greinwald, James Lai, Leonor Morin, and Karen Mojica, "Prevalence and Etiology of Hearing Loss in Rural Nicaraguan Children," *Laryngoscope* 117.3 (Mar. 2007):387–398.

97 Tania Barham, Logan Brenzel, and John A. Maluccio, "Beyond 80%: Are There New Ways of Increasing Vaccination Coverage? Evaluation of CCT Programs in Mexico and Nicaragua" in *HNP Discussion Papers* (World Bank, 2007).

98 PAHO, "Health System Profile Nicaragua," 13.

99 Ibid.

100 L. Blandón, L. Carballo Palma, D. Wulf, L. Remez, E. Prada, and J. Drescher, "Early Childbearing in Nicaragua: A Continuing Challenge," *Issues Brief* (Guttmacher Institute) 3 (Sep. 2006):1–24.

101 PAHO, "Health System Profile Nicaragua," 14.

102 Marianela Corriols, Jesus Marin, Jacqueline Berroteran, Luz Marina Lozano, and Ingvar Lundberg, "Incidence of Acute Pesticide Poisonings in Nicaragua: A Public Health Concern," *Occupational and Environmental Medicine* 66 (2009): 205–210; and Marianela Corriols and Aurora Aragón, "Child Labor and Acute Pesticide Poisonings in Nicaragua: Failure to Comply with Children's Rights," *Internation Journal of Occupational and Environmental Health* 16 (2010): 193–200.

103 Jeffrey K. McCrary, Mark Castro, and Kenneth R. McKaye, "Mercury in Fish from Two Nicaraguan Lakes: A Recommendation for Increased Monitoring of Fish for International Commerce," *Environmental Pollution* 141.3 (2006):513–518.

104 Joel B. Wickre, C. L. Folt, S. Sturup, and M. R. Karagas, "Environmental Exposure and Fingernail Analysis of Arsenic and Mercury in Children and Adults in a Nicaraguan Gold Mining Community," *Archives of Environmental Health* 59.8 (2004):400–409.

105 WHO/UNICEF Joint Monitoring Program (JMP) for Water Supply and Sanitation, www.wssinfo.org.

106 Magda Sequeira, Henry Espinoza, Juan Jose Amador, Gonzalo Domingo, Margarita Quintanilla, and Tala de los Santos, "Malaria in Nicaragua: A Review of Control Status, Trends, and Needs" (Seattle, WA: PATH, 2010).

107 GAVI Alliance "Country Hub: Nicaragua," available from www.gavialliance.org.

108 K. M. Plamondon, L. Hanson, R. Labonté, and S. Abonyi, "The Global Fund and Tuberculosis in Nicaragua: Building Sustainable Capacity?" *Canadian Journal of Public Health* 99.4 (Jul./Aug. 2008):355–358.

109 USAID in Nicaragua, http://nicaragua.usaid.gov; and Reynolds and Bongiovanni, "Nicaragua Health Program Evaluation."

110 Fernando Campos and Joseph Valadez, "The NicaSalud Network: Restoring Community Health Activities in Nicaragua after Hurricane Mitch: A Final Evaluation (December 1999–October 2001)" (Washington: NGO Networks for Health, 2002); and Federación Red NicaSalud, www.nicasalud.org.ni.

111 Collaborative Sahsa Health Initiative, available from www.med.unc.edu.

112 Hubert-Yeargan Center for Global Health, available from www.med.unc.edu.

113 Personal communication.

114 Foreign Project Database, University of Massachusetts Medical School, available from www.umassmed.edu.

115 Dartmouth Cross Cultural Education and Service Program (CCESP), available from www.dartmouth.edu, and Bridges to Community, www.bridgestocommunity.org, accessed Aug. 14, 2012.

116 Mayflower Medical Outreach, http://mmonicaragua.org.

117 Saunders et al., "Prevalence and Etiology of Hearing Loss in Rural Nicaraguan Children."

118 Paul E. Farmer and Jim Y. Kim, "Surgery and Global Health: A View from Beyond the OR," *World Journal of Surgery* 32 (2008):533–536.

119 Ibid.

120 Ibid.

121 David R. Welling, James M. Ryan, David G. Burris and Norman M. Rich, "Seven Sins of Humanitarian Medicine," *World Journal of Surgery* 34 (2010):466–470.

Suggested Reading

Belli, Gioconda. *The Country Under My Skin: A Memoir of Love and War*. New York: Anchor, 2003.

Cabezas, Omar. *Fire on the Mountain: The Making of a Sandinista*. New York: Crown Publishers, 1986.

Dix, Paul, photographer, and Pamela Fitzpatrick, ed. *Nicaragua: Surviving the Legacy of U.S. Policy*. Eugene, OR: Just Sharing Press, 2011. Available online at www .nicaraguaphototestimony.org.

Garfield, Richard, and Glen Williams. *Health Care in Nicaragua: Primary Care Under Changing Regimes*. New York: Oxford University Press, 1992.

Kinzer, Stephen. *Blood of Brothers: Life and War in Nicaragua*. Cambridge, MA: Harvard University Press, 2007.

Rushdie, Salman. *The Jaguar Smile: A Nicaraguan Journey*. New York: Picador, 2003.

Walker, Thomas, and Christine Wade. *Nicaragua: Living in the Shadow of the Eagle*. 5th ed. Boulder, CO: Westview Press, 2011.

6 Nicaragua II
Belinda Forbes and Gerardo Gutiérrez

This chapter complements material offered in chapter 5. It focuses on health themes specific to the Caribbean Coast region of Nicaragua, the condition of dental health in the country as a whole, and the role of faith-based organizations in development. The authors have worked for more than twenty years with the Nicaraguan ecumenical nongovernmental health and development agency Acción Médica Cristiana (AMC), which was founded in 1984 by young Nicaraguan health professionals during the Counter-Revolutionary (Contra) War. During that time, the revolutionary government had difficulty establishing health services in the war zones of the Caribbean regions due to ideological differences with the people, who resisted the imposition of Sandinista rule and forced relocations, and, with United States support, largely composed the Contra army. AMC founders followed a call of faith and social conscience to serve the vulnerable populations of the country in a context of war and disaster, and their banner of faith made for easier entry to these regions. Since that time, the organization has carried out community-based primary health and development models at the community level, and has contributed significantly to improving health indicators.

The Caribbean Coast of Nicaragua

The Northern Autonomous Atlantic Region (RAAN) and Southern Autonomous Atlantic Region (RAAS) formed part of the extensive Department of Zelaya until 1987, when they were divided to form the autonomous regions now known as the Caribbean Coast. Though various indigenous groups survive in small numbers throughout Nicaragua, the Caribbean Coast is home to the largest numbers of indigenous and Afro-descendant groups in the country (see Table 6.1).[1] The *costeña* people have a unique cultural, social, and economic history, and differ from the populations in the Pacific and central regions. Large areas of RAAN and RAAS are sparsely populated because of climate and topography that create difficult living conditions; many communities are accessible only by water of the still abundant Coco, Bocay, Maíz, and Indio Rivers.

Brief History

Christopher Columbus landed on the eastern seaboard of Nicaragua on September 12, 1502. The resistance of indigenous tribes prevented Spain from colonizing, which helped to preserve much of the rich cultural heritage to the present. However, in 1630 the English, as well as the Dutch and German Moravians, began to settle the region. The English established trade with the Miskito and Mayangna people, introduced English among the existing Spanish and indigenous languages, and created a protectorate, gifting weapons and "independence" to the Miskitos, who then dominated the region. A second cultural influence was the settlement of African slaves throughout Central America. The United States and England shared the wealth of the region until 1894, when Nicaraguan president José Santos Zelaya reclaimed the territory for the rest of Nicaragua.

Indigenous Populations

Resources and Social Conditions

The Caribbean Coast covers 59,566 square kilometers (see Table 6.2) and makes up approximately 46 percent of Nicaragua.[2] This region contains 35 percent of the country's cattle, 23 percent of its agricultural land, over 80 percent of its forests, 70 percent of its fish production, and 60 percent of its mineral resources. There is significant potential for hydrocarbon exploitation, and the country's 700 kilometers of coastline is located in one of the most renowned tourist areas in the world.

One might assume that natural resources, cultural diversity, and geography would ensure decent living conditions and allow the people to contribute substantively to the social, economic, and political life of Nicaragua as a whole. This has not been the case. The indigenous and African-descendant populations who settled on the banks of large rivers, lagoons, and seacoast areas experienced centuries of exclusion from the benefits of development elsewhere. Moreover, the impoverished mestizo farmers in the central part of the country, similarly caught in a cycle of poverty and marginalization, are now migrating east, attracted by the resources of the region. Between 1995 and 2005, the population in the autonomous regions doubled,[3] imposing new pressure on the land, environment, forests, and basic services. Finally, indiscriminate logging and the devastation caused in recent decades by hurricanes and flooding have dramatically changed the environment of the region.

All the municipalities of RAAN and most municipalities of RAAS live in poverty and extreme poverty,[4] which in turn reflects enduring disparity between the Caribbean and the already deteriorated and deeply impoverished remainder of Nicaragua. In Nicaragua, poverty defined by less than $1 US per day is

Table 6.1 *Population of the Caribbean Coast*

Population Groups	RAAN		RAAS		TOTAL	
	% Total Population	*Number*	*% Total Population*	*Number*	*% Total Population*	*Number*
Mestizos	35.68	63,999	60.0	44,590	42.82	108,589
Indigenous						
Mískito	57.3	102,806	10.0	7,398	43.46	110,204
Mayangnas	3.81	6,835	0.21	157	2.76	6,992
Ramas	0.12	208	1.67	1,239	0.57	1,447
Afro-descendants						
Creoles	0.95	1,711	22.38	16,607	7.22	18,318
Garífunas	0.05	89	1.48	1,095	0.47	1,184
Others	2.08	3,728	4.21	3,127	2.70	6,855
Totals	100	179,376	100	74,213	100	253,589
Total RAAN and RAAS population						432,965

Source: Data consolidated by Acción Médica Cristiana. AMC used population data from INIDE, "Censo 2005," Vol. 1. (Managua: INIDE, 2006), 30. Note that several other sources list higher populations for RAAN and RAAS, with up to a 30 percent variance compared to the 2005 census. The exact numbers of the Caribbean Coast population are not consistent even among organizations working in the region.

20 percent higher among indigenous and Afro-descendant populations compared to Euro-descendants.[5]

The Caribbean Coast has the highest percentages of rural population in the country: 72 percent for RAAN and 63 percent for RAAS (national, 59 percent). The national Human Development Index is 0.699, but the disparities are reflected in the HDIs of the regions: 0.454 for RAAS, and 0.455 for RAAN. Four of the poorest municipalities in the country are found in RAAN.[6]

Several legislative tools provide the legal framework for the protection of the unique attributions of the Caribbean regions and for regional coordination with the central government.[7] Despite this, the human rights of indigenous and Afro-descendant populations have not been fully respected. The Managua-based Nicaraguan government has historically demonstrated territorial, administrative/political, and ethnic exclusion of the Caribbean regions, as reflected in the absence of basic infrastructure, limited recognition of the autonomous governments, and the exclusion of the population from national economic and political agendas. The lack of accurate data about Caribbean Coast populations alone impedes a

Table 6.2 *Features of Autonomous Regions*

	RAAN	RAAS
Regional seat	Puerto Cabezas	Bluefields
Municipalities	Puerto Cabezas, Waspán, Prinzapolka, Rosita, Bonanza, Siuna, Waslala, and Mulukukú. Islands belonging to RAAN: Miskito Keys	Bluefields, Kukra Hill, Laguna de Perlas, Paiwas, Rama, Nueva Guinea, El Tortuguero, Muelle de los Bueyes, Desembocadura de Río Grande, La Cruz de Río Grande. Islands belonging to RAAS: Corn Island, Little Corn Island
Area (sq. km.)	32,159	27,407
Borders	North—Honduras South—RAAS East—Caribbean Ocean West—Jinotega, Matagalpa	North—RAAN South—Río San Juan East—Caribbean Ocean West—Matagalpa, Boaco, Chontales, Río San Juan

Note: The Prinzapolka River is a natural separation of RAAN and RAAS.
Source: INETER, "Mapa Turístico de Nicaragua, Geografía Dinámica de Nicaragua."
Los cayos Roncador and Quita Sueño are in litigation with Colombia.

comprehensive assessment of indigenous peoples, in particular women and children and their needs, and exacerbates the discrimination they experience.

In 2007, in an attempt to improve basic services to the marginalized indigenous sectors, a decree created the special regime zone,[8] separate from RAAN and RAAS, called Alto Wangki-Bocay. This zone encompasses part of the municipality of Waspam and the municipalities of Wiwilí and San José de Bocay in the Department of Jinotega. A multimillion-dollar development plan for all three regions was designed in 2009 to focus on social well-being, authentic autonomy, and institutional capacity building.

Health Policy and the Ministry of Health in Nicaragua

According to their constitution, all Nicaraguans have an equal right to health. It is the state's responsibility to establish the basic conditions for its

Table 6.3 *Social Indicators of the Caribbean Coast*

Indicator (% of population)	RAAN/ RAAS	National
Access to public water supply	18.6	63.1
Access to electricity	54.7	72.6
Access to sanitary services	15.7	26.2
Completed elementary education	37.5	59.4
Unable to cover Family Shopping Basket*	49	34

*The Family Shopping Basket or *Canasta Básica* of Nicaragua is a measure of consumer buying power that contributes to the calculation of minimum wage and to the assessment of poverty lines. The value of the Canasta Básica is the monthly sum needed to purchase fifty-three food, household, and clothing products for a family of two adults and four children. In March 2011, this sum was calculated at $418 US.

Source: UNDP, *Informe sobre Desarrollo Humano: Más allá de la escasez: Poder, pobreza y crisis mundial del agua* (New York: UNDP, 2006).

promotion, protection, recovery, and rehabilitation. The state is also responsible for directing and organizing programs, services, and activities for health, and for promoting popular participation in its defense. Citizens are obliged to comply with sanitary measures as determined by the law.[9]

To comply with this mandate, a General Health Law was passed in 2002, the first legal framework for health in Nicaragua. It defines the Ministry of Health (MINSA) as the body responsible for applying the law and evaluating its implementation.[10] The law also stipulates MINSA as responsible for coordination and supervision of all health activities, to be done impartially, in accordance with the provisions of special laws.

MINSA designs its health policy according to the General Health Law, the National Plan for Development, the National Health Plan 2000–2015, and external guides such as the MDGs. The slogan of the 2008 National Health Plan reads "Health, a right of all, an investment in development!" and states that the fundamental objective for health policy is to "develop a health system that guarantees the right of every citizen to health with equality, through which gender and generational practices will reduce existing inequalities and improve living conditions for the Nicaraguan population and the development of the country."[11] Three strategies are key for the autonomous regions: (1) to

Table 6.4 *Health Indicators of the Miskito Population of the Caribbean Coast*

Indicator (% of population)	RAAN–RAAS	National
Lack of access to prenatal care	29.3%	12.3%
Births in health facility	42.6%	72.3%
Chronic malnutrition in children under age five years	33.7%	19.6%
Population malnourished	12.8%	8.9%
Mortality rate in children under age five years per 1,000 live births	73.4	59.4

Source: PAHO, *Health in the Americas 2007*, *Vol. II*. (Washington: PAHO, 2007), 565.

bring health services to communities in extreme poverty and with difficult access, (2) to strengthen intercultural autonomous health models, and (3) to promote the traditional health system.

In 2008, the revised Model for Community Family Health (MOSAFC) included two health models specific to the autonomous regions: the Integrated Health Care Model for the RAAN (MASIRAAN) and the Integrated Health Care Model for the RAAS (MASIRAAS).

Health Outcomes and Disparities

The autonomous regions have the greatest health disparities in the country, with women particularly impacted by factors of inequality that limit access to health services.[12] In 2005, RAAN reported a maternal mortality rate 2.1 times higher than the national average, and indigenous communities reported higher fertility rates, as well as greater demand for family planning services that goes unmet.

There is a higher incidence of TB and malaria in the Caribbean regions, most commonly in indigenous populations. Access to mental health services is severely limited, with only one psychiatrist for the entire RAAN and RAAS. Estimates for human risk from disasters provoked by natural phenomena (61.6 percent for Miskito and 90 percent for Mayangnas) is much higher than the national average (31.8 percent).[13]

Geographical, linguistic, and cultural differences, lack of information, and economic marginalization are some of the barriers to healthcare delivery for indigenous and Afro-descendant communities. Health services are frequently provided by MINSA staff fulfilling their obligatory social service. These providers lack training specific to healthcare delivery in this geographic and multicultural context. Most are men who do not speak the local languages of the communities. This creates distrust among the people, especially the women, who avoid treatment as a result. In the autonomous regions, nurses and nurse auxiliaries, usually women originating from the region, represent 74 percent of the health workforce.[14] They have a more permanent presence, providing 88 percent of all outpatient visits, and are culturally oriented to the context. But they are the health staff with the least amount of formal training.

In the process of forming MASIRAAN and MASIRAAS, the social determinants of health were identified: a high degree of impoverishment, ethnic-racial discrimination, lack of adequate infrastructure (roads and communications), low rates of formal schooling, the advance of the agricultural frontier with high rates of deforestation and exploitation of natural resources, high levels of water contamination, the high-risk work model of fishing (especially for lobster), and the high rate of migration.

Maria Hamlin Zuniga, a global health worker and activist in Nicaragua with forty years of experience, signals a new factor likely to impact health of the regions: "Unlike the '70s when I worked on the Río Coco, today people are impacted by the drug trafficking and drug use that have become 'essential' for survival in some communities. This has resulted in dramatic changes within a single generation. What this means for the future of the region and its young people remains to be seen."[15]

Why are so many health and social interventions in the region unable to improve this reality? For years, health sector plans have been shaped according to the priorities of financing or implementing institutions, usually to serve a particular population group at the expense of some other, and often favoring one region over another or urban over rural areas. A less vertical restructuring of plans to guarantee health in indigenous rural communities is urgently needed. Global health workers must share knowledge and understanding to influence donors, and advocate strongly against top-down, donor-driven projects that are neither comprehensive nor sustainable, and do little to build local capacity.

Health Beliefs and Practices on the Caribbean Coast

When the Europeans arrived in the sixteenth century they brought more than disease to the Mesoamerican people. They also introduced the Hippocratic-Galenic humoral theory about illness, which they mixed with elements of popular Spanish medicine with its strong Arabic influence. Later, the African slaves contributed their health practices. The result is a traditional medicine system based on ancestral indigenous wisdom overlaid with influences from cultures on other continents. In all the indigenous and Afro-descendant communities of the Caribbean Coast of Nicaragua, traditional medicine has long been used as the most effective form of healthcare, and the health beliefs and practices of each subgroup are worthy of study. This section focuses on the worldview embraced by the Miskito people.

Two energizing and regulating factors guide life in a Miskito community: the unique worldview transmitted from generation to generation, and the harmony between human beings and nature where health of the people is understood within the framework of common historical experiences and a common spiritual vision of the world. This Miskito vision is a tapestry of myths, traditions, norms, and values that originated at the time of Miskut,[16] or the legend of Niki Niki,[17] which tells the creation story of the Wangki or Coco River. The elements of the vision include the river, wind, forests, animals, trees, stones, and good and bad spirits.[18]

The Miskito language has no word for disease, although the English word *sickness* is frequently used, or the phrase *saura takan*, which means "to be in disequilibrium with nature." Such imbalance is seen as harmful to the health of both individuals and community, as it undermines two strong cultural values central to the Miskito concept of health: happiness (understood as the sensation of well-being) and the capacity to work.

Health Providers in the Miskito Traditional Medicine System

Ukuly (prophets, meaning "maker of time and wind") are called to service by a cosmic ray known as the great spirit of space. The *Ukuly*'s mission is to prevent bad spirits from entering the community. This includes external ills, such as plagues on crops, as well as negative spirits that may lurk along the roadways.

Sukias are priest doctors empowered to remove bad spirits. They hold the highest authority in the traditional system, and are usually called to serve through a dream or vision. They are always inducted by another *sukia*. *Sukias* are not found in all Miskito communities, but mainly serve along the Coco River. In the absence of a *sukia*, the *curandero* (healer) or midwife is the next authority in the traditional system.

Urandero (healer, also called *uhura*) can cure diseases of a spiritual origin, but primarily heal physical illness through the use of medicinal plants grown in their own gardens.

Midwives offer special attention to women and children during pregnancy, childbirth, and the postpartum period, performing rituals and massages as well as coaching women during childbirth.

Herbalists cure diseases with medicinal plants, but have no capacity to cure disease of a spirit origin.

Most traditional providers cannot read or write; knowledge is learned and passed on orally.[19]

Health Perceptions of Miskito Communities

As documented in an ethnographic study, the Miskito people attribute both natural and supernatural causes to *saura takan*.[20] A common natural cause of disequilibrium is explained by the contradictory conditions of hot and cold.[21] For example, "It happened because he or she took a cold bath while agitated [overheated]." Other causes include infection, behavior such as laziness or slovenliness, and personal practices, such as frequent childbirth or childbirth in an unsanitary setting. The most common diseases in Miskito communities are identical to those diagnosed in the rest of the country: diarrhea, malaria, kidney problems, scabies, arthritis, and muscular pain.

The supernatural causes of disequilibrium are rooted in animism and magic. The elf, the spirit of the forest, the *liwa mairin* or sirena (mermaid or river spirit), or the *aubia* (forest spirit) can explain the suffering of one person or groups of people. A curse or witchcraft is often blamed for diseases, especially those difficult to diagnose or treat. Traditional diseases include fright, a spell, and *sontín* (possibly from the English word *something*) caused by spirit forces. Older generations of women, particularly midwives, attribute women's illnesses to the *liwa mairin*. An illness of cultural origin, *grisi siknis* (possibly from the English *crazy sickness*), occurs periodically in certain Miskito communities and is manifested by a collective hysteria among the population. It can last for several weeks or months, and involves young people in particular. It is expelled only through rituals performed by a *sukia* and never by a Western doctor.

In addition to animism and magic, religious beliefs influence the Miskito worldview. Often disease is understood as a result of sin, or as a punishment or test from God. The ill person may slide into resignation and accept the ailment in despair as inevitable. The church and its clergy play an important role in perpetuating a vision of an angry or providential God, one who punishes or promotes healing.

The Miskito people possess deep wisdom about basic diseases and the use of medicinal plants to cure them, although these are more widely used among older generations. Women play a fundamental role in the state of their family's health, most often diagnosing illness and deciding where to take a family member for healthcare. Younger indigenous and Afro-descendant generations are now more open to the official, Western-based health system, especially for common diseases such as high blood pressure, malaria, anemia, arthritis, and kidney problems.

In both indigenous and Afro-descendant populations, there is no contradiction in making use of both traditional and Western health systems concurrently, based on understanding the benefits and limitations of each. The people's choices are guided by information, efficacy, and experience, not by fidelity to a particular worldview.

In some Miskito communities, such as Alamikamba in Prinzapolka, traditional medicine remains a sustainable alternative. Difficult geographical access, social and cultural insularity, and extreme poverty limit the access and acceptance of Western medicine. Traditional medicine continues to meet the health needs of the population, and there is great demand for the services offered by traditional practitioners. In 2004, there was one midwife for every twenty women of childbearing age; eighteen trained healers for the total 7,470 inhabitants, equivalent to one healer per 415 people; and at least one herbalist per community. In contrast, the health post had one doctor and one nurse for the entire population. In Alamikamba, the community sees traditional practitioners as the main health providers, attributing to them the power to cure diseases that physicians cannot address.[22]

Health of Miskito Women

Internationally promoted gender equality has advanced the role, rights, and advocacy of women. Unfortunately, the focus on Nicaragua's Caribbean Coast has been limited to reproductive health, especially family planning, as if the principal health problem of women is childbearing. The development of interventions rarely draws on the input and experiences of women, especially indigenous women.

Miskito women are severely socioeconomically disadvantaged in contrast to men in their communities and to women in the nation. In 2004, Alamikamba was the poorest community in the nation. Of its population, 93.7 percent were rural and 77.1 percent lived in extreme poverty. A study showed that the average number of children per woman was 7.2 and that 64 percent of women had lost two or more children. Almost all women were indigenous and worked in the home, and 55 percent were illiterate.[23]

Discrimination and abuse, both physical and psychological, as reported by the Miskito women, is rooted in lack of respect and understanding in relationships. The commonly held perception is that boys are better than girls, "who will always be ordered around"; this is reflected in the pay of midwives, who charge more for their services if the newborn is a male. Domestic violence is accepted as a private family affair, and only when there are life-threatening consequences do authorities or tribal leaders intervene. Research documents the inequality and daily levels of violence to which Miskito women are subjected, their lack of access to both formal and informal education, and the subservient roles assigned to them by the community and their partners. The low self-esteem of Miskito women is the legacy of practices passed on from one generation to the next.

A prerequisite to any health intervention for Miskito women is a general understanding of their beliefs about health and illness, but especially their views about sexual and reproductive health, as well as pregnancy, birth, menstruation, family planning, diseases exclusive to women, and the woman's role in the family.

AMC has actively engaged in studying indigenous populations and applying results to the design and implementation of effective community health strategies, especially for women. Health interventions are aimed at food security, stability in the home, access to health information and family planning methods, and psychological support for women's self-esteem and overcoming domestic violence. All are offered in a context of respect for the deep-seated traditions and beliefs of the participating population. Trained midwives with technical skills in prenatal care and childbirth can identify high-risk pregnancies for referral to safe birthing conditions. Comprehensive healthcare for adolescents raises community awareness about sexually transmitted disease, especially HIV/AIDS prevention. As a result of using this culturally appropriate model in specific communities of RAAN, no maternal deaths were reported for a period of nine years, though maternal mortality in comparable communities has been reported to be three times the national average.[24]

The following case study of Miskito women can serve as an example of the unique history, worldview, wisdom, and health practices of indigenous communities.[25]

Sexual and Reproductive Health Beliefs of Miskito Women

GERARDO GUTIÉRREZ, MD, MPH

In Miskito culture, the perception of health and illness is linked to a sense of well-being (happiness) and capacity to work in the domestic labor and reproductive role assigned to women by society. A happy woman has food for her children and a man to provide security. Men consider a woman healthy if she can "attend to them in everything" and ill when she is "does not want to do anything."

Miskito women have little knowledge about their anatomy, particularly their sexual and reproductive organs, whose function they consider utilitarian and subordinate to the sexual satisfaction of men. Women refer to their reproductive organs as *tasba pis* or "piece of territory"—the place where a seed is planted and the "territory" that a man uses and owns. Contrarily, women value their organs and consider it their social obligation to offer their breasts for a man's pleasure or to breast-feed their children.

The origin of life for Miskito people is associated with bodily liquids: without blood, there is no semen or menstruation, no pregnancy, no breast milk. Older women consider menstruation as a gift from God. Younger generations associate menstruation less enthusiastically. For men, menstruation is a sign that women are healthy and "their bodies are working well."

Traditional Miskito women believe menstruation originates in various parts of the body, or that it is produced by a "bag" or a cup in the uterus that fills to overflowing, and is a trap that opens and closes. They understand absence of menstruation as pregnancy or an imbalance of humors (*resfrío*), often accompanied by fatigue or arthritic pain. For older women it is menopause. Traditional remedies are applied, but younger women seek Western medical care if they stop menstruating.

Miskito women live a juxtaposition of joy over and fear of pregnancy. They believe "the woman has one foot on the ground and one in the coffin; some die, and others come out okay." Family planning methods are available, but condom use is difficult to promote because men consider that it reduces sexual pleasure. A woman has little negotiating power over the sexual use of her body, even for its protection. Because men believe oral contraception gives a woman "license to be unfaithful," women seeking to limit pregnancies are forced to adopt the measure in secret or irregularly.

Misconceptions exist around sexually transmitted diseases, although some men will use a condom to prevent transmission or will seek treatment from the health center when infected. Women may engage in potentially dangerous behaviors like ignoring infection or intentionally passing on the disease, believing that intercourse will delay the advance of their own disease. Some men believe that having sex with a virgin will cure HIV/AIDS.

Miskito communities present high levels of teenage pregnancies because of considerable social pressure, especially on girls, to start sexual activity early.* The belief is "as long as she does not have sex she does not grow, but by trying it, she grows." Such attitudes create risks for young people whose ignorance about their own sexual and reproductive health leads to unwanted pregnancies, low birth weight of newborns,** risk of maternal and infant death from high-risk pregnancies, or induced abortions.***

NOTES

*Nicaragua has the highest number of adolescent births in the region: 109 births for every 1,000 adolescent girls. UNDP, *Regional Human Development Report for Latin America and Caribbean 2010: Acting on the Future: Breaking the Intergenerational Transmission of Inequality* (New York: UNDP, 2010), 69.

** Children born to women under age twenty in Nicaragua have an average of just over 3.2 kg. birth weight compared to 3.35 kg. born to women between ages thirty and thirty-nine. Ibid., 72.

***One-third of maternal deaths in Nicaragua occur in adolescents. (PNUD, "Valoración Común de País, Nicaragua" (Managua: PNUD, 2007), 63.

Organizations Working in the Autonomous Regions

Only a limited number of agencies choose to work in the Caribbean Coast because of the elevated costs for transportation and basic services, and the historic lack of political interest in indigenous and ethnic groups in Nicaragua. Many agencies that do exist are founded and led by indigenous and Afro-descendant groups. The Foundation for the Autonomy and Development of the Atlantic Coast of Nicaragua (FADCANIC) focuses on agriculture, the environment, and education. The Center for Human, Civil and Autonomous Rights (CEDEHCA) defends indigenous rights, contributing to a culture of autonomy and peace. The Association for the Development of the Atlantic Coast (Pana Pana), Association of Indigenous Women of the Atlantic Coast (AMICA), Association for the Development of Mayagna Communities (Masaku), and government agencies such as the Autonomous Regional Government and the Association of Municipalities of the Autonomous Regions of the Caribbean Coast of Nicaragua (AMURACAN), as well as diverse associations of local indigenous representation also contribute to the autonomy and development of the region and struggle for recognition by central government policy makers.

The two indigenous universities, University of the Autonomous Regions of the Caribbean Coast of Nicaragua (URACCAN) and Bluefields Indian and Caribbean University (BICU) work for authentic autonomy and development through cultural conservation, education, and research. The Bilwi Clinic (RAAN) and the Campaña Costeña Association (RAAS) specialize in HIV prevention and rapid tests, and in community health. The Sisters of Santa Inez have a decades-long presence in the region, focusing on education. The Social

Development Association of the Moravian Church implements community health and food security programs, and has added HIV/AIDS prevention to its church agenda. AMC is an example of an NGO of Pacific-region origin that has established successful permanent presence in RAAN and RAAS for more than twenty years. Research and practical experience has helped AMC evolve from a direct healthcare delivery organization to one that targets the social determinants of health in order to positively impact health indicators. Of AMC's current field staff, 90 percent are from the regions they serve. Many have been trained by AMC, and they bridge the traditional and official health systems.

Autonomous Health Models

The General Health Law of Nicaragua states that the autonomous regions have the right to establish their own models of healthcare, according to their traditions, cultures, and customs, but within the framework of policies, plans, programs, and projects of MINSA.[26] Measures have been incorporated into MINSA's autonomous health models to recognize, respect, and coordinate with traditional medicine practitioners and, as a right under the Statute of Autonomy, to recover, in a scientific manner and in coordination with the national health system, the knowledge of natural medicine accumulated through the course of history.[27] Despite this, the knowledge, beliefs, and traditional health practices of indigenous peoples and ethnic communities have not been fully respected, and there is still a limited degree of credibility and acceptance by the Western health personnel who consider the traditional system to be a risky alternative for the health of the population.[28]

Historically, the level of coordination between the two systems has been formative, and at a preliminary level of mutual recognition that both exist to resolve health problems. In 2006, more concrete efforts were made in RAAN by the central and regional autonomous governments to decentralize the health system and to create and implement a model of multicultural healthcare that articulates both official and traditional systems. The founding principles of the decentralization are shared responsibility, intercultural collaboration, equality in healthcare, and a gender focus. Expected results include the autonomous management of the system, the prevention of epidemics and disasters, better coordination among institutions, and traditional and Western health systems working together to improve health indicators.

During 2006–2008, collaboration among Nicaraguan organizations helped to launch the autonomous health model. Each partner had a defined role. The Regional Autonomous Council served as regulator of project goals and activities. MINSA restructured the regional health services for greater independence and incorporation of traditional medicine. AMC strengthened the existing community health system to better coordinate referrals between doctors and traditional healers. The Bilwi Clinic provided rapid HIV testing, and other agencies raised awareness about HIV/AIDS and its prevention. URACCAN carried out research to document the knowledge of medicinal plants and spirit-based diseases and their protocol for treatment. A northern partner (Horizont3000 of Austria) served to facilitate and finance the project and provide technical support. Each partner managed its own component, but all met regularly to assess the advancement of goals, review the budget, and plan. The Nicaraguan agencies worked in a spirit of collaboration, and the northern partner was recognized for its long-term vision and presence in the country, openness to dialogue, and respect of differences.

Decentralization has shown the following results: Western doctors and nurses are trained in traditional medicine; culturally based illnesses are treated in the official health system with a referral network. Traditional childbirth is institutionalized, and empirical midwives in RAAN are the only people in the country legally allowed to attend a birth in a health facility. Traditional healers are incorporated into the health assessment process at the community level. Youth, tribal leaders, educators, and religious and regional leaders are working together. A new focus specific to HIV/AIDS supports a regional health model aimed at prevention and treatment.

These results have limitations for several reasons: short, three-year interventions; political interests that often override the goals; and drug trafficking and migration into the autonomous regions, burdening already under-resourced health services. Despite this, southern partnerships as demonstrated in the decentralization project provide contextually appropriate efforts that allow vulnerable groups to be included in health strategies. These partnerships offer potential for institutional development for the groups involved, thereby contributing to broader-based development plans that recognize the contribution of poorer countries to global health issues.

The failure of many health projects is rooted in both vertical design and the lack of knowledge of the social and cultural principles of the population; as a result, interventions inadvertently trample on beliefs, traditions, and values, bringing consequences that foster rejection and frustration by all involved. Health professional training frequently focuses on the clinical, epidemiologic, and administrative aspects of health, and does not address the anthropological aspects of health and illness as well as the need for collaborative models.

Ideally, the resources for health in the autonomous regions should promote policies that strengthen the development of traditional medicine and ensure the health of indigenous people by respecting their culture, and by opposing *biopiracy* of traditional and indigenous knowledge and resources.[29] Global health workers should first and foremost believe in the capacity of the local agencies involved in health and development, and should seek ways to join forces, offering technical, material, and financial resources that are unavailable in Nicaragua.

AMC's Grassroots Model for Community Health

Community health in Nicaragua and as practiced by AMC is not merely the mobilization of clinical services outside a health facility, but a model in which the local population participates in identifying problems and planning appropriate solutions with the purpose of resolving health needs. Those who live in the local community may be poor farmers or indigenous people, but they have the capacity to address the first level of health in their community. They know the context and issues, and they have a moral commitment to attend to their own people. Health problems are not merely addressed on an individual level, but with a collective focus. Neither is health independent of the political, social, and above all, cultural context of the community. Most health problems have diverse and multiple causes; therefore, the community health system is a collection of integrated actions of disease prevention, health promotion, and healthcare delivery carried out with an inter-institutional approach in coordination with all stakeholders (state, regional, and local organizations) vested in improving health.

AMC's community health team is a multidisciplinary group made up of doctors, dentists, nurses, pharmacists, public health experts, sociologists, social workers, psychologists, educators, health communicators, hygienists, and agronomists; community health volunteers, who may be leaders, indigenous healers, midwives, first aid workers, teachers, pastors, health promoters, or farmers; and community organizations, such as water committees or indigenous and women's associations. Community health can improve health indicators by addressing issues such as clean water, HIV/AIDS, nutrition, sexual and reproductive health, health infrastructure, and access to healthcare.

Lessons Learned

In its first years working in the Caribbean Coast, AMC was staffed with young doctors and dentists who essentially fulfilled the role of MINSA in what was then a war zone, difficult for the 1980s revolutionary government to access. In the refugee settlement of Sahsa, RAAN, the infant mortality rate in 1989 was 200 per 1,000 live births.[30] A clinical response was mounted, and basic health indicators improved, but other problems remained dormant and unattended.

Through evaluations with the community and internal to the organization, AMC recognized that the Western-based medical approach had only limited impact on the health problems of the community, because it did not take into account the social and cultural characteristics of the population, whose world-view differs from that of the official health system.

In 1993, a cholera outbreak caused alarming death rates, and numerous fatalities occurred along the Coco River in RAAN. In response to the epidemic, AMC organized a campaign for Miskito communities called *Colerara Taka-skaia* (Stop Cholera) using health promotion and education techniques AMC considered effective: hand washing, boiling or chlorination of water, training for midwives and health leaders, and distribution of materials written in the local language.

Massive flooding of the river exacerbated the outbreak. The flooding de-stroyed crops and livestock, and left the population with no food sources and extensive water contamination from damaged latrines and wells. The popula-tion turned to other food sources, such as hunting deer and harvesting river shrimp, abundant in the receding waters. The cases of cholera grew.

AMC expected that the trained community leaders would put into practice preventive measures against cholera while AMC joined MINSA in treating ex-isting cases. But it did not happen that way. Midwives and leaders rejected the measures, exclaiming, "What cholera virus, what chlorine? This isn't a problem of cholera; what happened was that the spirits of the deer and shrimp are angry because people are eating too many of them without asking permis-sion." In Miskito culture, before hunting an animal, or cutting a tree or plant, permission must be requested of the spirit of each one, or a punishment will ensue.

AMC learned an important lesson from assuming that trained community members had sufficient ownership of serious public health issues from a Western standpoint. It was clear that AMC was just beginning to understand the indigenous worldview and how necessary it is to respect the beliefs that complement the work of the organization. Subsequent health campaigns openly recognized traditional beliefs and respectfully introduced Western-based strategies, resulting in more acceptance of collaborative methods and improved outcomes.

AMC next implemented a strategy for all projects based on the Participatory Action Research (PAR) method, a process that prioritizes the communities' analysis of their own problems, so they can then decide for themselves what to prioritize and what strategies and alliances are necessary to address the problem. In this way, AMC was able to promote investigative processes for understanding traditional knowledge worldview health promotion interventions that are respectful of and appropriate to that reality. AMC integrated complementary actions in health promotion, training *agentes voluntarias de salud* (community health volunteers) such as midwives, traditional health providers, and first aid workers, while strengthening community organizations such as community boards and health committees to respond to needs. Once the armed conflict was over, MINSA resumed its role as provider of clinical services.

This led to the current community health system, which includes the integration of the traditional and official health systems to address the multiple causes of health problems in a culturally appropriate way. Within the community health system, the health leader is the liaison between official and traditional systems, and may also be an herbalist or healer, although midwives can also maintain relationships with both systems. A concrete example of this integration was the publication of a manual for 546 medicinal plants. After careful documentation with traditional healers, a process only possible after years of building trust and the assurance that the knowledge would not be misused, AMC organized the scientific, Miskito, and Spanish names of each plant, along with the botanical description, medicinal preparation, use, and contraindications. To satisfy the scientific perspective, each plant was tested to identify and confirm its chemical and biological components, creating a resource useful to both systems.

It's important for readers to understand that AMC helped to launch, and continues to strengthen, this community system for primary healthcare, but its focus is *from* the community and *for* the community as a way to overcome models that focus only on health services. The community health system belongs to the community, not to outside agencies or institutions.

Later, activities involving water, hygiene, and sanitation began with latrines, wells, water systems, rainwater collection, and community cleanups combined with improved habits of personal and community hygiene. Building on previous work in improving healthcare, access to clean water helped infant mortality indicators drop to levels below the national average. Work in sexual and reproductive health improved the dismal indicators for maternal mortality, but the indicators for nutrition were poor and other problems emerged, such as domestic violence and HIV/AIDS.

AMC addressed malnutrition by introducing food security strategies combined with treatment for parasites. Vitamin supplements were then provided through family vegetable gardens, and mothers of malnourished children were organized in a mentoring model.

These efforts had some impact on nutrition, but many health problems were caused by social, political, and climatic determinants. Farmers planted one or two crops for only one seasonal cycle, and the repeated loss of harvest limited the food supply. Policy makers unfamiliar with the remote eastern region overlooked capital investment in social and agricultural programs. The potential threat of disasters caused by hurricanes, tropical storms, and flooding was constant.

The next level of evaluations led AMC to broaden its work to include food security by promoting sustainable food production through model farms, comprehensive pest control, and environmentally friendly agricultural practices. Additionally, AMC initiated the process of disaster preparedness. Where AMC has facilitated this type of preparation, communities are among the best prepared for an emergency. No deaths were reported in AMC communities after Hurricane Mitch (Oct. 29, 1998), and AMC led the emergency response committee after Hurricane Felix (Sept. 4, 2007).

Community organization efforts encouraged people to feel empowered and in charge of their own future. AMC's accompaniment in theological reflections also created a space for deeply religious communities to understand their health and development from a faith perspective, and to take further ownership of the community health system, deciding that God's will is not to punish people with sickness, but that people themselves can be agents of change for the abundant life that God promises. AMC's role by this time was shifting from protagonist to facilitator of processes of development.

A recent affliction in Caribbean Coast communities is HIV/AIDS. This disease has social, economic, cultural, and spiritual implications as well as an effect on gender relations, and is directly related to social phenomena such as discrimination, stigma, machismo, exclusion, and social inequality. Despite a law that protects their rights,[31] HIV-infected people may be rejected from their homes and shunned by their communities and peers, may have little opportunity for employment, or may be forced to live their HIV reality in secret. AMC affirms the campaigns carried out by MINSA and WHO/PAHO that have advocated globally in support of faithfulness, abstinence, or delay in sexual relations, as well as condom use as a method to prevent HIV and other sexually transmitted infections (STIs). On this basis, AMC as a faith-based NGO, familiar with church language, theology, and Biblical message, could approach different denominations and facilitate the formation of two pastoral networks of more than 6,000 church members willing to stand together against the injustice that discriminates against people living with HIV/AIDS and to promote acceptance of condom use in this context. The subsequent training of young health communicators and the formation of HIV/AIDS self-help groups serve as an oasis of hope and provide spiritual, material, and medical support to participants.

Churches, Faith-Based Organizations, and Community Development

TERESA BOBADILLA, DMD, MPH, AMC Founder and Current Executive Director. *Translation and edits by Belinda Forbes*

Poverty is not merely a lack of food, clothing and shelter, but has several dimensions: social (lack of opportunity to interact with others), political (lack of ability to influence people in positions of power), and spiritual (lack of relationship with God).*

Global health workers should not assume that Latin American development happens within a secular space separated from the divine, religious, or spiritual one. It is not necessary to believe in God to appreciate the tangible presence of beliefs about God in the collective self-identity that shapes the social life of a significant percentage of the region's inhabitants.

A providential vision of God predominates in Latin America, rooted in the Catholicism inherited from Spanish colonial times, but also expressed in the boom of charismatic Pentecostal Christianity. This vision has molded a pragmatic-resigned political culture that tolerates inequality and injustice as part of the divine plan. In a 2002 study, 79 percent of those polled stated that their belief in God rather than their own personal will was the force that determined the course of life and history.** In an AMC survey exploring perceptions about the cause of natural disasters, 80 percent of those polled stated it was God's punishment.

Nicaragua's largest religious representation is Christianity expressed through Roman Catholicism, an estimated 300 Protestant or Evangelical denominations, and numerous faith-based organizations.*** Churches and FBOs, using diverse doctrines and principles, and faith in God, seek to meet the needs of people. These institutions have an important role as agents of transformation in local communities, and as social stakeholders for human rights and policy making. In rural Nicaragua especially, religious leaders—pastors, priests, Delegates of the Word, Christian educators—are recognized as authorities and wield enormous influence over the beliefs and practices of the community, particularly around key social and health issues.

Unfortunately, the church and FBOs have often misinterpreted their mission to love and serve others. Many churches separate the spiritual and material aspects of life, perhaps from a dualistic view imported by missionaries.**** Few Christian education institutions teach the entirety of mission, so religious leaders lack the theological framework or skills to respond effectively to the needs of the poor in their communities, or churches use a paternalistic welfare approach, creating dependency by people on the church for charity. This latter approach may be useful in responding to short-term or emergency needs, but preferably, more empowering approaches that address long-term development exist. Some churches might abuse aid or social services by coercing people to convert to Christianity. Project beneficiary selection might be in exchange for regular attendance at church, or conversion to Christianity or a particular doctrine or denomination.

Across Central America, churches and FBOs have many advantages to be effective in development work. They have access to significant percentages of the population for transmitting health messages, and the moral grounding to promote justice and representation in many governmental and nongovernmental networks. However, there are challenges for churches and FBOs to overcome of which global workers should be mindful. Attitudes of condemnation of gays, lesbians, bisexual and transgendered people, and sex workers by church and FBO members circumscribes support that such organizations can provide to people living with HIV/AIDS or other STIs. There is no single organizational structure for faith groups, making coordination difficult; resources for community health are limited or sector-directed; and fundamental differences in values can exist between faith and secular organizations, limiting the critical capacity to collaborate. Key institutions and faith organizations need to offer greater mutual recognition of the unique and complementary strengths that each partner can contribute to health and development.*****

More and more churches and FBOs are taking up the call for comprehensive mission, defined as meeting the needs of people in a multidimensional way. In Nicaragua, a group of twenty church, pastoral, and FBO networks work collaboratively and ecumenically in support of health and community development. In recent years attention has been drawn to their pastoral care to HIV and AIDS patients, in helping to reduce discrimination against those living with the virus and preventing its propagation among youth. Several national NGOs participate: Acción Médica Cristiana, Apostolic Vicariate of Bluefields, Council of Evangelical Churches of Nicaragua, Interchurch Center for Theological and Social Studies, the Lutheran Church of Nicaragua, the Moravian Church of Nicaragua, Nehemiah Center, and international agencies such as Catholic Relief Services, Caritas, and St. Luke Association. The impact of these and other similar efforts may be reflected in reports that between 2006 and 2010, RAAS decreased from third to eleventh place in highest number of new HIV/AIDS cases.******

There are many positive experiences of churches and FBOs in Nicaragua that transcend healthcare or charity assistance: disaster risk reduction and climate justice, food security, clean water and sanitation, essential medicines, literacy, gender justice, and other long-term development issues. Indeed, these stakeholders have a responsibility to actively participate in fulfilling their mandate to build the Realm of God on Earth by caring for and being a voice for the most vulnerable populations.

NOTES

* Tearfund International Learning Zone, "Como asociarse con la iglesia Local," Roots 11 (Teddington, England: Tearfund, 2007), 10.

** "Nicas dejan su destino a la buena de Dios," La Prensa (June 16, 2002).

*** AmeriCorps, "Definitions of FBOs and CBOs," FACES AmeriCorps Applicants Toolkit, available from www.nationalserviceresources.org.

**** James Hastings, Encyclopedia of Religion and Ethics Part 9, ed. John A. Selbie (Whitefish, MT: Kessinger Publishing, 2003), 100.

***** Kathryn Pitkin Derose, David E. Kanouse, David P. Kennedy, Kavita Patel, Alice Taylor, Kristin J. Leuschner, and Homero Martinez, The Role of Faith-Based Organizations in HIV Prevention and Care in Central America, Rand Monograph Series, MG-891-RC, (Santa Monica, CA: Rand Corp., 2010):4.

****** MINSA, "Situación VIH y Sida Nicaragua Años 2006–2011" (Managua: MINSA, 2010).

Another successful community health initiative is the essential medicines network or Venta Social de Medicamentos (VSM). MINSA estimates that only 45.3 percent of the Nicaraguan population has access to medicines on a continuous basis, and that of the total amount spent by a family on health, 60 percent goes to purchasing medicines.[32] Designed for communities where commercial pharmacies are unavailable, this self-sustaining initiative improves economic and geographic access to medicines by the population through small pharmacies that then supply satellite pharmacies or *botiquínes* in surrounding communities. VSM also promotes rigorous quality control and the appropriate use of medicines, in keeping with legal requirements. A lasting impact of this effort is strengthened levels of community organization through local administration and staffing of the pharmacy. After ten years, the network is now sustainable, covers operating costs and salaries, and requires little outside financing.

AMC has learned to leverage the community's wisdom: working with all stakeholders, holding them accountable to their commitment to participate; and investing time and resources in shaping organizational structures and processes that build local capacity. No longer does the organization use quick-fix phrases like "If only they would . . ." or "They just need to . . ." to describe communities and the complex arena of development. It's crucial that global health workers assess their own cultural biases and the gross inadequacies of their own health systems before coming to judge the Nicaraguan reality and its people. Global workers should exchange a protagonist attitude for one of humility, and align themselves with effective models, learn from local experiences and recommendations, and support existing efforts that have proved successful. This leads to empowerment for all involved.

Vulnerability and Disasters on the Caribbean Coast

It is projected that climate change will impact every aspect of human existence: health systems, environmental and social conditions, and political systems will be affected by social discontent and economic instability caused by dislocations. Public health will be affected by diseases, especially those caused by vectors; by decreased access to quality water due to changes in ecosystems; and by decreased food security from low agricultural production. Loss of livelihood will be especially severe in rural areas, with likely deterioration of infrastructure such as roads and housing.[33] Climate change is a threat for poor countries, and threats added to factors of vulnerability define a population's risk for disaster situations. Nicaragua's geographic position exposes it to many such situations. It ranks second in the world for tropical storm impact and is among the top thirty countries most affected by earthquakes.[34] Nicaragua's Climate Risk Index (CRI)[35] is 16.17, placing it fourth for countries most affected by extreme weather events during the period 1990–2009.[36]

The Caribbean Coast has conditions that create higher risk than in other parts of Nicaragua. Threats include flooding that occurs almost every year in some parts of the region. Hurricanes have increased in frequency and intensity, for example, Hurricanes Beta (2005), Stan (2005), and Felix (2007). Hundreds of thousands or more hectares of trees were felled by Hurricane Felix,[37] posing the threat of wildfires each dry season, as well as increased runoff, erosion, and severity of floods. Strong winds and tsunamis threaten the seacoast, and there are frequent rat infestations.

The vulnerability factors in the region include fragile wood or bamboo housing that can't withstand the strong winds of a hurricane; time and money required for traveling the long, difficult distances between river or overland communities, making long-term projects in disaster preparedness and response difficult to implement; the state and regional institutions' lack of political will to respond; and the lack of regional economic development plans, aggravating poverty and disasters—for example, hurricane season coincides with the periods of highest agricultural production.

Humans contribute to the vulnerability factors for disasters in multiple ways. Deforestation and slash-and-burn agriculture (see Glossary) indirectly increase threats of extreme weather,[38] and they also increase vulnerability. Deforestation has been directly linked to increased flooding, soil erosion, and risk of landslides. Between 1990 and 2010, Nicaragua lost 31 percent of its forest cover and continues to lose 70,000 hectares or 1.55 percent of forest per year, mostly in the Caribbean region. Deforestation in the region is driven primarily by conversion of forests by colonist farmers to agriculture and then to pasture, though in some areas, forests have been razed to make way for monoculture plantations. The contribution by indigenous populations to deforestation is low compared to that of migrating groups. Other concerns include indiscriminate logging, the expansion of oil and mining industries, and firewood consumption.

Disaster Response

Successful national disaster strategies recognize links between poverty, the environment, and the risks posed by natural phenomena. A significant improvement in disaster management in Nicaragua is the 2002 law creating the National System of Prevention, Mitigation, and Disaster Awareness (SINAPRED) that gives responsibility to local authorities and stakeholders for prevention and risk management through the "formation of committees in departments, municipalities, and autonomous regions as elements of the National System." An environmental assessment process contributed across sectors, engaged government agencies, private sector representatives, and NGOs.[39] In 2007, the Inter-American Development Bank (IDB, IADB) approved a Disaster Risk Management Policy. However, Nicaragua is still ranked among the countries in Latin America with the least ability to respond and overcome the economic impact of disasters caused by extreme weather,[40] despite high levels of international participation in disaster response.

AMC became involved in disaster response simply by having development projects in RAAN and RAAS, which suffered the consequences of emergencies. Like other organizations in the region, AMC had experience in disaster response, but very little in how to reduce or avoid the devastating effects. Ultimately, prevention, mitigation, and food security efforts became key complementary strategies to ongoing community health projects. Along the Coco River and in RAAS, AMC installed early-warning radio systems, rain gauges, refugee centers, and trained promoters. Members of the community can organize evacuations, mobilize teams for crisis response, conduct risk analyses, and document experiences, as well as provide emotional recovery services to the population. AMC worked over two years to move the Coco River community, Tuskrutara, from a floodplain to safer ground where the community no longer loses its crops each year and now shows improved health indicators with lower risk for malnutrition. In other communities, land mines were removed along the river, eliminating one of the principal factors discouraging populations from relocating inland.[41]

Essential to all development work is the concept of crisis prevention: planning, risk mapping, land use, environmental monitoring, and poverty reduction, as well as efforts for adaptation to climate change. Fundamental to improving Nicaragua's capacity to both prevent and overcome emergency situations will be these factors: legislation; policy and projects that promote self-responsibility of all actors; decentralized planning and implementation to the local level; collaborative responsibility for implementation shared among public and private stakeholders; and rigorous accountability of those who create risks that threaten public well-being.

In summary, the Caribbean Coast, like much of Nicaragua, lives a contradiction—wealth of its resources, and impoverishment of its people. The 2005 Human Development Report for Nicaragua recommended that Nicaraguan society let go of historical separation and build a multicultural state that recognizes the richness of diversity without fear.[42] Autonomy of the Caribbean Coast is a courageous victory, a pending opportunity, and yet a potential challenge. Inhabitants of the Caribbean Coast want to make economic, cultural, administrative, and political autonomy the central means to achieve sustainable human development for them and for all of Nicaragua. To accomplish this, gaps in human development must be closed, and personal and collective capacity enhanced, particularly among historically excluded groups.

Dental Health in Nicaragua

Oral disease is a significant burden in all countries of the world.[43] There is hardly a community in Nicaragua where this burden is not visible. As in many developing countries, the most prevalent dental diseases are dental caries, responsible for 40 to 45 percent of tooth loss, and periodontal disease. Other maladies occur, such as tumors,[44] cleft palate, fluorosis, and increasingly, trauma from accidents; but the principal issues are found in primary care and can be addressed at the local level with successful interventions. Many Nicaraguans enjoy a wide mandibular arch and an even Class I occlusion, aiding in self-cleansing and nutrition, but this is not enough to prevent disease unless combined with other factors such as oral hygiene and access to dental care.

The epidemiological profile of dental caries and periodontal disease in Nicaragua shows high prevalence of each with the following characteristics: dental caries start at an early age (less than five years), and in twelve-year-olds the decayed, missing, or filled teeth (DMFT) value is 4 (Norway 1.4), increasing with age and demonstrating little difference between sexes. The average DMFT among adults is 10.25 and more prevalent in the rural areas. Periodontal disease is more prevalent among women and in the rural areas.[45]

Determinants for dental disease include geographic isolation; insufficient numbers of dental professionals, with most located in urban sectors and highly concentrated near the state dental school in León; and a government health system insufficiently resourced to make comprehensive oral health a priority. There is low dental health awareness by the population nationally, with low or no value placed on maintaining dental health; lack of association of consumption of fermentable carbohydrates with plaque production and ensuing dental disease;[46] historical and cultural patterns of tooth pain or loss and periodontal disease; and a delay in seeking out dental care. Economic limitations reduce access to restorative (filling) treatment, and even a toothbrush may cost more than the daily income of a person in the rural area.

MINSA has the responsibility for regulating services and promoting the prevention and rehabilitation of oral health of the population, but this health-care cost is largely paid for by patients themselves with no control for cost-effectiveness, and no objective evaluation of oral health problems of the population, especially for the most vulnerable sectors. A serious limitation for oral health in Nicaragua is the lack of data with respect to official epidemiological indicators. If popular awareness of oral health is expanded and strategies that address dental problems are implemented, the general health of the population will improve.[47]

Currently, the health system lacks budgetary and personnel resources, up-to-date equipment, and a dental health infrastructure. There are 0.48 dentists per 10,000 inhabitants in Nicaragua, and this drops dramatically in remote regions such as RAAN (0.19 per 10,000), where the highest levels of dental disease have been identified.[48] Of the 1,150 registered dentists in the country, only 257 are in the state health sector. Of the 1,091 health facilities in the country, MINSA has 189 dental units distributed among 145 health centers covering the fifteen departments and two autonomous regions. However, most units are located in the Pacific region's municipal or departmental seats, with no coverage of the rural areas where most of the population lives; and 50 percent of the units, as well as most of the accessory equipment, are in poor condition due to lack of periodic maintenance. MINSA has nine vans outfitted with dental equipment for travel to urban and semi-urban communities for one-day mobile clinics.

Only general dental services are provided in MINSA health centers. Specialty care is even more limited, with only one pediatric dentist and nineteen maxillofacial surgeons in government service, mostly located in hospitals in the capital, Managua. With a national policy of free healthcare, demand is up for dental services, but service is limited to emergencies and extractions. There is some emphasis on promotion and prevention.[49]

Dentists are the only dental health professionals in Nicaragua, and they are trained in five dental schools (one state and four private). There are only twenty-five dental assistants in the government system, but new programs for dental hygienists, assistants, and lab technicians are underway at UNAN–León. There is no required continuing education and little offered by dental associations or the government. An undetermined number of empirically trained dentists practice illegally in the rural areas, but they are not routinely penalized because they offer at least some level of services, however risky. Some private practices in Nicaragua now offer high-quality, sophisticated dental care, such as implants and full-mouth rehabilitation, to the wealthy population and are increasingly providing services for medical tourism. With these limitations, MINSA is unable to respond with ongoing broad coverage for dental health, but does provide limited attention through existing structures and programs.

Nicaragua is one of at least fourteen countries in Latin America with a proposed fluoridation program using salt as the vehicle.[50] A 1997 study by the faculty of dentistry at UNAN–León demonstrated that fluorosis is not a public health issue in Nicaragua. However, a more focused study in the community of Ticuantepe in the Department of Managua demonstrated cases of moderate to severe fluorosis thought to be a result of high levels of fluoride in the artesian well–water supply or in gases emitted from the nearby Masaya Volcano.[51] There are no water fluoridation programs in Nicaragua, and Managua water has been shown to have sufficient natural quantities of fluoride to aid in caries prevention. Research in this area is costly, but necessary to assess the need and impact of fluoride programs.

In general, Nicaragua falls short of PAHO's Ten-Year Regional Plan on Oral Health benchmarks to verify policies and programs for fluoridation, oral health promotion, and vulnerable populations with indicators on DMFT, published case studies, and the integration of an oral health plan into national health policy.[52]

To bridge this gap, international health teams offer services that the government or private efforts are unable to provide. Foreign dentists may practice in the country, and dental hygienists may do so under the supervision of a national or foreign dentist, each having MINSA approval. In 2010, MINSA registered 365 medical teams, 126 of which provided dental care. These teams visited numerous communities in the Pacific and central regions, rarely reaching the Caribbean regions, and provided short-term, intensive dental care; almost exclusively curative treatment in maxillofacial and pediatric care; and some preventive services, such as sealants, dental health education, and toothbrush distribution.

UNAN–León hosts five teams per year from universities in the United States or Spain in which the Nicaraguan and visiting dental students work together. Private businesses such as Colgate and local dental suppliers collaborate with MINSA and UNAN–León programs to provide some restorative and oral hygiene supplies and educational materials. UNAN–León is the leading institution for dental health research in the country.

According to public health dentist Dr. Yemira Sequeira, director of Nicaragua's National Oral Health Program, comprehensive initiatives to provide ongoing access to curative and preventive dental care, combined with replicable training strategies for health education and promotion, are the best option for preventing and reducing dental disease. Yet in Nicaragua, programs such as these are rare. Sustainable, supervised oral hygiene programs are comparatively inexpensive and can be carried out by educational personnel or community health volunteers without the continuous presence of a dental professional. The contribution of permanent or mobile teams of national or international professionals to such programs strengthens long-term efforts to improve dental health, and this is far more effective than just a "parachute" intervention with limited impact.

Since 2005, as part of its Community Health and Development Program, AMC has facilitated a successful dental health program in the municipality of La Dalia, Matagalpa, in a rural *comarca* of villages called Aguas Amarillas. The initial baseline survey showed a DMFT of 4 in the 150 elementary schoolchildren screened for the program. The nearest dentist is two hours by bus and costs more than a week's wages for most inhabitants. During five years of the program, nine local dental promoters were trained by dentist Belinda Forbes and Nicaraguan colleagues, with support from international health teams, to carry out monthly visits to eight schools. They reached 800 schoolchildren to teach and oversee oral hygiene, apply fluoride, and screen patients with the greatest need for clinical services from dentists during periodic visits. In many cases, three-to-five-year-old preschool children received their first toothbrushes through this program, leading to an early childhood caries risk-assessment component for mothers and toddlers, to address and prevent the devastating results of rampant caries in deciduous dentitions and their potential impact on nutrition and overall child development. In rural areas of Nicaragua, prevention is the best strategy because hospital pediatric dental services are practically nonexistent, and mobile care is limited for more complex rehabilitation.

Yearly evaluations of AMC's program document increasing oral health awareness, improved oral hygiene, increased demand for services, and expanded access to dental services from visiting teams. A permanent dental clinic was installed in the community and provides low-cost care paid for by patients in cash or with farm produce. The best results were in the schoolchildren who received all three levels of attention: dental education, oral hygiene practice in school, and curative services.

This model for integrated dental health is effective in reducing the incidence of caries. UNAN–León is currently conducting a study using the incremental system for schoolchildren, providing education, sealants on permanent molars, fluoride varnish, and regular toothbrushing. After the first year of the study, caries incidence dropped from the baseline of 4 caries average per child to 0 caries.[53]

In the Caribbean Coast, AMC coordinated with MINSA to train advanced dental promoters in RAAN to perform simple extractions. Of twenty-five promoters trained from 1992 to 1997, at least ten are still offering regular dental services in their communities as of this writing, for which they receive modest remuneration that replenishes their supplies. One promoter is sought after to travel a circuit of river communities, treating patients for several days at a time. In 2010 on a mobile medical team, Belinda traveled with two such promoters, who were both preferred by the population over her and the professionals on the trip because of their language skills (Miskito) and renowned ability in dental care. Their high level of technical training as well as compassionate care and cultural acceptance are fundamental to the success of the community healthcare system.

Global health volunteers interested in dental health have diverse opportunities for accompanying ongoing efforts to raise awareness and can contribute to improving dental health throughout Nicaragua.

ROLES AND RECOMMENDATIONS FOR DENTAL HEALTH VOLUNTEERS

Find a local partner to work with, preferably one with experience in
    community or public health programs.
Choose a target population, such as a school, to achieve measurable
    results that can be replicated.
Secure necessary authorization from relevant authorities (MINSA, MINED

[Nicaragua Ministry of Education], local leaders) to carry out interventions such as an oral hygiene program.

Work jointly with national dentists in local programs. Nicaraguan dentists not only have extraordinary skills in surgical extractions, but they have innovative experience to resolve even the most difficult cases in mobile clinic settings, and they can provide cultural insight into the dental health reality of the people. Programs that offer stipends and quality materials and equipment serve as incentives to national practitioners.

Offer continuing education for dentists: formal presentations, study group dialogues, hands-on training, and the introduction of new techniques and use of materials. Many dentists need simple refresher courses in radiographic technique, space-maintaining apparatuses, and diagnosis and treatment planning. Such two-way mentoring can make a lasting contribution to the dental profession in Nicaragua and the quality of care available.

Consider a joint investigation with Nicaraguan academic or government institutions in critical research areas such as dental caries, cleft palate, fluorosis, and trauma cases. A rapidly advancing area of research in industrialized countries is the oral-systemic disease connection,[54] an important area of research as Nicaragua's epidemiological transition shifts to include lifestyle-related diseases and cancers.

Remember that the use of expired medicines and materials is illegal in Nicaragua.[55] For the sake of the patients you may treat and the Nicaraguan dentists you may support, choose quality materials that can withstand hot, humid conditions and have at least one year of shelf life after they arrive in the country.

Approach any dental intervention with three driving principles of public health: disease prevention, disease surveillance, and health promotion.

Dr. Jorge Cerrato, tenured professor in the Department of Preventive and Social Dentistry and coordinator of social projects, UNAN–León, was asked what he would say to a potential global health volunteer considering work in Nicaragua. He shares, "Every contribution is an important one; we cannot do everything but can all do something. Keep a humanitarian spirit to help those with fewer opportunities. This experience can serve for your own professional development; you will learn a great deal."

List of Acronyms

AMC: Acción Médica Cristiana
BICU: Bluefields Indian and Caribbean University

CEDEHCA: Center for Human, Civil and Autonomous Rights

CEPAD: Council of Protestant Churches of Nicaragua

CIES-UNAN: Centro de Investigación y Estudios de la Salud, National Autonomous University of Nicaragua

FADCANIC: Foundation for the Autonomy and Development of the Atlantic Coast of Nicaragua

HDI: Human Development Index

IDB, IADB: Inter-American Development Bank

INIDE: National Institute for Development Information

MARENA: Ministry of the Environment and Natural Resources

MINSA: Ministry of Health

PHM: People's Health Movement

SINAPRED: National System of Prevention, Mitigation, and Disaster Awareness

UNAN: National Autonomous University of Nicaragua

UNDP: United Nations Development Program

URACCAN: University of the Autonomous Regions of the Caribbean Coast of Nicaragua

Acknowledgments

The authors thank AMC staff Francisco Gutiérrez, MD, and Licenciada Violeta Hernández for their support in researching this chapter; Dr. Lizzett Cortez for helping to secure dental health data in Nicaragua; and Marilyn R. Crocker, EdD, for her invaluable editing advice.

Notes

1 In the 2005 INIDE Census, indigenous and ethnic groups are listed as follows: Rama, Garífuna, Mayangna-Sumu, Miskitu, Ulwa, Creole (Kreyòl), Mestizo de la Costa Caribe, Xiu-Sutiava, Nahoa-Nicarao, Chorotega-Nahua-Mange, Cacaopera-Matagalpa.

2 The actual geographic parameters of the Caribbean region are not accurately stated in the Constitution of Nicaragua or in the Autonomy Law 28 passed in 1987.

3 INIDE, "Censo 2005," Vol. 1. (Managua: INIDE, 2006).

4 UNPD, *Nicaragua Informe de Desarrollo Humano 2005: Las regiones autónomas de la Costa Caribe ¿Nicaragua asume su diversidad?* (Managua: PNUD, 2005).

5 UNPD, *Informe Regional sobre Desarrollo Humano para América Latina y el Caribe 2010*, 36, table 2.5 cited from Busso, Cicowiez and Gasparini (2005) (New York: UNDP, 2010).

6 INIDE, "Censo 2005," 246.

7 Laws include Constitución Política, Artos. 5, 89, 90 y 91; La Gaceta No. 68, 2005 (1987/2005), Ley 162 Uso Oficial de las Lenguas de las Comunidades de la Costa Atlántica de Nicaragua; La Gaceta, No. 132, 1996; Ley 28 Estatuto de Autonomía de las Regiones de la Costa Atlántica de Nicaragua; La Gaceta, No. 238, 1987; Ley 445,

Régimen de Propiedad Comunal de los Pueblos Indígenas y Comunidades Étnicas de las Regiones Autónomas de la Costa Atlántica de Nicaragua y de los Ríos Bocay, Coco, Indio y Maíz; La Gaceta, No. 16, 2003; Ley 217, General del Medio Ambiente y Los Recursos Naturales; La Gaceta, 105, 1996. A bill for traditional medicine is currently in the National Assembly.

8 Decree 19–2008, Art. 1.

9 Cap. III, Art. 59.

10 Cap I, Arts. 2–4

11 MINSA, "Plan Nacional de Salud" (Managua: MINSA, 2008).

12 Nicaragua is in first position among countries that have the greatest losses in HDI due to inequality, and the greatest cost is in health.

13 PAHO, "Nicaragua" in *Salud de Las Américas, 2007, Vol. II–Países*, Scientific and Technical Publication 622. (Washington: PAHO), 565, 573.

14 Ibid.

15 Maria Hamlin Zúñiga, email message to author, May 31, 2011.

16 Avelino Cox, "Quienes somos, cuáles son nuestras raíces y cosmovisión," available from www.pto-cabezas.com.

17 The legend of Niki Niki concerns a Miskito chief whose son was lost while hunting. As Niki Niki searched, he threw pine nuts, his son's favorite food, on the ground. It is thought that the tears Niki Niki shed for his son gave birth to the Coco or Wangki River, and the pine trees in the region grew from the seeds. Taken from Rufino Lucas Wilfred, *Colección de Cuentos: Miskitos, Nicaragüenses* (Managua: CEPAD, 1997).

18 Alfonso Navarrete, "Caracterización fisiogeográfica y demográfica de la Regiones Autónomas del Caribe de Nicaragua" (investigative work, FADCANIC: 2000), 2–3.

19 Sofia Gutiérrez and Jessica Aguilar Moraga, "Traditional Miskito Medicine in Alamikamba in the Health Model Framework, RAAN" (MPH thesis, CIES–UNAN, 2004), 15, 34–37, 42, 44–45, 56.

20 Ibid., 15.

21 Alan Harwood "The Hot-Cold Theory of Disease," *JAMA* 216 (1971):1153–1158.

22 Ibid.

23 M. G. Gutiérrez, *Percepción de la Mujer Miskita en Alamikamba, sobre su Salud Sexual y reproductiva y las implicaciones en su atención, Salud enfermedad en Alamikamba.* (Managua: AMC, 2003), 26.

24 AMC Reports for RAAN Projects, 1995–2002.

25 In the studies carried out by AMC on women's health, the substantive theory used encompassed gender, ethnicity, and health, which are sociological and anthropological fields of study. The theme offered the exploration of women's views as the central focus of the research, but to do this, men were included as complementary informants.

26 Ley, 423, Ley General de Salud, Capítulo IV, Arto. 11, 2003.

27 Ley 28, Estatuto de Autonomía, Art. 11-B, 1987.

28 Gutiérrez and Moraga, "Traditional Miskito Medicine in Alamikamba," 56.

29 People's Health Movement, "People's Charter for Health," www.phmovement.org.

30 AMC archives.

31 Ley 238, Promoción Protección y Defensa de los Derechos Humanos ante el SIDA, 1996.

32 Acción Internacional por la Salud Nicaragua (AIS) promotional material (Managua: AIS, 2010).

33 Yvette Aguilar, "El cambio climático y sus impactos en la salud de las poblaciones humanas," presentation during the regional meeting "Retos para la Revitalización de la APS en las Américas" September 22–25, 2008, La Palma, Chalatenango, El Salvador, 68–69, 83.

34 Inter-American Development Bank (IDB), "Estrategia de País con Nicaragua 2008–2012" (Washington: IDB, 2008), 9, available from www.iadb.org.

35 The global Climate Risk Index (CRI), developed by Germanwatch, analyzes the quantified impacts of extreme weather events in terms of fatalities as well as economic losses.

36 Sven Harmeling, "Global Climate Risk Index: Who Suffers Most from Extreme Weather Events? Weather-Related Loss Events in 2009 and 1990 to 2009," debriefing paper (Germany: Germanwatch e.V., 2010), 6.

37 Centro Humboldt reports 718,000 hectares and MARENA reports 1.3 billion hectares.

38 Disaster Preparedness ECHO (DIPECHO), *II Documento País: Nicaragua.* (Managua: DIPECHO, 2007), 1966–1967.

39 Christian Bollin, Camilo Cárdenas, Herwig Hahn, and Krishna S. Vasta, *Natural Disasters Network: Disaster Risk Management by Communities and Local Governments.* IDB *Regional Policy Dialogue* (Washington: IDB, 2003), 1.

40 IDB, "Estrategia de País con Nicaragua 2008–2012" (Washington: IDB, 2008), 9.

41 Land mines planted along the Coco River during the 1980s armed conflict are thought to be almost entirely eradicated thanks to efforts by AMC and the civil defense in a 2004–2006 project for land mine removal.

42 UNPD, *Nicaragua Informe de Desarrollo Humano 2005.*

43 WHO, News October 2008, available from www.who.int.

44 Nicaragua has less than 2 ASR per 100,000 for oral cancer. WHO International Agency for Research on Cancer, "GLOBOCAN 2008 Fast Stats," available from http://globocan.iarc.fr.

45 Carlo Medina, Jorge Cerrato, and Miriam del Socorro Herrera, "Perfil epidemiológico de la caries dental y enfermedad periodontal, en Nicaragua, año 2005" (León: Facultad de Odontología, UNAN–Léon, 2005).

46 Per capita raw sugar consumption in Nicaragua was 41.3 kg in 2009 (United States 31.6, Brazil 63.7), WHO –Country Area Profile Project, available from http://www.mah.se/CAPP/Globalsugar/Risk-Factors/Sugar-Global-Data/Global-Sugar-Consumption/Sugar-Consumption-AMRO/.

47 Medina et al., "Perfil epidemiológico de la caries dental y enfermedad periodontal."

48 Daniel Vilchez, "Perfil epidemiológico de caries dental y enfermedad periodontal en el municipio de puerto cabezas (Bilwi)" (monograph for dental surgeon title, UNAN–León Facultad de Odontología, 2005), 46.

49 MINSA, proceedings from "Taller de Salud Bucal para las Americas," Mexico City, 2009, available from http://new.paho.org.

50 Saskla Estupiñán-Day, "International Perspectives and Practical Applications on Fluorides and Fluoridation," *Journal of Public Health Dentistry* 64.s1 (2004):40–43.

51 Lizzett Cortez, "Prevalencia de Fluorosis Dental y en la Comunidad de la Borgoña, Municipio de Ticuantepe, Departamento de Managua" (monograph for dental surgeon title, UNAN–León Facultad de Odontología, 2009).

52 "PAHO Regional Core Health Indicator Update" (Washington: PAHO, May 2009).

53 Jorge Cerrato, "Atención odontológica integral, aplicando el Sistema Incremental, en escolares de primaria, escuela 'La Esperanza,' barrio 'Mercedes Varela,' León, Nicaragua 2009–2014" (investigation in process).

54 Michael L. Barnett, "The Oral-Systemic Disease Connection: An Update for the Practicing Dentist," *Journal of the American Dental Association* 137.s2 (Oct. 2006): 5S-6S.

55 Internal regulation of Law 423, "General Health Law," Title VII, Chapter IV, "Foreign Provider of Health Services," Articles 81, 82, and 83.

Suggested Reading

Grigsby, William. "Caribbean Coast: Multiethnic, Multilingual . . . and Finally Autonomous?" *Envío* 266 (Sept. 2003). Available online from www.envio.org.ni.

Pérez Baltodano, Andrés. "The Ignored Contradiction between Modern State and Providential God." *Envio* 312 (July 2007). Available online from www.envio.org.ni.

Werner, David, and Bill Bower. *Helping Health Workers Learn: A Book of Methods, Aids, and Ideas for Instructors.* Berkeley, CA: Hesperian Health Guides, 2012.

Suggested Websites

AMC: www.amc.org.ni
BICU: www.bicu.edu.ni
CEDEHCA: www.cedehcanicaragua.com
Centro Humboldt: http://humboldt.org.ni
CISAS: www.cisas.org.ni
FADCANIC: www.fadcanic.org.ni
Global Health Council: http://www.globalhealth.org/
PAHO: www.paho.org
PHM: www.phmovement.org
UNDP: www.undp.org.ni
URACCAN: www.uraccan.edu.ni

7 Haiti

Natasha Archer and Phuoc Le

In this chapter, we elucidate the geopolitical determinants of Haiti's poverty, and how it and other factors such as water insecurity and the lack of access to medical care have contributed to the development of a chronically debilitated healthcare system. We also illustrate how the HIV/AIDS epidemic, the 2010 earthquake, and the ongoing cholera epidemic have exerted, and still do exert, devastating effects on the state of health in Haiti. Global health workers will be addressing health issues related to these three disasters in the decades to come. Knowledge of the past and an open mind to the future will serve all those who choose to work in this fascinating country.

Brief History

The first recorded European contact with present-day Haiti was in 1492, when Christopher Columbus landed near what is now the city of Cap-Haïtien, on the northern coast. The events that ensued over the next several hundred years in Haiti are similar to those that played out in other Caribbean colonies: in the first few decades of European rule, smallpox and other infectious diseases decimated the indigenous populations (in Haiti's case, the Taínos people). African slaves were then imported to create a new labor force, and colonial powers grew rich from exports off the backs of slave labor.

But in 1791, Haiti's history diverged from that of its Caribbean neighbors. A slave revolt against Haiti's French rulers that consumed the colony in a brutal war for thirteen years proved too much for a weakened Napoleon. In 1804, Haiti became the first black-led republic in the world and the second colony to become a sovereign nation (the first was the United States) when it gained its independence in a successful slave revolution. The first 100 years of Haiti's history as a nation were mired by repeated political upheaval. The fact that between 1844 and 1914, power changed hands a total of thirty-two times, and the majority of Haiti's rulers were either assassinated or forced from office, indicates how unstable the political environment was for the fledging country.

In 1915, US president Woodrow Wilson sent an occupying military force ostensibly to reestablish peace and order among the many foreign nationals living in Haiti involved in anarchy; but in reality, this was an attempt to prevent a possible German invasion of the country and the United States' precious Panama Canal. During the nineteen-year US occupation of Haiti, the United States assumed complete control of Haiti's finances and public works projects, thousands of kilometers of roads were paved, and hundreds of bridges, schools, and clinics were built. However, this time of tremendous improvements in Haiti's infrastructure came with profound costs, as repeated popular uprisings against the occupation were put down with lethal force by the US military. The expensive US military occupation of Haiti grew more unpopular among US citizens during the Great Depression. As a result, US president Franklin Delano Roosevelt withdrew from Haiti in 1934.

Since World War II, Haiti's modern history has been dominated by a combination of political oppression and violence. François "Papa Doc" Duvalier, most infamously known for his security team, the TonTon Macoutes (Volunteers for National Security), became dictator of Haiti in 1957. During his time in power, Haiti made no advancements in agriculture, health, education, or commerce. At his death in 1971, his son Jean-Claude Duvalier, also known as "Baby Doc," assumed power and only increased Haiti's debt further. During his reign, the HIV/AIDS epidemic began, further debilitating the economy. He was ousted in 1986. At that time, the Government of Haiti (GOH) wrote the 1987 Constitution of Haiti, which aimed to foster Haiti's independence, establish democracy, and restore equality among the Haitian people.

In 1990, Jean-Bertrand Aristide became Haiti's first democratically elected president, but in 1991, he was overthrown and forced into exile by a military coup d'état. On his return to power in 1994, he disbanded the Haitian Army, which to this day leaves Haiti exceptionally vulnerable. Aristide's presidential term ended when he ceded power after a coup in 2004. Since then, two presidents, René Préval (1996) and Michel Martelly (2011), have been elected and assumed power. To help ensure a stable environment, the United Nations has had peacekeeping missions in Haiti since 1994, now known as MINUSTAH (United Nations Stabilization Mission in Haiti).

Geography and Population

Haiti is situated in the Caribbean Sea, 600 miles (965.6 kilometers) off the coast of Florida. It occupies the western third of the island of Hispaniola, which it shares with its larger neighbor, the Dominican Republic. Slightly smaller than the state of Maryland, at 10,714 square miles (27,750 square kilometers), Haiti has a population of approximately 10 million, making it one of the most densely populated countries in the world. Approximately 2 to 3 million Haitians live in Port-au-Prince, while the majority live in rural settings. After the 2010 earthquake, hundreds of thousands of Haitians moved from the nerve center of Port-au-Prince to seek refuge with family and friends in other parts of the country, greatly straining already limited resources in health, agriculture, and business.

In addition, over 2 million more Haitians living overseas make up a politically and economically influential sector affectionately known as the Haitian Diaspora. Countries where large Haitian populations reside include the United States, Dominican Republic, Canada, and Mexico.

Language

Haiti has two official languages, Haitian Creole and French. Haitian Creole (*Kreyòl*) developed over several hundred years with influence from French, western African languages, Spanish, Taíno, Arabic, and English. Although the largest linguistic contributor to Creole is French, there are enough differences that most native speakers from francophone countries would find Creole unintelligible without additional training. Haitians who have attended sufficient schooling are bilingual in French and Creole, but the majority of Haitians speak only Creole. Formal meetings, presentations, and written reports are primarily in French, but everyday conversation even among the most highly educated people is in Creole. Along the border with the Dominican Republic, many Haitians, especially men, will also speak Spanish to a certain extent, given the large numbers of Haitian migrant laborers crossing the border to find work. English proficiency is becoming increasingly common among Haitians with higher educations.

Religion

Haiti has two official religions, Catholicism and *Vodou* (Voodoo or Vaudou). There is a saying that Haiti is 80 percent Catholic but 100 percent Vodou. The origins of Vodou lie in the integration of the worship of West African deities with Catholicism early in Haiti's colonial history. These deities, or spirits, are called *loa* (*lwa* or *loua*) and coexist with a supreme God. The practice of Vodou is characterized by ritual offering ceremonies intended to win favor with particular *loas*. Most Haitians who practice Vodou also consider themselves to be full members of the Roman Catholic Church. Vodou is also intimately connected to Haitian perceptions of health, and many Haitians consult Vodou practitioners to cure physical ailments before turning to Western biomedicine. Most foreigners have been exposed to Vodou only through the popular media, which typically associates Vodou incorrectly with sorcery, Satanism, zombies, and Vodou doll curses—all far from the reality of mainstream Vodou practices and rituals.

Environment

When Columbus first set anchor off Haiti's northern coast, he found a pristine island lined with mountain ranges blanketed by dense primary forest. Now, over 500 years later, only about 1 percent of Haiti's original covering remains, compared to 28 percent for its neighbor to the east, the Dominican Republic. The consequences of such deforestation are borne mostly by Haiti's poor, who live in the steep, hilly terrain and suffer from flooding and mudslides in the rainy season. There are weak harvest yields because of the loss of topsoil, leading to food insecurity. The causes of Haiti's near-complete deforestation include clear-cutting for farming, the lack of government initiatives to increase protected land, and the rural poor's need to cut the remaining trees for cooking fuel and supplemental income. Haiti's climate is also affected by deforestation, which via global warming results in warmer temperatures year-round. Temperatures average from the 60s Fahrenheit at night to the 80s during the day—though it often feels closer to 100 degrees Fahrenheit outdoors at high noon. Deforestation also leaves the country susceptible to deadly floods during both the rainy season (May to July) and hurricane season (August to October).

Economy, Debt, and Development

Haiti is often called the poorest country in the Western Hemisphere. What is not often understood is that Haiti is as poor as, or poorer than, most impoverished sub-Saharan African nations. It ranks 147 of 169 countries listed in United Nations Development Programme's (UNDP's) Human Development Index.[1] In 2010, the per capita income was $1,200 US, placing Haiti 207 of 228 countries with available data.[2] This is in stark contrast to its closest neighbor, the Dominican Republic, where the average person makes seven times more income.

About two-thirds of Haitians are subsistence farmers, working on small plots of scarce land. The majority of exports are in the apparel industry, but this accounts for only one-tenth of economic output. The largest source of gross domestic product (GDP) is in the form of remittances from the Haitian Diaspora that collectively make up about 20 percent of Haiti's economy. Since its birth as a nation, Haiti has struggled to rid itself of external debt; the largest amount was owed to France as restitution for the so-called losses that France suffered from Haiti's revolution. This unjust loan took 113 years to repay in full, but Haiti accrued more international debt during the three decades of the Duvalier dictatorships. In recent years, much of Haiti's debt has been forgiven as part of the Heavily Indebted Poor Countries (HIPC) initiative.

Planning Global Health Work in Haiti

Global health workers in Haiti will face the types of health risks that they would find in similar poor, tropical countries. Traveler's diarrhea is common. Dehydration can easily occur, given the hot sun and rare respite from shade trees. Drinking water needs to be either boiled or treated, or from a sealed bottle; and ice should be avoided. Malaria, a mosquito-borne infectious disease is endemic in Haiti and tends to surge during the rainy season. Foreigners are at risk, especially if they work in rural areas or do not take preventive medication. Global health workers should refer to the Centers for Disease Control and Prevention (CDC) website for the latest options for malaria prevention.[3]

Security

As in many developing countries, nonviolent petty crime is common, especially in heavily populated areas such as Port-au-Prince. Global health workers should take adequate precautions to lessen their chances of being victims of crimes like pick-pocketing. It's important to avoid wearing elaborate jewelry or clothing, and traveling in pairs or groups with Haitian friends or colleagues is recommended. There are often political protests, especially before and after local and national elections, which occasionally can become violent. Avoid all political protests as a precaution. In the weeks after the 2010 earthquake, kidnappings of foreign aid workers occurred in Port-au-Prince. Subsequently, most NGOs have instituted strict security protocols for their volunteers and employees, including curfews, and some even provided armed escorts for local excursions. Road traffic accidents are common, given the poor road conditions and lack of consistent traffic regulation enforcement. Most organizations that work with global health volunteers hire local drivers to navigate around the country. Any volunteer should request the security protocol specific to his or her organization before departure, and should ideally have a security briefing shortly after arriving in Haiti.

Healthcare System

Haiti's healthcare system is made up of the public sector, private-for-profit sector, nonprofit sector, and traditional sector, characterized by the Vodou described earlier.[4] The public sector consists of the Ministry of Public Health and Population (MSPP, Ministère de la Santé Publique et de la Population) and the Ministry of Social Affairs. The private-for-profit sector is composed of health professionals engaged in private practice. The nonprofit sector consists of MSPP staff who work in private facilities often established by NGOs or FBOs.

According to the most recent data published by WHO/PAHO in 2000, there were 371 *dispensaires* (health posts), 217 health centers, and 49 hospitals. Of the 49 hospitals, 31 were located in the West Department where Port-au-Prince is located. In addition, most of the medical training programs in Haiti are located in Port-au-Prince. The earthquake destroyed 70 percent of the physical healthcare infrastructure in the country. Forty percent of the only academic teaching hospital in Haiti, l'Hôpital Université d'Etat d'Haïti (HUEH), was destroyed during the earthquake. This includes vital structures, such as the medical and nursing schools, necessary for the future of the healthcare system in Haiti. At HUEH, the hospital buildings that were not destroyed bear the face of poverty, having been neglected for many years as the result of underfunding. Equally debilitated are the facilities and equipment within hospitals. This, coupled with chronically limited resources, leaves much of the healthcare system reliant on NGOS.

Healthcare Workforce

With only 0.25 physicians per 1,000 patients, one-tenth of the US figure, *task shifting*—the process of delegating tasks, where appropriate, to less specialized health workers—is a necessary approach to healthcare in Haiti. A family member will take the role of patient care assistant, a CHW or patient care assistant will take the role of nurse, and a nurse will take the role of doctor. Given the limited number of hospital beds in the country, 1.3 beds per 1,000 people or one-third of the US figure, hospitals that have removed the financial barriers to care (that is, user fees) are always full. As a result, even with task shifting, nurses and doctors working in Haiti are inevitably overwhelmed caring for patients and their families. Most of the time there are not enough doctors, not enough nurses, not enough medications, and not enough diagnostics. Haitian healthcare professionals work in regularly understaffed and under-resourced environments.

Even before the earthquake, there were few centers with the personnel to create specialized training programs. This is in part a result of the infamous brain drain: talented healthcare professionals from low- and middle-income countries emigrate to higher-income countries in the hope of a better livelihood. The lack of subspecialty care has contributed to the neglect of challenging infectious diseases as well as noncommunicable diseases. In addition to being overworked, Haitian healthcare providers and global health workers in Haiti still must watch their patients die senseless deaths, knowing that surgical and medical treatments that could save them exist but remain unavailable to the poor.

Water and Sanitation

Frustration is not just limited to medical obstacles, including the lack of general and specialized staff, stock-outs of key medications and supplies, and equipment failures faced on a daily basis. Those challenges are small compared to other obstacles to good health, including lack of access to potable water, lack of electricity, lack of sanitation, and lack of shelter—challenges that must be overcome to rebuild Haiti's healthcare system. A rural Haitian home typically consists of one room for cooking and sleeping. Most homes still don't have clean, running water, electricity, or indoor sanitation. In real-world statistics, 70 percent of Haitians living in rural areas do not have access to potable water, and 80 percent have only a rudimentary toilet or none at all. As of 2012, estimates suggest that there are still over half a million Haitians living in internally displaced persons (IDP) camps in Port-au-Prince, often sheltered from the elements only by tarps.

Poor sanitation and water systems have plagued Haiti for decades. In 1998, after determining that the water systems in most Haitian cities were deplorably inadequate, the Inter-American Development Bank approved a loan of $54 million US and a grant of $965,000 US to improve potable water and sanitation services and to establish a regulatory framework for developing waste-water services.[5] In 2001, that money was withheld after the United States voiced concerns, later felt to be political, about disbursing the loan—thus blocking the financing of clean water systems in the country.[6] A year later, Haiti was ranked 147 of 147 countries surveyed in the water poverty index (WPI), an international measure comparing performance in the water sector across countries.[7]

Leading Health Issues

As a result, by nearly all accounts, the health indicators of Haitians are far worse than those of their neighbors. Compared to other countries that make up the WHO Region of the Americas, Haiti's under-five child mortality rate and maternal mortality ratio are five times higher than the regional average. On average, ten times more cases of TB are diagnosed in Haiti per year, and the prevalence of HIV, at about 1.9 percent, far exceeds that of any country in the region.[8] The stark differences in health outcome statistics are similar when examining other indicators, such as neonatal mortality and diarrheal or respiratory diseases. There is also widespread food insecurity and childhood malnutrition. These dramatic disparities lead to an average life expectancy in Haiti fourteen years lower than others in the region (62 versus 76).

Paul Farmer, physician, medical anthropologist, and co-founder of Partners in Health (PIH), an NGO based in Haiti since 1983, has used the medical term *acute-on-chronic* to define Haiti's current healthcare system. When Dr. Farmer arrived in Haiti in the early 1980s, the health facilities serving the poor were nonexistent to mediocre at best. Even today, the lack of resources, including clinics, personnel, and medications, has left a system poorly equipped to address the health needs of a healthy population or address the challenges brought on by medical and natural disasters. As a result, acute catastrophes exert even more long-lasting effects on the chronically fragile system. Three examples of acute-on-chronic events that have greatly shaped the health of the Haitian people are the HIV/AIDS epidemic, the 2010 earthquake, and the subsequent cholera epidemic.

HIV/AIDS epidemic

In 1983, Jeffrey Viera published a report in the *New England Journal of Medicine* on ten previously healthy heterosexual Haitians in the United States with Acquired Immune Deficiency Syndrome, or AIDS.[9] Haitian immigrants were thus thought to be an at-risk group, which the CDC initially identified as homosexual men, heroin users, hemophiliacs, and Haitians. This became known as the "Four-H Club," and discrimination against Haiti debilitated the economy through a drastic decline in tourism and trade. Haitian providers caring for patients with AIDS founded the Groupe Haïtien d'Étude du Sarcome de Kaposi et des Infections Opportunistes (GHESKIO), a training, service, and research program established to combat the rapidly spreading and, at that time, mysterious AIDS epidemic. Within the same year that Viera published his results, some of the founders of GHESKIO described the first cases of AIDS in Haiti.[10] In this series, 80 percent of patients were men and often presented with weight loss, diarrheal illnesses, and skin diseases. They were found to have Kaposi's sarcoma or opportunistic infections such as Pneumocystis carinii pneumonia, central nervous system toxoplasmosis, genital herpes, disseminated cytomegalovirus, or cryptosporidosis—diseases that would soon be described as AIDS defining. Regardless of their presentation, all the patients died.[11]

With no existing form of primary healthcare to support this new population of young, severely ill Haitians, HIV/AIDS spread throughout the country, infecting members of all socioeconomic classes, with a disproportionate impact on the rural poor. In the context of poverty, many young women living in urban areas turned to transactional sex for financial security. Those not involved in the sex trade were often victims of sexual violence perpetrated by men in authoritative positions, such as police or husbands. Forced to migrate to and from major cities in search of economic opportunities, men and women from rural areas unknowingly brought the disease back home.[12]

The lack of knowledge about the disease, and the idea of fidelity being defined as having sex without a condom, led heterosexual intercourse to become the dominant mode of transmission by 1985. The unclear etiology of the disease, the universally morbid and fatal outcome, as well as the lack of access to clinics and medicines to treat HIV/AIDS and its opportunistic infections led to the stigmatization of people with HIV/AIDS, discouraging them from seeking medical care when symptoms arose.

As of 2009, it was estimated that 120,000 people in Haiti were living with AIDS with an adult prevalence rate of 1.9%.[13] This is a significant reduction from the HIV prevalence of 10% of the adults living in Port-au-Prince in 1989.[14] This decrease is largely due to the HIV prevention and care program within the country; yet these rates are still high compared to a prevalence of 1.1 percent in the Dominican Republic and 0.6 percent in the United States. Another disease of poverty, TB, which was already endemic (30 percent of population with latent TB) in Haiti prior to the advent of HIV/AIDS, only increased with the epidemic. HIV produces a progressive decline in cell-mediated immunity, altering the pathogenesis of TB and greatly increasing the risk of developing active disease in patients co-infected with HIV and latent TB. Indeed, an HIV-negative person has a 5 to 10 percent lifetime risk of developing active TB, and an HIV-positive person has a 10 percent annual risk of developing active TB.

The Earthquake

On January 12, 2010, at 4:53 (GMT - 5) on a sunny afternoon, a magnitude 7.0 earthquake struck Léogâne, just ten miles south of Port-au-Prince. For forty devastating seconds, people who were inside struggled to escape the buildings collapsing around them, and people on the streets fought to keep their balance and evade dangerous falling debris. The earthquake destroyed or severely damaged 90 percent of the buildings in Léogâne and 70 percent in Port-au-Prince, including twenty-eight of twenty-nine federal buildings and the National Palace. By 4:54 p.m., Haiti had suffered its worst earthquake on record, and humankind had witnessed one of the largest losses of life from a natural disaster. Instantly, more than 230,000 lives were lost, with hundreds more deaths in the following weeks from catastrophic injuries. Tens of thousands were injured, and over one-half of Port-au-Prince's population was left homeless. Among those killed were people that Haiti needed the most in its hour of greatest need—nearly the entire second-year class of nursing students was buried in classrooms at HUEH, one-half of Port-au-Prince's police force was decimated, hundreds of government workers did not escape their crumbling ministries, and dozens of UN personnel, including its chief of mission, died in their headquarters.

The earthquake left in its wake a new population of homeless people; those with chronic diseases such as diabetes and hypertension suffered the most. People who could afford medications lost them, and there was no pharmacy or money to replace them. In addition to the new homeless population, Haiti's healthcare system was now forced to confront two always present but ignored populations: the physically disabled and those with psychiatric disease. In a country already plagued with poverty and that had already demonstrated its vulnerability to disease and natural disasters, the *goudou goudou* (Creole colloquial term for earthquake) acutely exacerbated the scarcity of resources and highlighted the unidimensional nature of the nation's healthcare system, which had spent the last three decades focusing almost exclusively on HIV/AIDS.

Nongovernmental Organizations

When working in Haiti, it's essential to understand the role and scope of NGOs (here, we use NGO to represent both FBOs and CSOs [civil service organizations]) as they relate to the public sector. Namely, how does the organization's work align itself with the overall goals and objectives that the GOH has set for increasing development for the country as a whole? As of this writing, an estimated 10,000 NGOs are actively implementing programs in Haiti. That's the second-highest per capita ratio in the world.[15] Many public health practitioners would argue that the presence of so many NGOs may actually hinder, not help, development in Haiti because NGOs often are better than the Haitian government at attracting grant money from donors, thereby handicapping Haitians from being able to help themselves. For example, in 2007–2008, USAID spent all $300 million US allocated for Haiti on programs implemented by NGOs. After the earthquake, of the $2 billion US donated to Haiti relief efforts, less than 1 percent went directly to the government, while the overwhelming majority went to NGOs and private organizations. Much of this money went toward creating a parallel health system, as opposed to supporting Haiti's public sector, an act that not only undermines the current healthcare system but also the Haitian people. Without money and support from those trained in developing health systems, Haiti's health system will remain impoverished.

It is the responsibility and desire of the GOH to set national health priorities. Therefore, although at times it is much more challenging, global health workers are encouraged to communicate all projects being undertaken to the appropriate local ministry before beginning. Ideally, large projects would be carried out in partnership with the public sector and in support of the national health systems. In such an environment, one has an opportunity to train and serve Haitians while creating a lasting change within the country.

Working with the government is imperative, but it is also beneficial to partner with other NGOs. Collaborating not only diminishes redundancy, but can magnify efforts made to improve the health of the Haitian people. Many health-related NGOs currently working in Haiti have shown a long-lasting commitment to Haiti, and have recently enlisted global health volunteers to continue their work. These include Partners in Health, Hôpital Albert Schweitzer (HAS), Project Medishare, GHESKIO, St. Boniface Haiti Foundation, and Center for Rural Development of Milot Foundation (CRUDEM). In the rest of this chapter, we highlight the response of one of these organizations, Partners in Health, with which we have worked closely. In its work addressing the HIV/AIDS epidemic, the 2010 earthquake, and the cholera epidemic, PIH has taught critical lessons, including the importance of linking prevention with care, the value of long-standing relationships in effective global health delivery, and the significance of partnerships. We believe that global health volunteers should practice these lessons as they work in Haiti.

Partners in Health and Zanmi Lasante
Respond to the HIV/AIDS Epidemic

In 1985, Zanmi Lasante (ZL), the sister organization of PIH, started as a community-based health organization serving Cange, a squatter settlement in the Central Plateau, Haiti, formed by a population of peasants displaced by the construction of the Péligre hydroelectric dam. Two years later PIH was formed, in recognition of the need to establish long-term partnerships within Haiti and the United States to provide healthcare to this disenfranchised population. The members of the organization initially focused on HIV/AIDS patients in rural Haiti. In 1986, the first case of AIDS was detected in the Central Plateau. By 1988, Clinique Bon Sauveur offered free testing and counseling, and had launched an extensive HIV/AIDS prevention program. Despite the discovery and use of antiretroviral therapy (ART) to treat HIV patients in the United States starting in 1987, PIH providers watched helplessly for years as many of their friends, patients, and colleagues died from AIDS. Commonly cited arguments against using highly active antiretroviral therapy (HAART) in poor patients in resource-limited settings included that HAART is too expensive, there is inadequate health infrastructure to provide and monitor the medications, and the inevitable lack of compliance will lead to resistance.

In 1993, with the creation of the Institute for Health and Social Justice (IHSJ), PIH set out to advocate for decreased cost and increased access to the lifesaving ART available in resource-rich countries such as the United States. In 1995 zidovudine (AZT), a type of antiretroviral, was offered to HIV-positive pregnant women to prevent mother-to-child transmission of the virus. Three years later, through the HIV Equity Initiative, HAART was offered to patients with clinically advanced AIDS. This was revolutionary in that it linked prevention with the provision of care, activities previously considered mutually exclusive. The program enlisted CHWs—laypeople chosen by the community and trained to be health agents—to educate the community about the disease, to provide psychosocial support for patients, and to administer free HAART to patients daily. This became known as directly observed therapy-HAART, or DOT-HAART, modeled after the effective TB initiative.

The success of the HIV Equity Initiative at first rested in its ability to secure external funding through private donors to continue the efforts while working effectively and collaboratively with the MSPP in Haiti. Then in 2002, with the development of the Global Fund to Fight AIDS, Tuberculosis and Malaria (GFATM) as well as the US President's Emergency Plan for AIDS Relief (PEPFAR), PIH/ZL was able to scale up its activities to reach a larger population of patients.

PIH/ZL's continued success lay in its recognition that prevention and care are linked, and that care includes not only providing medicines, but also addressing structural barriers to care. In Haiti, structural barriers to care, including the cost of medical care and non-HIV/AIDS related medications, were eliminated. Testing and treatment for HIV, other sexually transmitted illnesses (STIs), and TB were offered as part of primary healthcare. People suffering from severe malnutrition were given nutritional support in the form of rice, cooking oil, and beans. Monetary stipends were provided to combat the prohibitive cost of transportation to and from follow-up appointments.

This approach to HIV/AIDS care strengthened not only HIV care but the healthcare system generally, forming a comprehensive healthcare system that provides free care to approximately 1.2 million people in Haiti's Central Plateau. This model of prevention and care has served as a model in the treatment of infectious diseases such as cholera, as well as in the treatment of noncommunicable diseases such as cancer.

Partners in Health and Zanmi Lasante Respond to the Earthquake

PIH/ZL was one of the first responders after the earthquake. For nearly three decades, PIH/ZL has partnered with MSPP to operate twelve hospitals in Haiti and, as of this writing, currently employs more than 6,000 local CHWs, who act as liaisons between patients and the healthcare system. Over the years, through its commitment to Haiti, PIH/ZL has built strong local, regional, and national relationships with Haiti's leadership.

So although PIH/ZL is not in itself a disaster relief organization, Haitians and the GOH have trusted it to help lead disaster relief efforts. As night fell on January 12, 2010, several PIH/ZL physicians were already in Port-au-Prince triaging and treating the wounded, despite minimal supplies and severely limited communication because power sources and cellular phone provider lines had all suffered heavy damage. Dozens of PIH/ZL staff from its rural hospitals set out immediately to bring desperately needed material and human reinforcements. Within days, teams from PIH/ZL headquarters in Boston and on the ground in Haiti were able to mobilize volunteer surgical missions from the United States, and had several fully functional operating rooms running twenty-four hours a day.[16]

Inside Port-au-Prince, PIH/ZL took an active role in caring for a large portion of the newly homeless population, which numbered well over 1 million. In collaboration with the public sector, PIH/ZL created mobile clinics in four spontaneous settlement camps and provided ongoing medical care to 100,000 victims. In addition, knowing the shortcomings of the Haiti healthcare system, PIH also expanded its mental health team to begin psychosocial outreach to this vulnerable population. PIH also set up a rehabilitation program with HAS. Within the first six months after the earthquake, dozens of patients with amputated limbs received prostheses and took their first steps in the physical therapy program. Outside Port-au-Prince, PIH/ZL rural hospitals prepared for the inevitable onslaught of patients. The hospitals, filled to capacity, had to think creatively about how to house an overwhelming influx of patients. One hospital took over the worship space of the church next door, and turned it into a full surgical ward with dozens of patient beds.

While hundreds of injured earthquake victims left Port-au-Prince and presented to PIH/ZL's rural hospitals in search of medical care, the majority of victims presented to HUEH, the largest public referral hospital in the country. Located just a few minutes' walk from the National Palace in downtown Port-au-Prince, the HUEH campus houses the nation's largest medical and nursing schools, and is home to the majority of residency training programs. As injured earthquake survivors struggled to seek care, hundreds made their way to HUEH, only to find that the hospital itself had suffered unthinkable losses. While many HUEH staff understandably left to search for and assure the safety of their loved ones, those who remained were overwhelmed quickly as the wave of patients poured in from throughout the city. To compound their seemingly insurmountable challenges, the nurses and doctors who stayed to provide clinical care those first few nights had to work without electricity, with no running water, and with virtually no material resources.

What happened next in the first few weeks after January 12, 2010, illustrates the successful, albeit imperfect, partnership created among HUEH leadership and staff, dozens of multinational NGOs, and private companies, and military forces from several countries. Working together around the clock to rescue limbs, treat infections, and relieve pain, the collective effort of this collaboration saved countless lives and provided hope for the survival of thousands of earthquake victims.

PIH's name acknowledges that without partners, it would be impossible to successfully combat the social and political determinants of poor health in Haiti. As a result, most of PIH/ZL's work has been done with the public health sector or other NGOs. From the early days post-earthquake until months later, when most of the NGOs had left HUEH, in order to minimize redundancy and maximize efficiency, the hospital's Haitian leadership had control over how the resources brought in from outside organizations should be allocated and used. To this end, the head of the hospital and his assistants met regularly with representatives from all of the NGOs present at HUEH to divide tasks, assess progress, collectively resolve problems, disseminate information, and request resources.

PIH/ZL was assigned the task of providing surgical teams to staff the two operating rooms that eventually ran twenty-four hours a day. It was also asked to provide a PIH physician to serve as liaison between HUEH leaders and NGOs; this led to improved communication between partners and expedited recognition of obstacles to clinical care. International Medical Corps (IMC) took the lead in staffing the emergency department, which in the first few months after the earthquake was housed in several large military tents, much like the majority of the other clinical wards. The Swiss Red Cross worked with Haitian physicians to operate the pediatric wards, while multiple NGOs, including PIH/ZL, recruited large surgical teams to care for injured earthquake victims. Other organizations, such as Bomberos Sin Fronteras (Firefighters Without Borders) and Operation Blessing, made it their objective to provide clean water. The US Air Force 92nd Airborne provided security, transport for patients who needed more specialized care not available at HUEH (to US Naval Ship Comfort or University of Miami field hospital, or evacuated out of the country), and direct patient care when requested. The Clinton Foundation stepped in to organize the supply chain and keep the new pharmacy stocked with medications and equipment. Private companies also made vital contributions to the medical care at HUEH. For example, a communications company donated dozens of high-end walkie-talkies to allow multiple medical staff to collaborate in real time. The entire tremendous effort depended on the leadership of the HUEH director and his deputies, and on the willingness of all NGOs working at the hospital to act as partners.

Cholera Epidemic

Cholera is an infectious disease acquired by drinking water in which the bacterium *Vibrio cholerae* has been introduced by the feces of an infected person. Many infections are asymptomatic or cause mild gastroenteritis. In severe cases there can be vomiting and profuse watery diarrhea resulting in electrolyte imbalances, profound dehydration, and death within just hours of the initial symptoms. Cholera is easy to prevent with access to clean drinking water and modern sanitation, and to treat with appropriate rehydration therapy and antibiotics. But when the outbreak began in Haiti, these resources were scarce. Prior to October 2010, cases of severe diarrhea in Haiti were assumed to be due to typhoid until proven otherwise, but this mindset suddenly changed.

On the night of October 19, 2010, five days after the first case of a patient with acute, watery diarrhea in Mirebalais, sixty patients suffering with similar symptoms presented to l'Hôpital de Saint Nicolas (HSN), a public hospital in the coastal city of St. Marc. Within four days, the National Public Health Laboratory in Haiti confirmed the presence of the El Tor biotype of *Vibrio cholerae* serogroup 01. Cholera had not been previously been reported in Haiti.[17]

Contamination by human feces of the Meye tributary of the Artibonite River initially resulted in the spread to residents along the riverbank in Mirebalais, but the cholera epidemic quickly grew to include residents from every department. Given PIH/ZL's presence at l'Hôpital de Saint Nicolas (HSN) since 2007, and its expertise in community-based health models in Haiti, the organization was well positioned to provide immediate care and to mobilize existing resources. Within eight hours of recognizing the epidemic, several physicians and nurses from other PIH/ZL sites in both the Central Plateau and Artibonite departments immediately traveled to St. Marc, the epicenter of the cholera outbreak, to begin treating patients. Within twenty-four hours, foreign doctors and nurses who had worked with PIH/ZL in Haiti previously also arrived to care for patients. Volunteers were involved in direct patient care as well as logistical planning.

PIH/ZL joined the UN health cluster, a forum for the GOH and NGOs in health, which convened daily to foster a synergistic team approach. At HSN, PIH worked closely with Médecins Sans Frontières, an organization with expertise in cholera epidemics. PIH/ZL collaborated with many other groups, including J/P Haitian Relief Organization (J/P HRO), which sent medical teams and provided workers to regularly disinfect the hospital, as well as medical teams sent by the governments of Cuba and Mexico.

PIH/ZL's experience as a community-based organization in Haiti made it particularly effective in the cholera relief efforts. In addition to providing care at HSN, PIH/ZL attempted to decrease the pre-care mortality rate using its previously successful model of CHWs as health agents. Within two weeks, PIH/ZL had trained 600 *accompagnateurs* in how to prevent the transmission of cholera, decontaminate homes, and care for the bodies of those that had died. These CHWs were given cholera treatment packets and went out to educate and treat their communities. The UN provided helicopters for the CHWs to reach distant villages, including those isolated from relief efforts because of overflowing river water or impassable roads.

CHWs informed the PIH/ZL leadership of areas that needed cholera treatment centers (CTCs) erected, to address the many critically ill patients who were dying before receiving any medical aid. A CTC is a contained space where severely ill patients can receive IV fluids and antibiotics, while those with mild disease can receive oral rehydration solution. Shortly after the outbreak, PIH physicians Louise Ivers and Paul Farmer partnered with Haitian ZL leaders Charles Patrick Almazor and Fernet Leandre to publish a report on five complementary interventions to slow cholera.[18] This emphasized the need to improve Haiti's water insecurity through public works projects and point-of-care water-purification systems. It also stressed the need to start using cholera vaccine, which was in very short supply when the epidemic began.

Today all healthcare facilities in Haiti have a plan in place to address cholera. The national approach is to treat patients with aggressive oral therapy and antibiotics while strengthening the water and sanitation infrastructure, and to vaccinate the country. By 2012 widespread oral cholera vaccination programs have begun. Yet people are still acquiring new infections, particularly during rainy periods. As of the two-year mark in October 2012 the cholera epidemic has killed more than 7,500 people and caused illness in more than 600,000.[19]

Conclusion

Haiti's weak economy, sparse healthcare workforce, limited medical supplies, poor water and sanitation systems, and political instability made it especially vulnerable to the HIV/AIDS epidemic, the 2010 earthquake, and the current cholera epidemic. In the case of the earthquake, weak economic opportunities elsewhere led millions of rural peasants to seek better opportunities in Port-au-Prince. This resulted in an overpopulated urban area that could not address the needs of its citizens. With poor road infrastructure, no emergency medical system, and limited medical care, the injuries and deaths from the earthquake exponentially increased. Cholera highlighted the decades of poor water and sanitation systems in Haiti as it spread rapidly throughout the country.

Although the personal rewards of helping those most in need are vast, frustration is inevitable in the face of human pain and suffering unrelieved because common medicines and medical equipment are unavailable. It's up to the GOH to continue to build supportive health systems and enact social change, but global health workers must continue to provide care and show a commitment to Haiti in the form of long-lasting partnerships, so that Haiti can build a healthcare system that responds to the needs of its citizens.

The Community Is Our Family

Guerre Maxin was born in Caracol, a commune of Lascahobas, Haiti. He did well in school and attended up to the eighth grade. At that time, his father died and his mother was too poor to continue to pay school fees. Guerre worked odd jobs and became a CHW in 2008, after being nominated by members of his hometown. He primarily serves pregnant women in Caracol. He also ensures that kids in his community through age five years receive their immunizations.

In response to the question "What does it mean to be an *accompagnateur*?" Guerre answers (translated by Joel Malebranche):

It means for me to watch and help the community. We are support. Patients feel self-confident because they have us as support. Some people are dealing with more than being sick. They are dealing with a family loss or a tough childbirth. We are ready to help because the community is our family. We live with them. Their pain is our pain. We work together on how we can improve the situation. Many patients are humiliated by their problems. We are the ones who know how they feel. Our job is to be on the ground and serve our people.

How to Strengthen Haiti's Health Infrastructure

Charles Patrick Almazor MD, MPH is the Director of Clinical Services Zanmi Lasante. He was born in Port-au-Prince and raised in Carrefour, Haiti. He decided to become a doctor as a high school student after being hospitalized with malaria in a public health facility in Haiti. He wanted to address the lack of access to medical services throughout the country. Charles attended medical school at Université d'Etat d'Haïti. He completed his one-year social service at Cange in Clinique Bon Sauveur, where he learned about PIH/ZL and its clinical work. He was then asked to head the PIH/ZL HIV program in Thomonde, Haiti. He remained HIV program director for two-and-a-half years, after which he took the over the MDR-TB program in Cange for the remaining year. As a Fulbright scholar, Charles obtained his masters in public health at the University of Alabama, and spent three months working in the HIV unit at PAHO in Washington, DC. In 2007, he returned to work with PIH as the regional director of programs in Rwanda. He returned to Haiti in 2009, where he has been a leader in HIV/AIDS care, post-earthquake efforts, and cholera prevention and care.

Charles writes:

Article 22 of the Haitian national constitution states that the GOH is obligated to create a health infrastructure that provides care to its citizens. To this end, the Haitian government has invested in training human resources, like doctors, nurses and other healthcare professionals, and in building health facilities. Despite the government's good intentions, there is insufficient funding to provide medicines and equipment for healthcare personnel to care for their patients. There is also not enough money to pay healthcare personnel competitive salaries. I will focus on low salaries, a complaint that often arises in Haiti, as that was particularly frustrating to volunteers during the earthquake recovery efforts and because of its significant effects on patient care.

In Haiti, an experienced professor is paid approximately $375 US a month. Due to this, the public medical education system does not attract very talented professors. This then results in substandard training of medical students, who, due to poor training, will go on to provide substandard, non-evidence-based care to their patients. Another unintended consequence is that doctors and nurses work several hours less than the mandated forty hours a week. This allows them to accept a second job with a private medical facility. Without healthcare personnel, hospitals and clinics cannot function. Haitian doctors and nurses want to care for their patients, but they also want to feed their families. Global health workers can help with medical training of our students and also help the government build a healthcare system that supports the work of our doctors and nurses.

Notes

1 United Nations Development Program, "Human Development Reports," accessed Jan. 21 2012, available from http://hdr.undp.org.

2 Central Intelligence Agency, *The World Factbook* (Washington: CIA), accessed Nov. 26, 2011, available from www.cia.gov.

3 Centers for Disease Control and Prevention, "Malaria," accessed Jan. 24, 2012, available from www.cdc.gov.

4 Pan American Health Organization, "Haiti," accessed Jan. 24, 2012, available from www.paho.org.

5 Center for Human Rights and Global Justice (CHRGJ), Partners in Health, Robert F.

Kennedy Center for Justice and Human Rights, and Zanmi Lasante. "Woch Nan Soley: The Denial of the Right to Water in Haiti" (2008).

6 Paul Farmer, Mary C. Smith Fawzi, and Patrice Nevil, "Unjust Embargo of Aid for Haiti," *Lancet* 361.9355 (2003):420–423.

7 Peter Lawrence, Jeremy Meigh, and Caroline Sullivan, "The Water Poverty Index: An International Comparison," Keele Economics Research Papers (KERP) 19 (Staffordshire, UK: Keele University, 2002), 1–24.

8 World Health Organization, "Countries: Haiti," accessed Jan. 24, 2012, available from www.who.int.

9 Jeffrey Vieira, Elliot Frank, Thomas J. Spira, and Sheldon H. Landesman, "Acquired Immune Deficiency in Haitians: Opportunistic Infections in Previously Healthy Immigrants," *New England Journal of Medicine* 308.3 (1983): 125–129.

10 Jean W. Pape, Bernard Liautaud, Franck Thomas, Jean-Robert Mathurin, Marie-Myrtha A. St. Amand, Madeleine Boncy et al., "Characteristics of the Acquired Immunodeficiency Syndrome (AIDS) in Haiti," *New England Journal of Medicine* 309.16 (1983):945–950.

11 Ibid.

12 Paul Farmer, *Aids and Accusation*.

13 UNAIDS, "Haiti," accessed Dec. 3, 2012, available from http://www.unaids.org/en/regionscountries/countries/haiti.

14 Warren D. Johnson and Jean W. Pape, "AIDS in Haiti," *Immunology* Series 44 (1989):65–78.

15 Madeline Kristoff and Liz Panarelli, "Haiti: A Republic of NGOs?" Peace Brief 23 (Washington: United States Institute of Peace, April 2010).

16 Tracy Kidder, "Recovering from Disaster—Partners in Health and the Haitian Earthquake," *New England Journal of Medicine* 362.9 (2010):769–772.

17 Centers for Disease Control and Prevention, "Emergency Preparedness and response," accessed Dec. 3, 2012, available from http://www.bt.cdc.gov/disasters/earthquakes/haiti/waterydiarrhea_pre-decision_brief.asp

18 L. C. Ivers, P. Farmer, C. P. Almazor, and F. Leandre, "Five Complementary Interventions to Slow Cholera: Haiti," *Lancet* 376.9758 (2010):2048–2051.

19 Partners in Health, "Haiti's Cholera Epidemic Reaches Two-Year Mark," accessed 4 Dec 2012, available from http://www.pih.org/news/entry/haitis-cholera-epidemic-reaches-two-year-mark/

Suggested Resources

History of Haiti

Girard, Philippe. *Haiti: The Tumultuous History—From Pearl of the Caribbean to Broken Nation*. New York: Palgrave Macmillan, 2010.

James, C. L. R. *The Black Jacobins: Toussaint L'Ouverture and the Santo Domingo Revolution*. New York: Vintage Books, 1963.

HIV/AIDS in Haiti

Farmer, Paul. *AIDs and Accusation: Haiti and the Geography of Blame*. Berkeley, CA: University of California Press, 1992.

Equity and Structural Violence

Farmer, Paul. *The Uses of Haiti*. Monroe, ME: Common Courage Press, 1994.

Partners in Health

Kidder, Tracy. *Mountains Beyond Mountains: The Quest of Dr. Paul Farmer, a Man Who Would Cure the World*. New York: Random House, 2004.

Creole Resources

Dartmouth College Rassias Center Accelerated Language Programs (ALPS): http://rassias.dartmouth.edu

Haiti Hub: www.haitihub.com

MediBabble (smartphone application for medical Creole translation): http://medibabble.com

University of Massachusetts Boston Summer Institute (three-week intensive Creole courses): www.ccde.umb.edu

Pimsleur Haitian Creole CDs

Heurtelou, Maude, and Fequiere Vilsaint. *English/Haitian Creole Medical Dictionary*. 2000.

Shapiro, Norma, and Jayme Adelson-Goldstein. *The Oxford Picture Dictionary: English/Haitian Creole*. 2008.

Turnbull, Wally. *Creole Made Easy* (with associated workbooks). 2000.

Valdman, Albert and Pierre-Henry Philippe. *Ann pale Kreyòl* (workbook and grammar primer). 2001.

8 Dominican Republic

Karen Sadler and Kim Wilson

The Dominican Republic is an island of contrasts and paradoxes. Luxury resorts on the coast lie next to communities living in extreme poverty. The country has one of the highest rates of economic growth in the region, yet has an ever-widening income disparity. Doctors, clinics, and hospitals are abundant, yet many woman and children do not receive the quality healthcare they need.

This chapter focuses on the health concerns of mothers and children. We discuss some of the social factors leading to wide disparities in health status and access to health services, and we explore some of the strengths and weaknesses of the current health system. We also describe examples of successful approaches to improving the health of women and children. The underlying principles and lessons learned from maternal child health can inform those working across all sectors of the health system.

Brief History

It's necessary to first appreciate how the Dominican Republic came to exist in order to understand what it is today. The answer to the question "What does it mean to be Dominican?" is still evolving. What follows is a thumbnail sketch of the history of the DR, emphasizing political and international relations.

The DR occupies the eastern two-thirds of the island of Hispaniola and shares its only land border with Haiti.[1] Hispaniola is located in the Caribbean between Cuba and Puerto Rico. The DR is the second-largest country in this region, in terms of population and land area (Cuba is first). Almost 10 million Dominicans live in a country slightly greater than twice the size of New Hampshire.

Hispaniola (originally named Quisqueya) was initially settled by native peoples who migrated from the tropical rain forests of South America to the Caribbean in roughly 3000 BC. There were Chiboneys, Arawaks, and Taínos, who became the dominant tribe. Driven to the northeastern part of the island by the aggressive Caribs, the Taínos numbered from perhaps 100,000 to possibly 2 million when Christopher Columbus first landed in 1492. Santo Domingo was not only the first European settlement and first capital in the

Americas, but it became Spain's headquarters in the New World. As in many countries, European presence led to the devastation of the native tribes, largely by disease, but also by migration, interbreeding, and murder. The Taínos, as a pure race, were extinct by 1865.

Bartholomew Columbus established the colony that became Santo Domingo (still the country's capital) shortly after 1492. His brother Christopher was buried there in 1506. A plantation economy was established, and West Africans were imported as slaves to support the crop-based economy. The population of Santo Domingo exploded, from 6,000 in 1737 to 125,000 in 1790. French buccaneers settled on the western part of Hispaniola when Spain was preoccupied with the Incas and Aztecs, and the western third of the island was ceded to France in 1697. This territory is the present-day Haiti.

In 1821, independence was won from Spain, but only nine weeks later, the Haitians (who had established independence from France in 1804) overran the new country. Haiti occupied the territory for twenty-two years, a fact that is still resented today by Dominicans. During this period, slavery was abolished; property was seized from both the wealthy and the Church, and was nationalized; and the economy was converted to a cash-crop model. Young Dominican men were enlisted in the army to such an extent that institutions of higher learning were abandoned. Many white Europeans fled the country. Dominicans were also forced to pay heavy taxes to Haiti.

After gaining independence in 1844, the Dominicans created a constitution based on the US Constitution. Turmoil ensued, and Pedro Santana, then leader, signed a pact with Spain reinstating the DR as a Spanish colony. Dissent followed within the DR, abetted by Haiti, and the Spanish abandoned the colony in 1865. The subsequent leader, Buenaventura Báez, requested colonial status from the United States. This was favored by President Ulysses S. Grant but rejected by the US Senate in 1870. The last decades of the nineteenth century saw relative peace and prosperity. Dominicans were able to improve their economy and to modernize the sugar industry, but the country was also plunged into debt. By 1902, Dominican autonomy was threatened by its European creditor nations.

By 1906, President Theodore Roosevelt saw a potential threat in greater European influence in the Caribbean. Worried about interference in shipping routes that would be created by the newly begun Panama Canal, he signed an agreement with the DR for American administration of all Dominican customs (revenue) and assumption of the Dominican foreign debt. Frustrated with the lack of a stable government over the next ten years, President Woodrow Wilson ordered an American occupation in 1916. This was widely opposed within the DR and was ended in 1924 by Wilson's successor, Warren

Harding, fulfilling a campaign promise. The occupation, though protested, allowed a revival of the economy, debt reduction, and the creation of physical infrastructure.

The year 1930 began the infamous Trujillo era, its scars still born by Dominicans today. Raphael Leonidas Trujillo ruled as an unconditional dictator from 1930 to 1961. Significant economic progress was made, including discharge of the foreign debt and the development of schools, clinics, and a pension plan. Trujillo and his cronies took total control of all economic enterprise and abolished personal and political freedoms. Once in power, Trujillo imposed his will through brutality, terror, and assassination. In 1937, he sought better control of the border with Haiti, and ordered his army to massacre 18,000 men, women, and children in an act of genocide while claiming it was a Dominican peasant uprising.

The four sisters from the Mirabal family and their husbands formed a group opposing the Trujillo regime, called the Movement of the Fourteenth of June. The sisters were known as Las Mariposas (the Butterflies). In the course of their political activism, the sisters and their spouses were repeatedly imprisoned. On November 25, 1960, three of the sisters were brutally murdered by Trujillo's men after visiting their husbands in prison. The Dominican people were enraged; the anti-Trujillo movement grew, and Trujillo was assassinated six months later. The Mirabal sisters became known as the Unforgettable Butterflies. To commemorate them, in 1981 the United Nations designated November 25 as International Day for the Elimination of Violence against Women. Memories of Trujillo's atrocities are still sharp in the minds of many older Dominicans.[2]

Trujillo's death signified the beginning of political democracy. United States president Lyndon Johnson intervened in Dominican affairs in 1965 in what was called Operation Powerpack, overseeing presidential elections—and attempting to assure that neither Cuba nor the "communists" would wield influence in the country. This brought Joaquín Balaguer to power, which he retained until 1978 as a military oligarch. Since then, the DR has had a succession of democratically elected leaders, though tainted by a legacy of corruption. Grassroots involvement in the political process is strong. The democratic process today is messy but genuine: campaign posters and billboards line the roads, and there is free and open political debate.

The People

As of this writing, there are about 10 million Dominicans living in the DR, which ranks it mid-size (82 of 193) among the world's countries. It has an annual population growth rate of 1.5 percent, and 40 percent of Dominicans are under age fifteen. Santo Domingo is the largest city, with over 3 million. Sixty-five percent of the population is urban.[3]

The DR is a mixed-race society. Sixteen percent of the population is Caucasian and 11 percent black. The majority, approximately 73 percent are a multiracial mixture of European, African, and Taíno ancestry. The DR inherited from Spain a race-conscious class structure, and racism is pervasive in Dominican society. Although 90 percent of Dominicans have some West African blood, most do not identify themselves as black. Far from being color-blind, Dominicans have many words to describe skin tones (and unfortunately, darker-skinned individuals are at a cultural disadvantage). Those of Haitian descent have experienced discrimination and social exclusion. There is also the complex issue of the legal status of "nonresidents" who have lived in the DR for a significant amount of time and yet are "stateless." That said, in 2010 the Dominican people and their government were generous toward Haitians injured by the earthquake.

Roman Catholicism is practiced by 70 percent of Dominicans, and 18 percent are Evangelical. Abortion is illegal under all circumstances, even those that threaten the life of the mother. Education is free and compulsory for ages five to fourteen, though not accessible by many in remote areas of the country. Higher education is not possible for many poor Dominican children. Wealthy Dominican children are often sent to private schools, many of which are nonsecular.

Economics

The DR has the second-largest economy among Caribbean and Central American countries, ranking as an upper-middle-income developing country. In comparison to the 2010 per capita GDP of $47,000 in the United States and $1,200 in Haiti, that of the DR is $8,600. However, there is a skewed distribution of income, with the upper 20 percent receiving 55 percent of the total income. The service industry (tourism and free-trade-zone manufacturing) is the largest employer; agriculture is second. Textiles, tobacco, sugar, coffee, and beverages are the main export products. The United States is the DR's largest trade partner: 58 percent of exports are bound for the United States. Haiti and Western Europe are also significant partners.[4]

Practical Insights
Dominican–United States Ties

The Dominican-American relationship goes back at least 150 years, and remains an important force in modern Dominican society. The Dominican community in the United States is estimated at 1.2 million, which is over 10 percent of the entire population within the DR. Remittances from overseas Dominicans account for 10 percent of the country's GDP. Dominican communities in the United States are concentrated in the Northeast (in New York, New Jersey, and Massachusetts), with a second concentration in Florida. Of the Dominicans in the United States, about 73 percent are non-US citizens. New York is by far the largest community, concentrated in the Washington Heights section of Manhattan. The 70,000 Dominicans living in New England are mainly located in Boston's Jamaica Plain neighborhood and in areas north of Boston.[5]

There have been three large waves of emigration: in 1961 after Trujillo's assassination, from 1966 to 1978, and in the 1980s, spurred by high rates of unemployment and inflation.

Many Dominican immigrants view their time living in the United States as temporary. Their typical immigration pattern involves cycles of immigration and repatriation, with families often split between a home village in the DR and a Dominican community in the States. In her book *The Transnational Villagers*, Peggy Levitt documents the depth and strength of these connections in an analysis of the socioeconomic, family, and cultural ties between a Dominican community outside of Boston and a village near Baní.[6] She documents a remarkably free flow of family members, repatriated money, cultural practices, media, and merchandise between the two communities. Likewise, these transnational Dominicans often receive healthcare services in both the Dominican and the US systems. Time spent in the States also has an effect on the family and community dynamics of Dominicans. In Levitt's study, families traveling between the Dominican Republic and the United States were less likely to include extended family members, and were more likely to be headed by a female and be better educated.

The close ties between the United States and the DR can be of potential import to health workers. Economically, US communities represent a significant source of repatriated funds and potential sources of philanthropic funds. Socially, extensive migration and family separation increases the importance of the extended family and community. The widespread introduction of American cultural influence, from fast food to baseball, has had a dual impact. Close ties to the United States lead to a generally warm and friendly response to American workers. On the other hand, poor nutritional influences most likely contribute to increasing rates of obesity and to a low breast-feeding rate. Strong ties to the States can both help and hinder access to heath services, with some duplication and disruption of services as families migrate between the two countries. In an example of a positive influence, the maternal newborn NGO Infante Sano grew around the service to migrating patients shared between pediatricians in the United States and in the DR.[7]

Haitian Immigrants and Batey Communities

A population of special concern lives and works on the sugar-cane plantations, commonly known as *bateyes*, of the Dominican Republic. Batey communities generally include a central administrative office, a sugar mill and refinery, the fields of cane, and barracks housing the field workers. Due to seasonal spikes in the need for labor and a historic reluctance by Dominicans to perform this work, the DR has relied for more than seventy years on a migrant labor force from Haiti. Haiti, with a poverty rate of 80 percent (and an abject poverty rate of 54 percent) and a per capita income of less than one-sixth of its only neighbor's, is a steady supplier of young men eager to work.

Until 1986, Dominican heads of state paid a finder's fee for migrant workers.[8] More recently, many landowners pay *buscones* (headhunters) to round up the labor supply. These headhunters often promise young Haitians a "work permit" and also extract a fee from the prospective immigrant for the work. Haitians are often stripped of their Haitian identity cards and find themselves working long hours in challenging conditions for extremely low wages. Racial discrimination makes it difficult to leave the bateyes for better work (though some people do, and find work in tourism, agriculture, and domestic jobs), and the Haitians remain in poverty, "stranded" in a country that is not theirs. Because their homeland provides little in the way of a better opportunity, many choose to stay in the DR beyond the six-month harvest period. Over the years, a year-round and stable population has arisen, numbering at least 800,000. Yet these communities remain stateless and marginalized from Dominican society. Only 5 percent are documented and, because they are considered "persons in transit," no path to citizenship has ever been available to this population or to their children—or to subsequent generations—even those born on the batey who identify themselves as Dominican rather than Haitian.

A 1999 survey of the bateyes found remarkably stable communities. Ninety-seven percent of the residents lived in the bateyes year-round, and two-thirds of households had both parents. One-third of residents were under age five; one-half were under age fifteen. Only 6 percent were born in Haiti, and two-thirds of mothers identified themselves and their children as Dominican. Only one-half knew any Kreyòl (the language of Haiti).[9] Without birth certificates, these Haitian-Dominicans have limited access to government services, from schools to clinics. According to a 2007 report by Amnesty International, two-thirds of batey dwellers have no sanitation, one-third are illiterate, and only 7 percent have a clinic or dispensary on their bateyes.[10] Ostensibly, these services should be provided by the State Sugar Council, but few, if any, are. Because healthcare is nationalized in the DR (thus requiring an identity card to access), preventive services are often denied to this population. Privately offered services are too expensive. In the past, world outcry has been met with aggressive deportation campaigns by the Dominican government.[11]

The economic situation of Haitians living in the DR is worse than that of the poorest one-fifth of Dominicans. Not surprisingly, healthcare indices here are significantly worse than those of the DR as a whole. As estimated by the Batey Relief Alliance, 40 percent of batey children under age five are chronically malnourished. One-third are stunted (a linear growth deficit caused by chronic undernutrition), and *kwashiorkor* (a state of malnutrition involving severe protein deficiency) is still seen in the bateyes because sugar cane is used to pacify hunger. Immunization rates are difficult to ascertain, though they are significantly less than national rates. Diarrhea and parasites are rampant.[12] The most common conditions in children include gastrointestinal and parasitic disease, skin infections, upper respiratory infections, asthma and allergy symptoms, and symptomatic anemia.[13] The majority of children present with chronic medical problems and multiple complaints, reflecting the general lack of access to primary and preventive health services. Among adults, diabetes mellitus, hypertension, and gastrointestinal complaints are major causes of morbidity, though the most frequent complaint at clinics is pain (back pain in men from the work of cutting sugar cane, and headaches and abdominal pain in women). Dental decay is prevalent, from the habit of sucking on sugar cane. Cataracts from long hours working in the bright sun are universal in men over age fifty.

HIV prevalence in the bateyes has been reported as greater than 5 percent, in contrast to a 1.1 percent prevalence among adults in the DR.[14] Poverty in the bateyes promotes the spread of HIV, due to lack of education and access to preventive strategies such as condoms. The ratio of HIV between men and women is 1 to 1, which reflects heterosexual transmission as well as a growing sex trade. HIV-positive batey residents remain a relatively untargeted population. Unfortunately, although foreign aid organizations and NGOs are active in the bateyes, efforts remain decentralized and uncoordinated.[15]

Larger economic issues also threaten the viability of the batey population. Although plantations once numbered around 400,[16] the decline in the sugar industry has led to a reduction in plantation size and number. As the economic importance of the sugar industry declines, and as the country transitions to a tourism and service economy, the future of the already disenfranchised batey population may be in greater peril.

Recent advocacy efforts have improved the plight of migrant Haitian workers and their families with increased wages, improved access to water and sanitation, and increased legal protection from deportation, as well as changes in birth registration practices. Despite this, Haitians living and working in the bateyes remain a highly vulnerable group, with significantly more poverty and notably worse health.

Haiti and the Dominican Republic: A Comparison

Flying over the island of Hispaniola provides the first striking comparison between the two countries that share this island: Haiti is 98 percent deforested, while the hills of the Dominican Republic remain lush with tree cover (28 percent of DR land is covered by forest).* The border, even from the air, is clear. Ancestry, too, is sharply different. Dominicans consider themselves Latino, of Spanish blood, while the majority of Haitians carry the features of their West African ancestors. Decades ago, the countries pursued divergent economic strategies, with Haiti being the more insular. Many years of political instability have had a tremendously negative impact on the people of Haiti, highlighted by a comparison of health indicators. Malaria is uncommon in the DR and still rampant in Haiti. The life expectancy in the DR exceeds that in Haiti by twenty years. Cholera has resurfaced in Haiti, leading to a significant epidemic, while transmission within the DR has been limited.** A well-established Dominican health infrastructure exists; not so in Haiti. A relatively stable, democratically elected government in the DR has allowed the tourist industry to flourish, bringing in large revenues.

The commonalities between the HIV epidemics in Haiti and the DR include poverty, gender inequity, and stigma.*** One notable NGO, the International Family AIDS Program, serves as a regional center for HIV care in the eastern DR, providing services to families with HIV, with outreach to high-risk populations including sex workers and batey residents.**** Through the United States President's Emergency Plan for AIDS Relief (PEPFAR) both Haiti and the DR have received extensive financial support to implement a national HIV/AIDS response.*****

NOTES

* MDG Monitor, accessed Jan. 11, 2012, www.mdgmonitor.org.

** Centers for Disease Control and Prevention, "Update on Cholera—Haiti, Dominican Republic, and Florida, 2010," *Morbidity and Mortality Weekly Report* 59.50 (Dec. 24, 2010):1637–1641, available from www.cdc.gov.

*** Daniel T. Halperin, E. Antonio de Moya, Eddy Pérez-Then, Gregory Pappas, and Jesus M. Garcia Calleja, "Understanding the HIV Epidemic in the Dominican Republic: A Prevention Success Story in the Caribbean?" *Journal of Acquired Immune Deficiency Syndromes* 51 (2009):S52–59.

**** International Family AIDS Program, accessed Jan. 11, 2011, www.global health.columbia.edu.

***** The United States President's Emergency Plan for AIDS Relief, "Partnership to Fight HIV/AIDS in the Dominican Republic," accessed Dec. 19, 2011), available from www.pepfar.gov.

International Aid Collaborations

A distinguishing feature of health service work in the Dominican Republic is that one will not be alone. In close proximity to the United States, the DR receives an abundance of philanthropic aid and support from volunteers. Over 4,300 Peace Corps volunteers have served since 1962. Major development organizations, such as USAID, support projects targeting HIV and maternal mortality. In addition, there are many faith-based health initiatives, reflecting the importance of religion, particularly Catholicism, in the local culture. Numerous small NGOs and medical mission groups provide local and episodic services, ranging from surgical specialty care to rural primary care clinics. Coordination among these efforts can be challenging, and it is crucial to coordinate with local services to prevent duplication and to improve effectiveness of services. Strategies for maximizing effectiveness when working with short-term medical aid trips include defining a common mission, establishing strong community collaborations, serving community-driven needs, learning from and with international colleagues, and developing a capacity-building sustainable intervention.[17]

Healthcare System

The health of women and children in the Dominican Republic epitomizes important strengths as well as critical weaknesses of the healthcare system as a whole. Like much of Latin America, the DR is an emerging middle-income country. It has a Human Development Index of 94 and one of highest rates of economic growth in the region. Yet these gains have not been fully translated into an anticipated improvement in health, in part because of very low social spending (lowest of the Latin American countries per GNP), leading to a variety of structural issues in health and educational services. Although there have been some gains in health status and infrastructure, the system is plagued by underfunding and mismanagement. The most vulnerable groups in the DR have not benefited from the improvement in living conditions; the country has one of the highest levels of income disparity in the Western Hemisphere. As mentioned earlier, the wealthiest 20 percent of the population receives 55 percent of the income; and the lowest 20 percent receives only 14 percent.[18] Over 16 percent of Dominicans are classified as living in extreme poverty.[19] This wide heterogeneity in distribution of economic growth has led to large disparities in health indices and in access to health services.

The majority of the population uses the Dominican Republic's existing infrastructure for government health services, although as is often noted it is underfunded and poorly managed. There are no significant environmental or geographical barriers to accessing healthcare, although ethnic and racial barriers persist. Health facilities, ranging from primary clinics to district, provincial, and regional referral hospitals, service most regions; 75 percent of Dominicans report access to health services less than 2 kilometers from their homes.[20] Human resources for health generally exceed recommended standards, with more than 18,450 physicians (20 per 10,000 people and increasing), eighteen universities offering careers in health sectors, and graduate education available in more than forty medical specialties.[21] The number of nurses is low and declining (3.9 per 10,000 people). Public health services are coordinated through the Ministry of Health and a public health organization called SESPAS (Sociedad Española de Salud Pública y Administración Sanitaria); these include immunization outreach, reproductive health services, and safe water and sanitation campaigns. Despite this infrastructure, there have been concerns about the quality of care delivered. In 2005, a strategic plan for restructuring national health services addressed the challenges.

Low Public Health Expenditures

Public health expenditures have fallen recently, from 1.9 percent of GNP in 2002 to 1.2 percent in 2006.[22] This decrease in funding has resulted in government facilities that often lack basic equipment, supplies, medication, and management.[23] Water and electric systems malfunction. Supplies intended to be disposable are reused, often with limited attention to infection control. Despite an adequate number of health workers in the country as a whole, public facilities are functionally understaffed as clinicians juggle multiple jobs. In addition to their work in the public hospitals, physicians also work in the private sector (which provides higher-quality services and better pay). Primary health facilities and district hospitals often have limited services and hours of operation.

High Out-of-Pocket Health Expenses

Out-of-pocket costs account for close to 50 percent of all national health expenditures.[24] Patients receiving care in a government hospital are often required to pay a fee, and to purchase essential supplies and medication, ranging from IV antibiotics to blood for transfusions. Some families, concerned with the quality of care at government facilities, use the private health sector. Given the high out-of-pocket costs, many people avoid seeking care. Unexpected medical emergencies can easily deplete family savings.

Disparities in Access to Care by Region, Income, and Race

Physicians and other health workers are concentrated in the urban and affluent areas, often not serving the needs of more vulnerable groups or those in more remote mountainous regions. Other populations, such as the more than 800,000 Haitians and others living on the bateyes, face even greater challenges, including the ongoing effects of long-standing discrimination, which continues to pervade the health system.

Health Status of Children and Women

Government-sponsored public health services have resulted in some notable improvements in health over the past few decades.[25] Infant mortality rates have fallen 44 percent, from 48 per 100,000 in 1990 to 27 per 100,000 in 2009. Successful public health campaigns have reduced morbidity and mortality from many communicable diseases, with less than 0.1 percent annual reports of vaccine-preventable disease. Although rates of dengue and malaria have risen, this is generally believed to be due to improved surveillance. Dominican children continue to suffer high rates of diarrhea and pneumonia, in part because of limited access to quality primary care, particularly among marginalized populations. Nationally, only 57 percent of children with suspected pneumonia receive antibiotics, and only 55 percent receive appropriate treatment for diarrhea. Average HIV sero-prevalence rates in the adult population are 1.1 percent, with considerably higher rates reported in some groups, again reflecting the wide disparities of health in the region.[26] In the country's estimated 100,000 female sex workers, HIV sero-prevalence has been estimated at between 2.5 and 12.4 percent.[27] Malnutrition across the country is improving, and manifests most commonly as stunting in 18 percent of children as well as micronutrient deficiency.

Similar to many middle-income countries, the DR is in a state of epidemiologic transition. Declining mortality and morbidity from infectious disease is being replaced by an emerging burden of noncommunicable disease with an increasing prevalence of cardiovascular disease, cancer, mental illness, and injury. Although perinatal mortality does remain unacceptably and paradoxically high (see next section) for women, chronic diseases such as hypertension and obesity are of increasing importance.

There is also a growing and unmet need to focus on preventive healthcare, including the environmental and social determinants of disease. A high burden of disease from cervical cancer exemplifies the consequences of limited preventive care. Latin America and the Caribbean have an extremely a high incidence of cervical cancer (30.8 cases per 100,000 women compared to 8.9 in the United States), and cervical cancer is ranked as the second most common cause of cancer in the DR, following breast cancer. Estimates of more than 1,000 new cases diagnosed per year grossly misjudge prevalence, as many women are unable to access care, and over 50 percent of diagnosed women die from the disease. Some factors contributing to this high prevalence include low health literacy regarding prevention and need for screening, cultural factors including low rates of condom use and higher numbers of sexual partners, and lack of access to health services such as the HPV vaccine, early diagnostic screening, and treatment regimens.[28]

Other common health concerns facing women include high rates of adolescent pregnancy, increasing substance use, and high reported rates of gender- and sex-based abuse. Common chronic health issues for children include asthma, epilepsy, and developmental concerns, which are often undertreated due to lack of access to both primary-level health and educational services.

Maternal and Child Health: A Case Study

The health and nutritional status of the mother is a key factor in determining the health of the newborn and young child. The following case illustrates a multigenerational cycle of poor health and disability.

Janeil was born at a low birth weight of 1,850 grams (4 pounds) to Sara, a fifteen-year-old single teenager. Sara had attended several prenatal visits. She was noted to have an elevated blood pressure at thirty weeks of pregnancy, but she did not make her follow-up visit at the high-risk clinic at the local hospital. She presented with eclampsia (uncontrolled hypertension of pregnancy) and in premature labor at approximately thirty-three weeks. Janeil was delivered by cesarean section, blue and not breathing, and after a delay while the doctor completed the cesarean section, she was resuscitated. In the newborn period, Janeil suffered from respiratory distress that was treated with antibiotics and oxygen. She also had a seizure and low muscle tone in her first month of life. She survived the newborn period, and in infancy and early childhood she continued to have chronic health concerns, including asthma, epilepsy, and developmental delay.

Janeil and Sara lived in Baní, a middle-income city with multiple public and private clinics, a regional hospital, and many schools. Despite this, Janeil received fairly limited services. As a child, she had frequent asthma flares and received emergency treatment in the local hospital, but medications to control and prevent her symptoms were not available. Although Janeil was seen by a specialist in Santo Domingo for her epilepsy, her family couldn't afford the medication he prescribed. Janeil attended school for a few years, but with no special educational service available to support her special needs, she quickly dropped out. She was cared for by her family, and sought healthcare as needed at the local public health clinic, which was often staffed only in the mornings by an inexperienced doctor completing a mandatory post–medical school year of service.

As Janeil grew into a young woman, she gradually gained weight, and by her teen years she became significantly overweight. She became pregnant. The pregnancy was complicated by gestational diabetes and hypertension, and she delivered, in a repeat of her own beginning, a low-weight, premature son.

Janeil's story is notable because many of her lifelong health problems could have been mitigated with some fairly basic interventions. Babies like Janeil, who weigh less than 2,500 grams (5 pounds 8 ounces), are considered low birth weight, regardless of gestational age at the time of birth. They are at risk for complex, ongoing health issues, ranging from developmental delay and respiratory problems in childhood, to obesity and hypertension as adults. Experience in more developed settings has demonstrated that access to even basic levels of educational, medical, and preventive services can result in profound benefits in physical and emotional well-being. Developing and implementing these types of services will continue be important for the DR in this stage of epidemiologic transition.

Strategies to Reduce Deaths in Mothers and Newborns

The Dominican Republic has lagged significantly behind the region and below expectations in perinatal health (the health of women and babies before, during, and after birth). This is somewhat surprising because access to critical perinatal interventions is excellent. For instance, over 95 percent of women receive the recommended four antenatal visits, and over 97 percent of women deliver in a hospital with a skilled attendant or physician.[29] Emergency obstetric care is readily available in most regions. The distance to and between facilities is short, roads are good, and transportation is generally available.

Other regions in Latin America (for example, Costa Rica and Venezuela) that deliver this level of essential maternal newborn health services have had significant improvements in maternal and newborn health, with many reporting maternal mortality ratios lower than 50 per 100,000 live births and newborn mortality in the single digits.[30] Yet in the DR, maternal deaths remain surprisingly high, with a maternal mortality rate of 150 per 100,000 live births. Similarly, while child mortality and infant mortality have improved, newborn mortality has not fallen as expected, remaining stable at 17 deaths per 1,000 live births.

Complex factors contribute to this paradox between access to healthcare and health outcomes; reflection sheds light on some of the challenges faced by the health system as a whole. The Three Delays model is one way to understand factors contributing to maternal and newborn mortality in low-resource settings.[31] This model describes three tiers of barriers that women face in receiving services across the continuum from individual to community to facility-based care:

1. *The first delay addresses the barriers an individual woman faces in the decision to seek care for herself or her newborn, including a lack of awareness of danger signs and a lack of faith in health services.* The culture of the DR generally supports seeking care, and most women and communities do accept the need for antenatal care and facility-based births. Countering this is a lack of faith in the quality and humanity of services, with many women reporting experiences with poor quality of health services. In addition, vulnerable groups, such as Haitians, must weigh the need for healthcare against concerns about discrimination and deportation. For those living in poverty, high out-of-pocket expenses associated with hospital care may lead to delays in deciding to seek early treatment for perinatal emergencies.

2. *The second delay involves barriers in reaching appropriate services because of difficulty with transportation or other socioeconomic obstacles.* For most women, transportation barriers to a primary facility are minimal because the DR has good roads and adequate public transportation. However, due to an overly centralized health system, most primary facilities do not provide maternal services, and most district hospitals provide only basic maternal newborn care. Only referral hospitals provide emergency obstetric care, HIV testing, and medications to prevent mother-to-child HIV transmission. These facilities are often difficult to reach. Communication and referrals between facilities is often uncoordinated, slow, and at the expense of the patient. Vulnerable groups in rural regions and in bateyes, and those living in extreme

poverty, may face even greater financial or social barriers to reaching needed health services.

3. *The third delay arises from a failure to receive appropriate, high-quality services at health facilities, and is the most significant.* Important issues leading to low quality in maternal healthcare have been reported by S. Miller and others.[32] Issues include the following:

- Facilities lack basic medications, supplies, and equipment.
- Marked out-of-pocket expenditures limit access to quality care, as the families of women in labor are asked to finance emergent blood transfusions or cesarean sections.
- Facilities are functionally understaffed. Physicians are concentrated in more urban areas, and are not always present when and where they are needed (or where they are supposed to be). Much of the care is provided by nursing staff, and there is a relative shortage of RN-level nurses. There are no midwives or mid-level providers (nurse practitioners or physician assistants) in the DR.
- The knowledge base and skills of perinatal health workers are often inadequate. Multiple sources describe examples of facilities that are unable to consistently deliver key evidence-based interventions for mothers and newborns.[33] There is often inadequate monitoring of vital signs and labor progression, lack of attention to infection control, and delayed recognition and treatment of maternal and newborn complications. There is an over-medicalization of the birth, with an extremely high cesarean section rate, often for unclear indications. Episiotomies are routine. For newborns, observers report limited or delayed newborn resuscitation; limited access to ongoing care for low birth rate and ill newborns; poor infection control practices; high rates of sepsis; and limited support for breast-feeding, with low breast-feeding rates of only 10 percent. Early discharge from a facility after birth is also frequent.
- Some additional issues include lack of respect, dignity, and privacy in facilities, as well as poor coordination and communication between facilities.

Partnerships for Change

Infante Sano, a Maternal Newborn Health Initiative

Multiple initiatives have aimed at improving the quality of and access to maternal and newborn services across the continuum of maternal and child health. One initiative, Infante Sano, illustrates some of the challenges and successful strategies for health workers seeking to address these complex issues.[34] Infante Sano developed from preliminary collaborations between US physicians and DR clinicians, and sought to improve maternal and newborn health services in the province of Peravia in the Dominican Republic. The project addressed challenges across the continuum from community- to facility-based care.

At the community level, Infante Sano targeted two high-risk communities with vulnerable populations. Infante Sano collaborated with local providers to support primary health services for mother and children, and trained CHWs in outreach and health promotion for high-risk mothers and newborns. At the facility level, the program aimed to improve the quality of care. Strategies included training physicians and nurses in essential interventions for maternal newborn health, such as using a partogram to monitor labor and newborn resuscitation. In addition, the program worked to improve hospital systems, including facility renovations, equipment upgrades, and improvements in management and medical records systems. Infante Sano collaborated with local teams and used a standardized quality improvement tool to focus on the areas of care that most needed improvement.

Some measures were more successful than others, and the lessons learned may be informative for other health workers.[35] Key lessons include the following:

- *The importance of local ownership of changes.* At the community level, health committees of community members led the initiative, including setting health priorities, choosing the physician and CHWs, and participating in ongoing management of health-related activities. At the facility level, hospital leadership was supported in forming quality improvement committees and in identifying local champions for implementing change.
- *The importance of a multidisciplinary approach and flexible task-shifting.* The Dominican health system is strongly hierarchical, with strictly defined tasks for nurses, doctors, and other ancillary health workers. Working with administration to allow nurses to monitor vital signs and to begin newborn resuscitation was critical in achieving change.
- *The fact that improvements in knowledge don't necessarily translate into changes in practice.* Various organizations, including the Ministry of Health and SESPAS, PAHO, and various NGO and international development organizations, have provided extensive in-country training to clinicians. Training initiatives have included the Integrated Management for Childhood Illness, newborn resuscitation, and a maternal quality improvement training. Even in facilities where many providers trained, recommendations were not being implemented.

This highlights the need to combine training with interventions to improve facilities, health information, and management systems.

- *The challenge of obtaining maternal newborn health data.* Monitoring and evaluation are clearly critical to effective programs, yet existing perinatal data systems are limited. Data routinely collected from birth logs may often be inaccurate, with some under-registration and misclassification of maternal deaths, as well as misclassifications of stillbirths and newborn deaths. Medical records are often incomplete and difficult to access. Outpatient records and testing are not linked to facility-based services. Data systems for perinatal health may improve as the national policy mandate for maternal mortality review is increasingly implemented.

Elizabeth Seton Nutrition Center

In 1979, Sister Catherine McGowan, a Catholic nun from Nova Scotia with a nutrition degree from Cornell University in her pocket, was posted to the Dominican Republic. There, she started a nutritional rehabilitation program for desperately malnourished children in the slums of Santo Domingo. By 1995, Sister Catherine felt her work within the Dominican capital was completed, and she moved her center (called the Elizabeth Seton Nutrition Center) to a *barrio* (slum) of Baní called La Saona. This barrio held 2,000 people who lived without an electric grid, schools, clinics of their own, or basic sanitation.

Over the next fifteen years, through determination and extraordinary dedication, Sister Catherine built a multiservice center for the children and families of La Saona. First and foremost, the center serves as a nutritional recovery program for severely wasted children. Some mothers hear about the center and come seeking help, but the center also conducts a census project each year, recruiting infants and young children found to be in poor nutritional shape. Fifty children yearly receive two protein-rich meals five days a week, and free healthcare and multivitamins. Their mothers are asked to come to the center one day a week to receive nutrition and parenting education. The food comes partially from a garden at the center. (Sister Catherine is famous for her "green soup," using the leafy tops of root vegetables to make a nutritious and very green concoction.) Growth is monitored, and most children are no longer malnourished within six months. So far, free of charge, more than 1,500 children have been served in this way.

Other services include a day care, which provides a safe and enriching environment for children whose mothers have found work. There is a preschool for more than 100 children between ages four and five years, at a cost of only $5 US per month. The teachers at the center are supported while seeking advanced education certificates. The success of this effort can be summed up with this fact: although children from La Saona rarely go to school, *all* of the children from this preschool program are sent on to elementary school by their families.

The center also has a clinic. Initially supported internally and through NGO partnerships, it is now staffed by the Dominican public health sector and gives this barrio access to a doctor, dentist, social worker, lab, and pharmacy at minimal cost. Lastly, the Elizabeth Seton Nutrition Center actively engages the community. Its Parent Project teaches parenting skills and nutrition. A group of residents volunteer to guard the center at night, as the barrio has a very high crime rate. For years, service groups visited the center from America and Canada to contribute, and to learn about the poverty that exists so close to American shores. College students have painted murals, trimmed the garden, and built a safe playground surface. High school students have brought soccer and baseball equipment. A group of oral surgeons from Buffalo came faithfully for decades, setting up a portable "operating room" and improving the dental health of children and adults.

In anticipation of Sister Catherine's retirement in 2011, a local board of directors was formed to continue to support the center and to assure its sustainability. Members include local politicians, a lawyer, and a local shop owner who for years has donated milk to the children. Most members have never before been on a board, and are on a learning curve themselves. In addition, an American sister board and foundation was created as a fundraising and support entity for this bright and far-reaching program.

Kids to Kids: Youth Lead Development Projects

EMILY AND SARAH NUSS, Co-founders, Kids to Kids

Kids to Kids was started in 2006 by four young people after accompanying their parents during a health-related project in the Dominican Republic. The group began by building a relationship at Espiritu Santo, a school near Baní, and gaining a personal understanding of the life and culture of youth in the DR. The group sent supplies and donations to the school, and also made service trips to work with local youth on projects linked to sports and education. The members of Kids to Kids realized that their work had resulted in many positive changes for them as well as for other children, and they decided to expand their efforts. Looking to work with people living in-country at the community level, the group partnered with the Peace Corps, and developed a program to provide grants to Peace Corps workers leading projects to help children. They focused their mission on improving the educational, athletic, and artistic opportunities for youth around the world.

With its youth advisory board, Kids to Kids has grown, now involving more than 1,000 other US-based youth. The program has given over $80,000 US in grants to more than 200 Peace Corps workers in nine countries. The youth team is still involved with the initial school, through visits and Facebook, and with a recent trip to work collaboratively on a community garden. The team has also learned the value of partnerships in helping to make a positive difference.

Health Reform

In 2001, to address some of these health services problems, the Dominican Republic enacted laws that laid the foundation for the development of a national health and social security system. Little changed immediately, but in 2005, the government developed a strategic plan to implement much-needed health reform. Key goals for reform include addressing disparities in equitable access to healthcare and decentralizing services by creating health networks. There are also provisions aimed at strengthening leadership and management of the health system. Providing universal health insurance to improve access and decrease out-of-pocket expenditures is another important change.[36]

With an eye to fulfilling the MDG health targets, the Ministry of Health adopted a zero-tolerance policy toward reducing the incidence of priority health issues including vaccine-preventable illness, malaria, dengue, TB, and HIV/AIDS. Reducing maternal and infant mortality remains a key target issue, and the strategic plan for health reform includes provisions for maternal mortality reviews and decentralization of essential maternal child services in order to improve equitable access.

Conclusion

Although global health work is stimulating, enriching, and worthwhile, each country brings unique challenges to the effort. The Dominican Republic has a stable, democratic government and relatively easy access for global health workers. Extensive travel vaccines and precautions are not necessary, and crime is relatively minimal. A fairly well-developed healthcare system accessed by most Dominicans provides ample opportunities for collaboration and partnership.

Given these factors, and the warm relations between the two countries, the DR remains a welcoming host country for US health workers.

Insight into Dominican culture and the country's health status and challenges will facilitate more effective work. Dominican customs and values in relationships, in family and gender expectations, and in religion are important to understand. Communication styles are often less direct, and an overly assertive approach may make locals uncomfortable. An understanding of recent improvements as well as ongoing challenges in the health system provide important context for US health workers planning to travel to the DR. Change is more permanent when Dominican healthcare workers are instrumental to that change. The roles of nurses and physicians are quite separate, and flexibility is required when new tasks are introduced. A good command of Spanish is needed to be effective at the grassroots level. Finally, many different types of groups from the United States are working in the DR with distinct agendas. Awareness of existing efforts, from within the country and abroad, is important in order to avoid duplication and to optimize results.

Notes

1 Central Intelligence Agency, "Dominican Republic" in *The World Factbook* (Washington: CIA), accessed July 8, 2011, available from www.cia.gov.

2 DRI, "Dominican Republic History: 1492–1821," accessed Jan. 11, 2012, available from http://dri.com. US Department of State, "Background Note: Dominican Republic," accessed Jan. 11, 2011, available from www.state.gov.

3 Pan American Health Organization, "Dominican Republic" in *Health in the Americas, 2007*, 290–303, accessed Jan. 11, 2012, available from www.paho.org.

4 CIA, "Dominican Republic." US Department of State, "Background Note: Dominican Republic."

5 City of Boston, "Imagine All the People: Dominicans in Boston," *New Bostonian Series* (June 2009):1–9, accessed Jan. 11, 2012, available from www.bostonredevelopmentauthority.org.

6 Peggy Levitt, *Transnational Villagers* (Berkeley, CA: University of California Press, 2001).

7 World Connect, accessed Jan. 11, 2012, www.worldconnect-.us.org.

8 Amnesty International, "Dominican Republic: A Life in Transit—The Plight of Haitian Migrants and Dominicans of Haitian Descent" (Mar. 21, 2007), accessed Jan. 11, 2011, available from www.amnesty.org.

9 Inter-American Commission on Human Rights, "Situation of Haitian Immigrant Workers and their Families in the Dominican Republic," *Report on the Situation of Human Rights in the Dominican Republic* (Oct. 7, 1999), accessed Jan. 11, 2010, available from www.cidh.oas.org.

10 Amnesty International, "Dominican Republic: A Life in Transit."

11 International Rescue Commission (IRC), "IRC Expresses Concern for Haitian Immigrants in the Dominican Republic and Caribbean Region" (Oct. 3, 2005), accessed Jan. 11, 2011, available from www.rescue.org.

12 Batey Relief Alliance, "The New Situation Inside Those Bateyes," accessed Jan. 11, 2012, available from www.bateyrelief.org.

13 Heather L. Crouse, Charles G. Macias, Andrea T. Cruz, Kim A. Wilson, and Susan B. Torrey, "Utilization of a Mobile Medical Van for Delivering Pediatric Care in the *Bateyes* of the Dominican Republic," *International Journal of Emergency Medicine* (2010):227–232, doi: 10.1007/s12245–010–0198–4.

14 PAHO, "Dominican Republic" in *Health in the Americas.*

15 Batey Relief Alliance, "The New Situation Inside Those Bateyes."

16 Amnesty International, "Dominican Republic: A Life in Transit."

17 Parminder Suchdev, Kym Ahrens, Eleanor Click, Lori Maclin, Doris Evangelista, and Elinor Graham, "Model for Sustainable Short-Term International Medical Trips," *Ambulatory Pediatrics* 7.4 (2007):317–320.

18 World Health Organization, "Dominican Republic Country Brief," accessed Jan. 11, 2012, available from www.who.int.

19 PAHO, "Health Systems Profile: Dominican Republic," (2007), available from www.lachealthsys.org.

20 WHO, "Dominican Republic Country Brief."

21 WHO, "Dominican Republic Country Brief."

22 PAHO, "Health Systems Profile: Dominican Republic."

23 Gerard La Forgia, Ruth Levine, Arismendi Diaz, and Magdalena Rathe, "Fend for Yourself: Systemic Failure in the Dominican Health System," *Health Policy* 76.2 (2004):163–188.

24 PAHO, "Health Systems Profile: Dominican Republic."

25 MDG Monitor. WHO, "Dominican Republic Country Brief." UNICEF, "Infant Mortality in the Dominican Republic," accessed Jan. 11, 2012, available from www.unicef.org.

26 Crouse et al., "Utilization of a Mobile Medical Van." CDC, "Update on Cholera."

27 WHO, "Dominican Republic Country Brief."

28 Kymberlee Montgomery and Owen C. Montgomery, "The Development of a Cervical Cancer Prevention Program for Underserved Women in the Dominican Republic," *Oncology Nursing Forum* 36.5 (2009):495–497.

29 MDG Monitor.

30 Ibid.

31 Joy Lawn, Kenji Shibuya, and Claudia Stein, "No Cry at Birth: Global Estimates of

Intrapartum Stillbirths and Intrapartum-Related Neonatal Deaths," *Bulletin of the World Health Organization* 83.6 (2005):409–417. Deborah Maine, "The Strategic Model for the PMM Network," *International Journal of Gynecology and Obstetrics* 59.s2 (1997):S23–S25, doi: 10.1016/S0020-7292(97)00144–6.

32 S. Miller, M. Cordero, A. L. Coleman, J. Figueroa, S. Anderson, R. Dabagh et al., "Quality of Care in Institutionalized Deliveries: the Paradox of the Dominican Republic," *International Journal of Gynecology and Obstetrics* 82.1 (2003):89–103. D. Mavalankar, "Quality of Care in Institutionalized Deliveries: the Paradox of the Dominican Republic: A Commentary on Management," *International Journal of Gynecology and Obstetrics* 82.1 (2003):107–110. Kim Wilson, Dominika Siedman, and Rachel Bremen, "Partograph Use and Compliance with Maternal Labor Protocols," poster presented at Institute for Healthcare Improvement (IHI) 20th Annual National Forum on Quality Improvement in Health Care (Nashville, TN, Dec. 9–11, 2008).

33 WHO, "Dominican Republic Country Brief."

34 DRI, "Dominican Republic History."

35 Wilson et al., "Partograph Use and Compliance with Maternal Labor Protocols." Dominika Siedman, "Implementing Use of the Partograph" (honors thesis for MD degree, Harvard Medical School, June 2009).

36 PAHO, "Health Systems Profile: Dominican Republic."

Suggested Reading

Alvarez, Julia. *In the Time of the Butterflies*. Chapel Hill, NC: Algonquin, 2010.

Díaz, Junot. *The Brief Wondrous Life of Oscar Wao*. New York: Penguin, 2008.

Llosa, Mario Vargas. *Feast of the Goat*. New York: Picador, 2002.

Pons, Frank Moya. *The Dominican Republic: A National History*. Princeton, NJ: Markus Wiener Publisher, 1998.

Glossary

Animism   A belief system that gives a living soul and powers to nonhuman entities, such as plants and animals, and to objects of nature, such as rocks or rivers.

Beasts of burden   Animals that are used by humans to do heavy labor, such as carrying a load or pulling a cart; they include donkeys, mules, horses, and oxen.

Biopiracy   The use of wild plants by commercial interests to develop medicines without compensating the peoples or nations from which the plants were discovered and taken.

CAFTA-DR   A free-trade agreement between the United States and five Central American countries and the Dominican Republic. Its features include tariff reductions, quotas, changes in "rules of origin" for apparel manufacturers, and more generous treatment of foreign investment.

Cardiomyopathy   Any disease of the heart's muscle that prevents it from functioning properly, usually producing symptoms of heart failure or irregular heartbeats. Some of the many possible causes include genetic diseases, heart attacks, and heart infections, such as Chagas disease.

Central America   A region of southern North America extending from the southern border of Mexico to the northern border of Colombia. It separates the Caribbean Sea from the Pacific Ocean, and includes seven countries (Honduras, Nicaragua, Guatemala, Belize, El Salvador, Costa Rica, and Panama) and many small offshore islands.

Chagas disease   A disease of the heart or gastrointestinal tract caused by the parasite *Trypanosoma cruzi*, which is spread through the feces of the reduviid bug that lives in thatched roofs and mud walls. The infection can also be transmitted through blood transfusion and from mother to infant. Most of those infected are asymptomatic, but 25 percent develop heart or gastrointestinal disease in the late stages. Affects primarily the poor living in rural areas.

Child mortality   The number of deaths in a population, usually counted as number of cases within 1,000 members of that population; for example, infant mortality was 250 per 1,000 live births.

Cholera   An acute infectious disease of the small intestine, caused by the bacterium *Vibrio cholerae* and characterized by profuse watery diarrhea, vomiting, muscle cramps, severe dehydration, and depletion of electrolytes.

Communicable disease   Also called an infectious disease. It can be transmitted from a human to another human, from an animal to another animal, from an animal to a human, or from a human to an animal. The disease can be caused by a bacteria, as in tuberculosis, or by a parasite such as hookworm.

Conditional cash transfer program   A social safety net program that provides cash to beneficiaries only if they meet certain criteria, such as attendance in health and nutrition programs, school, and follow-up in government clinics.

Conquistador A Spanish adventurer involved in conquering the people of the Americas.

Corruption Refers to dishonest practices such as bribery and cheating, which undermine democratic institutions, slow economic development, and contribute to governmental instability.[1]

Cost-sharing Sharing the costs of a program among the various people involved. In healthcare delivery, this usually means that patients are charged an insurance premium before getting care, or are charged a fee once they receive care.

Curandero A general term for a traditional folk healer in Latin America. Some *curanderos* emphasize herbal treatments, and others emphasize the spiritual causes of illness and have shamanic properties. *Yerberas* are herbalists; *hueseros* are bonesetters and treat musculoskeletal conditions; and *parteras* are midwives, sometimes called *comadronas* in Guatemala.

Dengue Also called dengue fever; a viral infection known as "break-bone" disease or fever because of severe headaches and joint pains. The most severe form, dengue hemorrhagic fever, can be fatal. The mosquitos that transmit dengue bite during the day, as opposed to the mosquitos that transmit malaria, which bite at dawn and dusk. Dengue is more commonly spread in urban areas than rural ones, and because there is no treatment (other than symptom management), prevention is particularly important.

Diaspora People who disperse from their ancestral homeland and often hope to return. For example, the long-term expatriates from Haiti are referred to as the Haitian Diaspora.

Disappearance (forced) A crime that occurs when a person is secretly imprisoned or killed by agents of the state or by people acting with the authorization or acquiescence of the state.

Disparities Any difference between two groups, as in income, rank, health outcome, or living standard.

Drug cartel An association between various drug traffickers and drug dealers that controls the production, distribution, and sale of illicit drugs.

Ecumenical A movement in the worldwide Christian Church (ecumenism) that celebrates the unity of all believers in Christ, transcending differences in creed, liturgy and ecclesiastical nature, and promotes dialogue among churches, unity in witness, and service to the world.

Ejido system Landholding cooperatives in Mexico in which decisions about the land can be made only through the consensus of all founding members. The negatives of the ejido system are that it tends to be inefficient, and families often must divide their land between sons, leaving each future son with a smaller and smaller plot. The main positive is that the collective power of the ejido system prevents the land from being easily taken from the poor. This is most relevant now that mining companies (mostly Canadian) have received many concessions to mine in ejido territory, but they can't start until the ejido agrees as a whole. In the ejidos where this collective decision-making power was dismantled by the program called PROCEDE, each ejidario can sell its land as if it were private property.

Encomienda system   Grants of land, as well as the indigenous people to work that land, that were given to the Spanish conquistadors.

Epidemiologic transition   A shift in the pattern of disease from largely infectious diseases to noncommunicable diseases.

Equity   Health services should be available to all people, whether living in rural, urban, or indigenous communities. When inequities in health systems exist, the poor generally suffer greater consequences. (See also *health inequity*.)

Evangelicals   Born-again Christians in Latin America whose Pentecostal Protestant churches promote messages of individualism, hard work, and sobriety.

Expropriation   The process of taking over private property for public use if that property will assist the country's welfare. Many agree that the original owners should be adequately compensated for their losses.

Faith-based organizations (FBOS)   Nonprofit religious organizations; distinguished from governmental or public organizations that are secular.

Fecundity   Fertility, and how it translates to the number of offspring one has.

Food insecurity   Lack of access to enough food to meet a person's basic needs at all times.

Garifunas   African-descendant people living on the Caribbean coast of Central America whose language and culture more closely resemble their roots in the Caribbean.

Gini coefficient   Also called Gini index. A number between 0 and 1 that describes the level of inequality within a population. Countries with a high number will have more wealth skewed toward the rich instead of the poor. The Gini coefficient is useful because the better-known Human Development Index can mask marked inequality.

Gross Domestic Product (GDP)   Also called GDP per capita, and GDP adjusted for purchasing power parity (PPP). The total dollar value of all goods and services produced within an economy over a given period of time. GDP per capita is that total amount divided by the total population, and reported as a money amount per person. PPP helps understand what type of lifestyle that GDP per capita buys in the country, based on the exchange rate and the cost of commonly used items.

Health   "[A] state of complete physical, mental, and social well-being and not merely the absence of disease or infirmity": As defined in the preamble to the Constitution of the World Health Organization as adopted by the International Health Conference in 1946, and available at www.who.int.

Health disparities   Differences in health states that do not necessarily imply the presence of injustice.

Health inequity   The inequitable distribution of disease and early death between rich and poor.[2] Refers to the unfair, avoidable, and remediable differences in the health status of different groups of people within and between countries.

Healthy migrant effect   A phenomenon observed in some countries, in which migrants into the host country have better health outcomes when compared to others in that country. Often considered a paradox, because migrants are normally socioeconomically disadvantaged, so they should be sicker. Some factor is making or keeping migrants healthy, though this factor may not be recognized or fully understood.

Health outcomes   The change in the health status of an individual or population after an intervention is implemented.

Heart failure   Also called congestive heart failure. The medical condition caused by inefficient pumping of the heart. Associated symptoms include shortness of breath on exertion or while sleeping, leg swelling, and abdominal swelling. Can be managed with a combination of medications.

Heavily Indebted Poor Countries (HIPC) initiative   Founded by the International Monetary Fund and World Bank in 1996, the HIPC initiative was intended to reduce the foreign debt burden of the world's poorest countries. To be eligible, the country must have unsustainable levels of external debt despite multiple attempts at traditional debt relief.

Holistic mission   Refers to the satisfaction of basic human needs, including the need for God, but also the need for love, food, shelter, clothing, physical and mental health, and a sense of human dignity.

Human Development Index (HDI)   A composite scale that combines the measurements of several different development themes (a long and healthy life, access to knowledge, and a decent standard of living) to rank countries as having either very high, high, medium, or low human development. Critics of HDI say that because it is limited in what it measures, it gives only a partial vision of human development.

Indigenous   People with historical ties to ethnic groups that lived in the territory prior to colonization. They self-identify themselves as indigenous, use indigenous language in daily speech, and may be active in indigenous community affairs or religious ceremonies.

Informal sector   Refers to a variety of different tasks in contrast to the *formal sector* of waged jobs in industrialized nations. Examples include vendors doing street and bus selling, domestic service, and casual labor.

Infrastructure   In healthcare, this implies physical infrastructure, such as healthcare centers and hospitals, as well as the trained staff who provide high-quality service.

Internally displaced persons (IDP)   Those who have fled or lost their homes due to armed conflict, generalized violence, human rights violations, or natural disasters. Unlike refugees, IDPs have not crossed an international border.

International Monetary Fund (IMF)   Specialized agency of the UN formed in 1945. It works to promote monetary stability among its 187 member countries through technical and financial assistance to promote growth and reduce poverty.

Kaposi's sarcoma   A vascular cancer that is most commonly seen in patients with advanced HIV/AIDS. Although the tumor can be located in any organ, most patients are diagnosed when the cancer affects the skin.

Latent tuberculosis   Inactive or dormant infection caused by *Mycobacterium tuberculosis* in a person who has been exposed to TB but does not show symptoms of TB. Those who have low immune function (for example, with HIV/AIDS) have a manyfold greater risk of getting active TB if the latent TB is not treated.

Latin America   Areas of America where the official languages are derived from Latin, including Spanish, Portuguese, and French, and also Creole, derived from

French. Includes South America, Central America, and certain islands in the Caribbean (Cuba, the Dominican Republic, and Puerto Rico). In the United States, the term Latin America often is used more broadly to apply to all the nations south of the Rio Grande, including all the islands of the Caribbean.

Liberation medicine   The conscious, conscientious use of health to promote social justice and human dignity. Involves people learning how to liberate themselves and to accompany others in their liberation (rather than how to liberate others). Liberation medicine has an interdisciplinary approach, drawing on the synergy of medicine, public health, health and human rights, community-oriented and community-based primary care, ethics, history of medicine, liberation theology, cultural competency, medical humanities, health literacy, art, and anthropology.

Machismo   A cultural attitude of Latin American masculinity that reflects an exaggerated male dominance and virility. A general theme is that men show aggressive behavior and hypersexuality through promiscuity, and that women are naturally submissive and dependent.[3]

Malnutrition   A condition that occurs when the body doesn't get the right amount of nutrition needed to be healthy. Caused by undernutrition, which results in poor growth and low weight, or by overnutrition that results in obesity and related diseases such as diabetes and hypertension.

Maquiladoras (commonly abbreviated as *maquilas*)   Assembly plants run by transnational companies that take advantage of low wages and lax environmental laws in underdeveloped countries. The components are imported into the factory, and the finished product is returned to the original market.

Marginalization   The process of being put on the margins or edges of society, which limits opportunities and development. Can be quantified in a variety of ways, including literacy, scholastic achievement, earnings, housing with basic needs such as a non-dirt floor, electricity, and plumbing.

Mesoamerica   A cultural area where once over 50 million people lived; roughly contiguous with the modern nations of Mexico, Guatemala, Honduras, Belize, and El Salvador.

Mestizo   A person with mixed European and indigenous ancestry who has adopted the dominant Hispanic social values. The term *mestizo* is used generally in Latin America, and the mestizos in Guatemala and Chiapas are known as *Ladinos*.

Micronutrient   One of the vitamins or minerals that is needed only in small amounts for normal body function; micronutrients include iron, folic acid, iodine, vitamin A, and zinc.

Millennium Development Goals (MDGs)   A group of eight development goals agreed to by 189 nations at a UN conference in the year 2000. The MDGs include the eradication of extreme poverty, universal primary education, improvements in gender equity and maternal health, reduced child mortality, treatment for key diseases such as HIV and TB, environmental sustainability, and global partnerships.

Multidrug-resistant tuberculosis (MDR-TB)   Tuberculosis that is resistant to the two most powerful first-line antibiotics available for TB, isoniazid and rifampin.

MDR-TB is more challenging to treat because the second-line medications are less effective, more toxic, and more expensive than the first-line drugs.

Neglected tropical disease   One of a group of chronic infectious diseases that, despite being some of the most common and severe of all diseases that poor populations experience, have traditionally received inadequate attention. Their control is now recognized as a major goal for the attainment of the MDGs.

Neoliberalism   Also called the Washington Consensus. A political theory that emphasizes strong private property rights, free markets, and free trade. Deregulation of markets and privatization of state-owned enterprises are key features.

Nepotism   The practice of giving jobs to friends and family, regardless of their abilities.

Noncommunicable disease (NCD)   An illness that is not spread by an infectious disease. NCDs include chronic conditions such as cardiovascular disease (heart attacks, stroke) chronic respiratory disease, diabetes, and cancer, and are caused by a combination of risk factors including unhealthy diet, physical inactivity, alcohol, and tobacco. Management of NCDs requires frequent contact with patients over time as well as prevention strategies that emphasize lifestyle and health-promoting behaviors.

Nongovernmental organization (NGO)   A nonprofit agency, organization, or foundation that is organized outside of government to realize a specific social objective, such as human rights, or to serve a particular constituency, such as indigenous people. NGOs maintain their own funding and are independent of central or municipal government.

North American Free Trade Agreement (NAFTA)   An agreement between Canada, the United States, and Mexico to lower trade barriers and promote increased economic activity between the countries.

Oral rehydration solution (ORS)   Refers to pre-measured packets of sugar and salt that are diluted with one liter of clean water and can be taken at home to treat dehydration. ORS packets are inexpensive and readily available. They are frequently used to treat fluid losses from diarrhea, which is a leading cause of death for infants and young children in developing countries.

Out-of-pocket   Medical expenses that are paid for directly by the patient, usually with cash.

Pan American Health Organization (PAHO)   International public health agency that works to improve health and living standards of the countries of the Americas. It is part of the WHO and UN system.

Paramilitary group   A force whose function and organization are similar to those of a professional military, but which is not considered part of a state's formal armed forces. Usually refers to militias or private armies with a political purpose.

Participatory Action Research (PAR)   The focus of this kind of research starts from the interest of the population and not the researcher. The population is the principal stakeholder of any social transformation, and any effective change in living situation depends on the people's active collaboration. PAR rejects top-down aid programs implemented by a benefactor, a social institution, or technical professionals.

Pathophysiology   The study of how normal processes in the body become diseased.

Point-of-care   The point of contact between the patient and the medical system. Often used to describe a moment when patients are available; lab tests, payments, and other parts of the medical transaction usually happen at this time.

Ready-to-use supplementary food (RUSF)   Supplementary foods, containing a modest amount of calories and a range of vitamins and micronutrients, and often in the form of spreads or pastes, which can be eaten straight from the package without the need for preparation. Unlike traditional grain-based food supplements, RUSFs typically derive the bulk of their calories from milk powder, peanuts, sugar, and oil. They do not require cooking or refrigeration, and they are useful in preventing chronic malnutrition.

Remittances   Grassroots financial aid, consisting of private financial transfers from migrant workers, regardless of their immigration status, to recipients in their country of origin. The value of remittances often exceeds that of any source of foreign aid by governments.

Selective primary healthcare (SPHC)   A concept of healthcare priority setting and delivery that was developed at the Bellagio conference hosted by the Rockefeller Foundation. In contrast to the concept of *comprehensive primary healthcare*, as described in the UN conference at Alma Ata, SPHC does the minimum necessary to achieve key aspired outcomes for priority diseases while controlling costs in the process; comprehensive healthcare focuses on the broader risks and processes involved in keeping people and communities sick or healthy, and then considers the investments needed to achieve priority goals.

Slash-and-burn agriculture   The vegetation of a plot of land is cut and burned, then cultivated until the soil is depleted, and subsequently left fallow to recover before the cycle is repeated again.[4]

Smallpox   Highly contagious viral infection that causes fever, rash, and blindness. Smallpox decimated native populations in the Americas soon after European settlers arrived; it was declared eradicated in 1980 after a worldwide vaccination campaign.

Social determinants of health   Refers to health inequities that arise from the societal conditions in which people are born, grow, live, work, and age.

Social gradient   At all levels of income, health and illness follow a social gradient in which the lower the socioeconomic position, the worse the health.

Social medicine   Seeks to understand how health, disease, and social conditions are interrelated, and to foster conditions in which this understanding can lead to a healthier society.

Structural violence   The social, economic, and political conditions that harm individuals and populations, and keep them from their full potential. Term coined by Johan Galtung and liberation theologists in the 1960s and linked to the concept of social injustice.[5]

Stunting   In a child, low height compared to age. Abnormally short children usually have suffered chronic malnutrition. Of the two forms of child growth failure—length and weight—that of length, or stunting, is three to six times more prevalent in Latin America and the Caribbean. Underweight can be reversed, but stunting is permanent. Children with stunted growth are at increased risk for becoming overweight as adults, which increases their risk of developing chronic diseases.

Task-shifting   Where there is a shortage of healthcare workers, tasks are delegated to health workers with less training than those traditionally assigned to do the job. Tasks traditionally performed by doctors may be shifted to nurses, and nursing tasks may be shifted to or shared with trained community health workers.

Transnational migrants   Migrants who belong to two societies at the same time, and live their lives across national borders. They may move back and forth, and their kin and friendship networks can span both locations.

Transnational corporation   Entity that does business, ranging from agriculture to manufacturing, in two or more countries. The format can be a single company or a merged conglomerate of companies.

Tropics   Region between Tropic of Cancer and Tropic of Capricorn characterized by a hot climate with no dramatic change in seasons because the sun is consistently high in the sky throughout the year. There are two major seasons, dry and rainy, and temperatures vary with elevation.

Tuberculosis (TB)   Bacterial infection, usually of the lungs, that causes a chronic disease characterized by cough, night sweats, and severe weight loss. TB is fatal if not treated, and is one of the most common causes of death worldwide. (See also *latent tuberculosis* and *multidrug-resistant* TB.)

Upstream determinants   In public health, this term refers to seeking the causes of disease and disability and addressing the problem through prevention rather than treatment (the downstream effect).

USAID   United States Agency for International Development, a branch of the government that promotes US foreign policy goals by funding economic and social development throughout the world. Provides grants and technical assistance to governments, NGOs, and international agencies.

Vertical programs   Efforts that focus on preventing or treating individual diseases or working with specific populations (for example, vaccinations), in contrast to *horizontal* efforts that focus on a health system delivering comprehensive care with a primary care provider at the core. Vertical programs usually have a specific outcome focus and are managed by a separate funding stream. Vertical is also used metaphorically to refer to top-down decision making, as oppsed to horizontal processes in which all team members have input.

Wasting   Low weight compared to height. Wasting usually indicates a sudden loss in adequate nutrition, as in an acute famine.

Water poverty index (WPI)   A standardized, calculated measure to assess the link between household welfare and water availability. WPI is a composite of available statistics, including factors such as environment, capacity, use, resources, and socioeconomics.

World Bank   An international institution, owned by 187 member nations, that provides assistance to developing countries in the form of technical support, loans, credits, or grants.

NOTES

1 United Nations Office on Drugs and Crime (UNDOC), "UNDOC's Action against Corruption and Economic Crime," accessed 28 Feb. 2012, available online at www .unodc.org.

2 Lawrence O. Gostin, "A Framework Convention on Global Health: Health for All, Justice for All," *JAMA* 307.19 (2012):2087–2092.

3 Duncan Green, *Faces of Latin America*, 3rd ed. (New York: Monthly Review Press, 2006).

4 Robert M. Carmack, Janine L. Gasco, and Gary H. Gossen, *The Legacy of Mesoamerica: History and Culture of a Native American Civilization*, 2nd.ed. (Upper Saddle River, NJ: Prentice Hall, 2007).

5 Paul E. Farmer, Bruce Nizeye, Sara Stulac, and Salmaan Keshavjee, "Structural Violence and Clinical Medicine," *PLoS Medicine* 3.10 (2006):e449.

Contributors

Ryan Alaniz, PhD (sociology), MA (Latin American studies), grew up on a farm on the central coast of California. The son of a Mexican-American father and white mother, Ryan's interest in bridging cultural understanding and economic opportunity started when he was young. At fourteen, on a trip to build homes for the impoverished in Tijuana, Mexico, Ryan saw the disparity of wealth between the two nations; this encouraged him to address poverty in Latin America, and to find ways to effect positive change while bringing lessons of social health back to the United States.

After college, Ryan volunteered at Nuestros Pequeños Hermanos orphanage from 2001 to 2002. It was there that he was inspired to start the Fútbol Project, a nonprofit that provides soccer equipment to orphaned and underprivileged children after they complete a service project for their community. It was also where he decided the future trajectory of his life: teaching in higher education. Ryan believes that informing university students, who he enthusiastically calls "future leaders of the world," about their privilege empowers them to find ways to effect positive change. In this way, he attempts to motivate students to bridge the ivory tower with the dirt roads, and to learn theory by engaging in praxis. Many of his former students are now volunteering throughout Asia, Latin America, and Africa.

Ryan is assistant professor at California Polytechnic State University, a Fulbright Ambassador, and a board member of Restorative Partners. He has published with United Nations University and the Social Science Research Council, and is finishing a manuscript titled *How to Be a Conscientious Gringo: Twelve Ways to Effect Change in Yourself and the World*. His current academic research investigates the long-term social health (for example, trust, low crime, and participation) of post-disaster planned communities. More specifically, Ryan focuses on seven Honduran communities eleven years after Hurricane Mitch (1998), highlighting not only how residents and sponsoring NGOs work together to create community, but the interactions and contradictions that are born from this process. When asked about his development philosophy, Ryan usually refers to the fishing analogy. "It is good to give a person a fish. And we know it is even better to teach him or her how to fish. Engaged academic research provides the tools for us to examine why the person did not have a fish in the first place, and then address that issue. Our role as committed scholars is to understand when and how to accomplish all three."

Natasha M. Archer, MD, was born in Queens, New York, to Haitian emigrants. She was raised in a strong Catholic household in Queens. As a child, Natasha never traveled to Haiti but always had an interest in her parents' home country. She went to Yale College in New Haven, Connecticut, where she majored in molecular, cellular, and developmental biology. She also worked as a tutor for New Haven youth, and a biology tutor for Yale College underclass members as part of the Science, Technology and Research Scholars (STARS) program.

After graduating, Natasha pursued further teaching opportunities as a Yale-China teaching fellow; her interest in working in resource-limited settings began while she was teaching English as a teaching fellow in Changsha, Hunan. There, she first witnessed the social and political barriers to delivering healthcare to the disempowered. While still in China, Natasha applied to medical school and matriculated at Yale University School of Medicine in 2002.

The atmosphere at Yale was both encouraging and instructive. At this time she began volunteering with Concerned Haitian Americans of Illinois (CHAI) in Cap-Haïtien, Haiti, where she helped to develop and maintain three clinics. After her first medical mission and first trip to Haiti, Natasha enrolled in the Directed Independent Language Study (DILS) at Yale that allowed her to study Haitian Creole in order to better communicate with her patients. She returned to Haiti annually throughout medical school. From this experience, Natasha realized her responsibility as a physician to challenge the current health system within which she now worked, and to develop healthcare strategies that not only are accountable to the people they serve, but also address the broader social forces that perpetuate disease.

Natasha moved to Boston as a resident in the combined Harvard Medicine-Pediatrics Residency Program and the Global Health Equity Residency Program. Through the Global Health Equity Residency Program, Natasha has spent the majority of her time abroad at Partners in Health sites in Haiti. Immediately after the earthquake, she spent six weeks in Port-au-Prince as the volunteer coordinator for PIH and as liaison between PIH and Haiti's largest hospital, l'Hôpital Université d'Etat d'Haïti. She was also one of the first responders after the cholera outbreak in the Artibonite.

As this book goes to press, Natasha is in her second year of a hematology-oncology fellowship at Boston Children's Hospital and the Dana-Farber Cancer Institute. She plans to help start both a sickle cell program and an oncology program in Haiti after completing her fellowship.

Linnea Capps, MD, MPH, was born in Kansas and grew up in the Midwest. She earned her MD from the University of Missouri. From the beginning of her studies, her goal was to be a primary care doctor. She decided to pursue training in an urban public hospital and completed her residency in internal medicine at Harlem Hospital in New York City. On finishing her residency, she expected to spend her career in Harlem as a primary care doctor in a neighborhood health center.

Linnea studied public health soon after finishing her residency, with the idea of learning about community-oriented healthcare as a supplement to her traditional medical education, which had been almost entirely about treating sick individuals. Meeting colleagues working in developing countries, as well as being involved in organizations in solidarity with El Salvador in the years of that country's civil war, led her to volunteer to work in a small rural clinic and train village health workers in El Salvador in the mid-1980s. She lived in the rural Department of Chalatenango for two years, and worked as a part of the health program of the Archdiocese of San Salvador.

In 1987, Linnea returned to New York and took a position as medical director of a network of community clinics associated with Columbia University Medical Center. In 1990, she returned to Harlem Hospital to work in the Harlem AIDS Treatment Group, which was participating in community-based research with people living with HIV/AIDS. She later became associate director of the Department of Medicine and director of the Internal Medicine Residency Program. She was also coordinator of the internal medicine rotation at Harlem for Columbia University medical students.

Linnea continued to work with solidarity organizations, supporting the struggles of people in Latin America, and served on the board of directors of three health-related NGOs. One of these was Doctors for Global Health. In 1998, she spent the year as a DGH volunteer at Hospital San Carlos in Chiapas, Mexico, and has been a member of the DGH board of directors since 2000. She returned to work at Columbia University and Harlem Hospital in 1999, but continued to spend time each year in Chiapas.

In 2012 Linnea accepted a position at Montefiore Medical Center in the Bronx where she is a member of the faculty of the Primary Care/Social Internal Medicine Residency Program and has a faculty appointment at Albert Einstein College of Medicine. Her work includes teaching Montefiore residents and Einstein students in a global health program based in a rural community hospital in Uganda. She is the president of DGH and continues to work with the DGH project in Chiapas.

Peter J. Daly, MD, completed his undergraduate studies at the University of Notre Dame, then his medical school at Mayo Medical School in Rochester, Minnesota. He stayed on at Mayo Clinic for his orthopedic surgery residency, in the Mayo School of Graduate Medical Education, finishing in 1991. From 1991 to 1992, he completed a shoulder and sports medicine fellowship at Harvard University's Massachusetts General Hospital. He is board certified by the American Board of Orthopedic Surgery, and subspecialty certified in orthopedics sports medicine. He admits to being strongly influenced by his wife and best friend, LuLu Romano Daly, RN, who has worked tirelessly for humanitarian medical efforts as a pediatric oncology and hospice nurse. LuLu's motto, "I can't do what you do, you can't do what I do, but together we can make a difference" (Mother Teresa), prompted them to work as a team. Together with their four children, they have worked as a family volunteering with Orthopedics Overseas, and subsequently with Nuestros Pequeños Hermanos™, an organization that provides extensively for orphaned, abandoned, and disadvantaged children in Latin America and the Caribbean.

After visiting several NPH homes in Mexico, Nicaragua, Haiti, and Honduras, the Dalys began taking in—to their home in St. Paul, Minnesota—patients who required complex surgical care not readily available in their own countries. One of the NPH Honduras children lived with the Dalys for one year, and prompted them to build a surgical center at the NPH Honduras home in 2006. They now split their time between Honduras and St. Paul. While in Honduras, Peter and his family continue to work toward complete staffing of the Holy Family Surgery Center by Honduran personnel, and toward making it an integral component of Honduran healthcare delivery, specifically targeting indigent Hondurans who would not receive care otherwise. While in St. Paul, Peter and his family procure used equipment for Honduras, and also facilitate several medical/surgical brigades to Honduras to support the efforts of the Honduran staff at the surgery center. Peter has continued his academic interests with multiple publications, and he works as a clinical assistant professor at the University of Minnesota Medical School. He also maintains a private orthopedic surgical practice with Summit Orthopedics.

Anne Kraemer Díaz, MA, began her path to Guatemala as a child intent on visiting the ancient Maya ruins. She traveled to Guatemala in late 2003 to begin her master's research in anthropology, studying the lack of collaboration and communication between archaeologists and indigenous Maya peoples in Guatemala. Tecpan, the hometown of her Kaqchikel professor, was where Anne's real understanding of Maya culture, language, and history began. Interviews with Maya daykeepers, or traditional Maya spiritual leaders, revealed the daily struggles of being indigenous in Guatemala.

Anne has returned to Guatemala every year since then for extended visits to research and volunteer. For several summers she lived in a rural community in southwestern Guatemala to study the impact of a community archaeology project and its involvement, interaction, and collaboration with the local community. It was here, among the coffee plants growing on top of 2,000-year-old Maya ruins, while watching K'ichee' men excavate the history they rarely knew as their own, shoeless and wearing torn t-shirts donated from the United States, that Anne was overwhelmed by the negative impacts of development, foreign aid, community archaeology, and the abandonment of the Maya people by the state and NGOs. From that point forward, Anne focused on access to services for Maya peoples and the paucity of cultural and linguistic services available for the majority of Guatemala's population.

At a Kaqchikel field school, Anne had the good fortune of meeting Peter Rohloff, along with other linguists, anthropologists, and medical professionals. Together, they began developing ideas and a methodology on medical care delivery and access to services based on their experiences living in Maya communities. In 2007, as a Fulbright scholar, Anne began a yearlong research study to understand the impact of development and archaeological projects in Guatemala. For twenty months she lived in rural communities, collaborating with and learning from the local people about the real problems that plagued their everyday lives. The common thread was the continual failure of the state and local and foreign NGOs to reach the people in their culture and language.

Since the founding of Wuqu' Kawoq in 2007, Anne has served in several roles: first as treasurer; then as project manager in the field; and, since 2009, as executive director. Anne travels to Guatemala as often as possible to support the work of Wuqu' Kawoq and to learn more from the families who taught her so much in the southwestern piedmont. Currently, Anne oversees the operation of the organization in the United States and Guatemala, with financial and risk management, fundraising, volunteer supervision, and the organization of clean-water initiatives.

Belinda Forbes, DMD, was born in the United Kingdom and raised in the United States. After completing her high school years in Scotland, she earned her BA in biology and Spanish at American International College in Springfield, Massachusetts, and her DMD from Tufts University School of Dental Medicine in Boston. Belinda attributes her path to a health profession to her parents: her father, a physician and ob/gyn; and her mother, a dentist. After her father's untimely death, Belinda's mother influenced her awareness of the struggle of women to make a place for themselves in a male-dominated profession—for fifteen years Belinda's mother was the only female dentist in the city of Springfield. She also set an example of using one's profession for social service, as she worked in a mental hospital for several years.

During Belinda's years in dental school, she felt an impulse to use her education for an alternative career path, but in the mid-1980s the choices were few, and any inkling for public health seemed to be undervalued at her university. Even the classes for nutrition and prevention were taken lightly, with more focus on advanced technical skills in restorative and prosthetic dentistry to be used in private practice and to generate income. Despite this, Belinda emphasizes that she graduated from Tufts in 1988 with the best dental professional education available in the United States.

Belinda's first employment was as an associate in a private satellite office in East Boston, a sector of the city with a large population of immigrants. There, she used her Spanish daily and honed her skills in dentistry, treating patients from Latin American, Asian, and Eastern Bloc countries, as well as low-income Caucasian patients. She became aware of the implications of costly healthcare for immigrants who worked three jobs and barely had time or resources to pay for dental care, and the limitations of government healthcare for the unemployed. Her yearning to do something more with her training persisted. She volunteered in the dental clinic of Bridge Over Troubled Waters, a resource organization for runaway and street youth, and became more active in her local United Methodist Church. Through the church, she pursued a short-term volunteer service in a Spanish-speaking country as a way to explore alternatives to full-time private practice. An opportunity existed in Nicaragua, where her church worked with a partner church in social justice projects and programs.

So with her quality training, considerable educational debt, and a faith call, in early 1991 Belinda set off for what was supposed to be a year's volunteer work in Nicaragua. She lived in a community house, hosted visiting church delegations, and helped the local church develop its first program for dental health—training school teachers to provide dental health education and oral hygiene practice for students, and offering dental healthcare in rural mobile health teams and through a subsidized treatment plan in the Acción Médica Cristiana clinic in Managua that made basic services available at low cost to the population. She was also supported by US-based activist organizations such as the Training Exchange and the Committee for Health Rights in the Americas.

After the first six months of working in community health, Belinda realized that this diverse use of her skills was what she had been looking for. To be sure that Nicaragua was the right place to pursue this path, she returned to the United States for three more years, working in private practice and sending out curricula vitae and cover letters to diverse international agencies and organizations. The resulting opportunities were either short-term (one month or less) service work in clinics or high-level public health positions requiring further training. There appeared to be little or no opportunity for a full-time, remunerated career in global health. Belinda felt her skills were best used at the community level, so she became a full-time missionary and returned to Nicaragua.

Belinda collaborated with the local church for ten years, continuing to develop the small, primary care dental health program that later integrated into a comprehensive health program and focused on health promoter training, health education in schools, and mobile clinical care. In Managua, Belinda worked at AMC's multispecialty medical and dental clinic, treating Nicaraguan and expatriate patients alike. From her arrival in the country, Belinda worked closely with Nicaraguan professionals, many of whom were trained during Nicaragua's revolutionary period and also felt a call to use their education in service to the population. Belinda has organized continuing education events for Nicaraguan dentists and hosted US dentists in AMC's projects. The mutual learning that has taken place during twenty years of dental health practice has helped Nicaraguan colleagues expand their knowledge and practice base, and has helped Belinda to understand the complexities of delivering healthcare in a poor, developing country while finding ways to be effective in that context.

After handing over the first dental health program to a Nicaraguan colleague, Belinda moved to AMC full-time, where she currently collaborates in dental and community health as well as in diverse areas such as partnership development, intercultural exchange programs, and becoming an information resource and liaison for health to visiting teams from the United States and Europe.

Her work in dental health at AMC led to the design and implementation of a dental health program based on the first one she developed, but in the remote region of Matagalpa, where dental health services are geographically or economically inaccessible for most of the population. Besides dental promoter training and health education, the program offers clinical dental care from visiting mobile teams and also in a permanent dental unit that was installed on one of AMC's model farms. Evaluations leave no doubt that this effort by Belinda and the AMC staff has led to a greater awareness of dental health and use of services. But the model cannot work independently from other efforts in health and development. Belinda has learned that in any intervention, the community must participate to the full extent, and that all social stakeholders—NGOs, government, international donors—must also have a level of commitment that guarantees success.

Belinda was fortunate to have mentors in her faith journey, as well as the support of her family and colleagues, who, if doubtful at times about her career choices, in general accept that her life in Nicaragua is enriched and that she is making a difference in the world. Belinda also recognizes that learning Spanish and becoming an intermediate-level translator was key to opportunities that would lead to a career in global health. Belinda's expanded skills also allow her to represent the US-based organization Global Health through Education, Training and Service, and she facilitates a pioneering occupational health project between a university and a union confederation.

In 1996 Belinda married Gerardo Gutiérrez, a medical doctor specializing in public health and on staff at AMC. They live in Managua, have two daughters, and work together as part of AMC's multidisciplinary team to promote global health issues and contextually and culturally appropriate responses. Belinda's biggest personal challenge has been to address a debt of thousands of dollars on a missionary's salary, a task that took more than sixteen years and many sacrifices for her and her family. This achievement strengthened her commitment to use her privileged professional formation in service to vulnerable populations in the world. She considers her specialty to be "access," making services and knowledge about dental health available to populations who would otherwise not have it.

Belinda is comfortable in urban private practice, but she also feels at home with opportunities to be in the *campo* working alongside AMC staff, community leaders, and local people as they struggle with daily living and overwhelming needs. She went to Nicaragua thinking she would solve all of the dental problems there, but has since expanded her understanding to know that any work in dental health must be integrated into comprehensive plans for empowering local people to determine their own future. She has a saying, "Every missionary should work themselves out of a job," and tries to live up to that, working to build local capacity, hand over any project or program to Nicaraguan leadership, and play the role of accompaniment and consultant rather than protagonist. The results continue to be satisfying.

Gerardo Gutiérrez, MD, MPH, is a mestizo Nicaraguan born in 1964 as the eldest of three children whose parents were *campesinos* and barely literate. He grew up in the small city of Diriamba south of the capital Managua, and attended public school. He filled afternoons with soccer and weekends with church activities.

His high school years coincided with a tremendous social upheaval in Nicaragua: the Sandinista Popular Revolution, which inspired great expectations for the social development of the country. In 1980, when he was a teenager, Gerardo participated in the five-month National Literacy Campaign, through which he taught fifteen *campesino* men, women, and children to read and write. As an active member of a local church in Diriamba, Gerardo participated in and later coordinated a missionary campaign to various rural communities surrounding Diriamba. By this time, in the early 1980s, Nicaragua had entered into the Counter-Revolutionary War and suffered from the economic blockade imposed by the US government.

These significant social experiences, set in a context of severe social and economic challenges, gave Gerardo the opportunity to live with *campesino* families in conditions of extreme poverty, and led him to consider choosing a vocation that would benefit the poor. He considered either a religious career or one related to health. Supported by his strong academic performance, Gerardo classified for the degree in medicine at the National Autonomous University of Nicaragua (UNAN) in its newly established Managua campus. The challenges involved in pursuing this course of study were extreme. Texts were often photocopies, sometimes written in English rather than Spanish. Unable to afford bus fare, Gerardo resorted to hitch-hiking to and from medical school during his five years of study. Despite the limitations, he frequently volunteered to attend communities affected by disasters and participated in church programs ministering to those suffering from war and scarcity.

From 1989 to 1990, as he was concluding his intern year, he volunteered with AMC's projects serving indigenous groups on Nicaragua's Caribbean Coast, first with the Rama and then the Miskito communities. These experiences with AMC provided contacts that would later shape both his personal and professional choices and give him a broader vision about his country and its needs. Moreover, they gave him the opportunity to put into practice his desire to combine a faith call to service with a profession in health.

Gerardo shares his first encounter with different culture and world views on health:

When I was recently graduated as a medical doctor, I went to Tasba Pri (Bilwi [Puerto Cabezas], RAAN) for my social service. Because of the armed conflict, the health ministry could not have a presence, so I went with Acción Médica Cristiana, a nongovernmental organization establishing projects in this region.

Like every new doctor, I had my head full of ambitious ideas (like being a great clinical doctor) and with a mind full of scientific reason. I was thinking that I could solve every health problem in that community. On the other hand, I was there as a representative worker of a Christian organization, so I had to maintain certain values, attitudes and behaviors.

On my first day in the community, a neighbor knocked on my door, and when I opened it, I asked him, "May I help you?" He said, "Doctor, I'm coming to you to ask you a favor: my daughter is sick because she is being attacked by bad spirits, so I need your truck to take her to Waspam. In Waspam there is a witch or *sukia* who can take care of her." I was speechless and told him, "I'm sorry sir, I can't help you, because as a medical doctor I don't believe in bad spirits, and as a Christian person I cannot allow you to use our truck to take your daughter to a witch."

The man and his family left, and from that moment no person in the community talked to me. I asked other people what was happening, and someone told me, "They are very angry with you because you offended their culture and beliefs." Luckily for me, three days after that situation, the girl ran away with her boyfriend. Then the family realized that she was pretending to be sick, so they forgave me. I started to pay more attention to the Miskito indigenous beliefs and worldview about health.

Another experience happened later that same year. I attended a difficult birth in the company of Doña Florencia, the indigenous community midwife, who offered the expectant mother massage, medicinal plants, and a prayer ritual. A baby boy was finally born, after which Doña Florencia received the placenta with great respect and carried it away to bury outside. I nodded in approval, assuming burial was a good way to dispose of biological waste in a community with limited water and sanitation. Later, in conversation with her, my Western assumption about infection control and hygiene was unexpectedly called into question.

"You see, Doctor," said Florencia, "I went to bury the placenta because it represents the baby's root—the same as the roots of a tree. A tree with superficial roots will be weak, and surely end up as nothing more than firewood. A baby whose placenta is buried deep will grow strong and healthy. If the placenta is buried near the surface, it can be unearthed and eaten by animals; that person will be sick and die young, unable to overcome disease."

Thus began my transformation as a health professional to consider the social and cultural aspects of women's health and to research the sexual and reproductive health of Miskito women. I worked very hard for one year, and after attending around 15,000 people, I observed that there were no changes in the health situation of the population. So with AMC I began to work more in primary healthcare—health education and promoting a healthy lifestyle—instead of simply treating diseases. Out of that experience, I chose to focus my career on community health and training people, and taking into account their belief systems. And my dream about becoming a great clinical specialist was replaced by a dream to develop healthcare models based on the people's needs and not on the capacities or requirements of medical institutions.

The Miskito worldview on health continues to fascinate and motivates Gerardo to work toward developing public health models that are appropriate to the culture, context, and expectations of local communities. His academic knowledge obtained in university and hospitals has been enriched with the popular knowledge of midwives, *sukias, curanderos*, health leaders, and the population in general. His interest in primary healthcare, and in particular community health, is driven by his interest in deepening knowledge about what the population believes and practices in health and sickness. Gerardo has participated in diverse research, has collaborated on writing manuals and other publications on community health in Nicaragua, and has represented AMC in diverse national and international events where this knowledge and experience can be shared.

From 1994 to 1995 he carried out his first investigation, "Traditional and Popular Illnesses in the Communities of Alamikamb and Laguna de Perlas," which he also successfully presented as the monograph to complete his degree in medicine. His respect and appreciation for women and his desire for health interventions targeting this population group to be successful led him to conduct his MPH research project titled "Perceptions of Miskito Women on their Sexual and Reproductive Health and the Implications for Medical Care," which served as the basis for a book with the same title.

Gerardo has held various positions within the structure of AMC. When he concluded his social service in Tasba Pri, he became project manager of AMC's RAAN projects for the next fifteen years, and in 2006 he was named director of the Health and Community Development Program, the principal avenue by which AMC implements health strategies on the Caribbean Coast and in other departments of Nicaragua. He is also a member of the five-member directors' council of AMC, a leadership group within which the most important decisions of this organization are shared: strategic plans; general evaluations; review of mission, vision, and policies; and negotiation with key national and international agencies and authorities. He recently served on the commission responsible for selecting AMC's new executive director.

In 1996 Gerardo married Dr. Belinda Forbes, dentist and missionary of the United Methodist Church, with whom he is raising two daughters. Belinda and Gerardo work as a team at AMC to host visiting health volunteers and build partnerships between the organization and its numerous partner agencies in North America and Europe. Gerardo's career in global health is led by a desire to continue training in social and anthropological health, and to advance the knowledge of popular, indigenous, and *campesino* cultures, contributing to the improvement of their conditions and quality of life.

Benjamin Jastrzembski is a student at Harvard Medical School and from Hanover, New Hampshire. He first visited Nicaragua in 2005 as a college sophomore through Dartmouth's CCESP program. Visiting Nicaragua sparked his interest in medicine and in Latin America. As an undergraduate, he majored in Latin American and Caribbean studies, writing a thesis about undocumented Mexicans working on Vermont dairy farms. He also continued his involvement with Dartmouth's Nicaragua program, leading an exchange that brought a group of Nicaraguan university students to Dartmouth in July 2007. After graduating from Dartmouth in 2008, Benjamin spent a year in Nicaragua on a Fulbright scholarship, studying the history of the gold-mining town of Siuna. He also has collaborated with Dr. James Saunders and a team at Dartmouth on research investigating the potential health effects of heavy metal exposure in Nicaraguan mining communities.

Jennifer Kasper, MD, MPH, was born in a small town in Indiana. She received a combined BA/MD with honors from Boston University and Boston University School of Medicine and an MPH from Boston University School of Public Health. She completed her pediatric residency at Boston City Hospital, where she was taught that everyone has a right to timely, high-quality healthcare regardless of his or her ability to pay. During her training, She had numerous mentors who practiced the Mother Jones saying, "Pray for the dead and fight like hell for the living."

Jen became interested in global health after completing her chief residency in pediatrics at Boston City Hospital in 1996. She planned on being a volunteer in a Spanish-speaking country for two months and then returning to the United States to work as a bilingual primary care pediatrician. Her two months turned into two years, as she volunteered with Doctors for Global Health and worked alongside *campesinos* in rural El Salvador. There, she learned about the US government's role in the Salvadoran civil conflict. She gained firsthand knowledge about the social determinants of health and how they impacted the well-being of impoverished, underserved Salvadorans. She also witnessed the creativity and commitment of the *campesinos* as they strove for equity, optimal health, and human rights. It was a transformative experience. Ever since then, Jennifer has had one foot in the United States and one foot overseas, working for equity, health, and human rights for marginalized populations, for those who have been silenced.

Jen is currently in the Division of Global Health in the Department of Pediatrics at Massachusetts General Hospital. She is also instructor at Harvard Medical School, and pediatrician at Chelsea HealthCare Center. For the past fifteen years, she has been a board member of DGH, serving as chair, vice president, and president. She is currently chair of DGH's International Volunteer Committee. Her academic pursuits include the use of innovative technologies to address educational needs of healthcare providers overseas; the role of academic institutions in addressing human resource constraints in resource-limited settings; rural community development; and training healthcare providers in pediatric HIV/AIDS. She has worked in El Salvador, Nicaragua, Honduras, Mexico, Haiti, India, Mozambique, and Uganda. She has published works on the human rights of children; immigrants and hunger; child labor; orphans and vulnerable children in the context of HIV; Doctors for Global Health; and human resource constraints in resource-limited settings. In her daily domestic and international health work, she strives to practice the following quotation from Lao Tse (700 BC): "Go with the people. Live with them. Learn from them. Love them. Start with what they know. Build with what they have. But of the best leaders, when the job is done, the task accomplished, the people will all say, we have done this ourselves."

Margo J. Krasnoff, MD, was born in New Jersey and graduated from Dartmouth College in Hanover, New Hampshire, with an AB in biology. In 1982 she received her medical degree from the Geisel School of Medicine at Dartmouth on a full scholarship through the National Health Service Corps. She completed a residency in internal medicine at Dartmouth-Hitchcock Medical Center in Lebanon, New Hampshire, and to fulfill her scholarship, she worked for three years as a solo primary care physician in a medically underserved rural community in Vermont. She subsequently specialized in geriatrics and in hospice and palliative care. Margo was on the faculty of the State University of New York at Buffalo for six years, where she took care of an inner-city population with many Latina patients. She is currently associate professor of medicine at Geisel School of Medicine at Dartmouth, where she has maintained a longitudinal primary care practice for twenty years, taking care of adults as well as teaching medical students and residents. Her practice includes making house calls to homebound seniors, and she is involved in initiatives to reduce falls and to improve end-of-life care.

The dream to "someday" become involved with global health became a reality in 2004 when Margo read a newspaper article about a locally based NGO that had a long-standing alliance with the village of El Rosario in Honduras. She was attracted by the mission, which was to promote sustainable programs for health, education, and development in collaboration with the host community, and to foster cross-cultural understanding. On her first morning in Honduras, the trip leader, a distinguished physician with years of international health experience, gave Margo a list of frail seniors that he wanted seen in their homes. These encounters were transformative. In addition to seeing patients in clinic, Margo learned a great deal from her mentor, the other team members, and especially the Hondurans. The benefits of the sustainable development approach over time (economic, water, sanitation, education, and health) were even more obvious when the team traveled to treat an indigenous community located just a short distance away yet suffering from extreme deprivation.

Although Margo had learned Spanish at a local community college, her stay in Honduras inspired her to improve her language skills. The following year she spent two weeks in Quetzaltenango, Guatemala, at a medical Spanish program where she was able to combine intensive language classes with clinical care and a homestay. She then volunteered in Belize educating healthcare workers, in Mexico, and in Nepal. Her appreciation for Latin America continued to grow.

In 2007, Margo was invited to help lead a group of Dartmouth College undergraduate and medical students on a two-week service trip to Nicaragua. She has done this three times, in different villages near Siuna, located in the RAAN region. Her roles included helping to prepare the students to understand the socioeconomic and political context; supervising patient care; working with Nicaraguan physicians, nurses, and community health workers; and fostering critical self-reflection by the team. As a result of her experiences at home and abroad, Margo is committed to working collaboratively and respectfully with each patient she encounters.

Phuoc Le, MD, MPH, was born in rural central Vietnam in 1976, shortly after the end of the American War. When he was four, Phuoc's mother and older sister fled Vietnam as part of the refugee movement known as the Boat People. They eventually ended up in a refugee camp in Hong Kong, where they lived for a year before being accepted by the United States. Phuoc's family was placed in Wichita, Kansas, but subsequently found extended family in Sacramento, California, where he spent most of his childhood. He went on to Dartmouth College, where he majored in Chinese and biochemistry. During college, Phuoc took an additional year to study acupuncture in Beijing, China, and spent several months as a health volunteer in an indigenous area of rural Costa Rica. These experiences solidified his desire to practice medicine and public health.

Phuoc went on to complete his MD at Stanford University and his MPH at the University of California–Berkeley, focusing on global health. His master's project took him to Lhasa, Tibet, where he conducted research on traditional Tibetan medicine, and on health communication among rural Tibetan women. These experiences confirmed his commitment to serve in resource-poor settings, and to think broadly about the upstream determinants of health. After graduating from Stanford, Phuoc entered a combined residency in internal medicine, pediatrics, and global health equity at Harvard University.

For the next five years, Phuoc had the opportunity to spend three or four months a year working with Partners in Health, in their rural clinical sites in sub-Saharan Africa. In addition to caring for hospitalized patients and making home visits, Phuoc spent several months in Malawi working with local colleagues to tackle noncommunicable diseases such as diabetes and epilepsy. He helped to develop a chronic care clinic model in which mid-level providers used detailed protocols to provide longitudinal care for the most common NCDs.

After the Haiti earthquake of January 2010, Phuoc was sent by PIH to the General Hospital in Port-au-Prince to coordinate the transfer of critically ill earthquake victims and to oversee teams of expatriate medical volunteers. He also was an early responder to help with the cholera response at the PIH hospitals in St. Marc and Hinche, Haiti.

After completing his residency in 2011, Phuoc joined the faculty at the University of California–San Francisco (UCSF) as assistant professor. Clinically, he practices as a hospitalist on the teaching services in internal medicine and pediatrics. He recently has become a founding director of the Global Health Hospital Medicine Fellowship in the Division of Hospital Medicine at UCSF. He continues to volunteer in Haiti for PIH, based in St. Marc, for about three months a year. His work focuses on capacity building by training Haitian medical students and residents.

Daniel Palazuelos, MD, MPH, is a physician at Brigham and Women's Hospital, an instructor in medicine at Harvard Medical School, and clinical director for the Partners in Health projects in Mesoamerica. PIH is a Boston-based NGO working in some of the poorest places on the planet to provide high-quality healthcare in solidarity with those who need it the most. In Mexico, Dan works with the Mexican branch of PIH, Compañeros en Salud, in the Mexican state of Chiapas. In Guatemala, he works with EYESC (Technical Team for Education and Community Health), the Guatemalan NGO supported by PIH. When in Latin America, he lives in isolated communities in the Sierra Madre Mountains, training local community health workers and young doctors, providing medical care, conducting research, hosting medical student projects, and creating original curricula. A graduate of the Program in Liberal Medical Education at Brown University, where he majored in English and American literature and studied poetry at Oxford University, he later graduated from Brown University Alpert Medical School, completed a residency in global health equity and internal medicine at Brigham and Women's Hospital, and completed an MPH at Harvard School of Public Health.

Reflecting on his career path, Dan writes:

I never planned to work in global health, but yet so much of what I did beforehand actually led me to it. As a child, I was attracted to the idea of being a doctor because it seemed like an engaging and challenging job where you can use concrete skills to directly help people every day. On the other hand, I was also interested in the arts because I experienced early on that the creative moment makes me feel renewed; to be involved in some creative process helps me engage with and make meaning of my surroundings. This led me to perform improv comedy in high school, write poetry in college, and spend more time on photography than was good for my sleep schedule in medical school. By the time I entered my internal medicine residency at the Brigham and Women's Hospital, I was not entirely sure how I was going to make all these seemingly disparate interests fit together. Global health became that solution.

Born in Mexico, but raised in New York, I spent a year in Mexico during medical school doing independent social sciences research. This was before global health as a field had been branded, so any work outside of the traditional medical system was called "international medicine." Since I already knew Mexico so well, it didn't really feel international per se. When I was later accepted into a global health equity residency that allowed me to spend even more time in Mexico, it seemed like just another way of returning home. Once I got on-site, however, I understood that I had come home in more ways than one: in the mountains of Chiapas, there are problems that ache for justice, questions that necessitate innovative solutions, challenges that demand consistent dedication, and colleagues who inspire me because we know that good work will always be our greatest compensation. The sensation of being at home comes from being comfortable in your own skin; this is why I became a doctor instead of what is traditionally considered an "artist," and why I do global health and not international medicine—to help be a part of the change I'd like to see in the world.

Now, a few years out of residency, I split my time between work as a physician in Boston and work as an *acompañante* (someone who accompanies a process) for the PIH-supported projects in Mesoamerica. The two worlds I live in fortify each other: from the brilliant fluorescent halls of a hospital in Boston to the endless green mountains of Chiapas, I learn lessons in both places and try to apply them wherever I go. Above all else, I've learned that even though the world is in a precarious situation, whole teams of people want to help improve it.

Students often ask me how to forge a career in global health. I respond that this is a hard question to answer because global health is still a young field that needs time to be defined; it's really only a collection of problems slowly being addressed by a nascent, yet growing, delivery science. In the meantime I tell my students, "Don't look for a project you can help; rather, look for partners with whom you can work to tackle the issues you care about." If the problems we face are approached with creativity, mindfulness, dedication, patience, and a yearning for justice, I believe we can all make a difference. Making that change, however, is a process of creatively finding solutions to unsolved questions. It never ends, the work renews me every day, and I can't imagine ever stopping.

Peter Rohloff, MD, PhD, began his path to working in Guatemala accidentally. When he went to Guatemala for the first time, he was just finishing his PhD work at the University of Illinois at Urbana-Champaign, where had been working in a laboratory whose goal was to research orphan diseases such as malaria, trypanosomiasis, and leishmaniasis. As he prepared to begin his medical studies, he was looking for an opportunity to improve his Spanish and also to gain some volunteer medical experience in a developing country.

Over several years, Peter returned each year to Guatemala for extended stays, working as a volunteer with several medical organizations and learning about the health-care system in Guatemala. One of the most important elements of discovery for him was learning about the Mayan culture and Mayan languages. He began to realize how closely Maya ethnicity was tied to healthcare disparity, and how few organizations, governmental or nongovernmental, were taking this reality seriously.

Consequently, he returned to Guatemala in 2005, where he spent a year conducting research with Kaqchikel-speaking midwives and learning Kaqchikel Maya. In this setting, he began working with community leaders to address some simple community problems, principally the lack of access of elderly Maya to healthcare for chronic disease. At the same time, he had the good fortune of meeting other like-minded anthropologists, linguists, and medical researchers, including Anne Kraemer Díaz.

Throughout 2006, Peter, Anne, and others worked hard to lay the foundations for what would become a new medical nonprofit, Wuqu' Kawoq, which was incorporated in 2007. Peter served as executive director of Wuqu' Kawoq from 2007 to 2009, when he became the medical director. He continues to work actively in Guatemala, spending about half of his time there. Currently, he manages Wuqu' Kawoq's medical programs and oversees in-country staff, while also coordinating Wuqu' Kawoq's medical and linguistic research efforts and technology innovations.

Karen Sadler, MD, finished her residency in the early 1990s and began a career combining academic medicine and primary care in an affluent Boston suburb. Three years later, she left the 'burbs for a job at one of Boston's neighborhood health centers, serving an inner-city, largely immigrant, and underserved population. During her eight years there, she helped found and run their first teen clinic, which still flourishes.

Karen's interest in immigrant populations and multicultural issues grew, and she jumped at the chance to join her friend, Kim Wilson, on her trips to the Dominican Republic as Kim worked through the nonprofit she had started to reduce disparities of healthcare for transnational Dominican children. Initial efforts were toward educational events for local Dominican healthcare staff, then extended to outreach efforts as a course was developed to train community outreach workers. Karen remains active in the DR today through a microbusiness project begun in 2008 with poor women in the area around Baní.

Reflecting on her work in the DR, Karen writes:

In 2008, while working with Infante Sano as a volunteer in community outreach efforts and specifically with the clinic at the Elizabeth Seton Nutrition Center, I decided to leave my medical skill set (and comfort zone). I saw a group of mothers and grandmothers eager to improve their lives and the lives of their families. Many families in La Saona are headed by single women: the fathers either are not involved, or are off in New York or Boston. Drugs from South America sweep through this southern Dominican city on their way to North America or Europe, devastating families and increasing crime in their wake.

I wondered whether there could be another way to help these women in addition to enhancing healthcare, and I posed a question to a group of them: would they be interested in creating locally inspired crafts, if I was willing to bring them back to America to sell? We agreed that I would sell the crafts wherever and for whatever I could, and bring 100 percent of the profits back to the women. Oh, were they excited! Sixteen of them sat down and decided that the first task was to find a name. They chose the Artisans of La Saona, or Las Artisanas de La Saona.

Then came the hard and interesting part: How would they organize? Who would be the leader? How would they police themselves (the first shipment of white t-shirts I sent was stolen in an "inside job")? Who could read and write? Who knew how to sew? How would they catalog what they made? And what, exactly, could they make? The last question proved the hardest to answer. What was truly Dominican in a country more eager in the past few decades to imitate the culture of the United States than to develop its own?

Since 2008, after *much* trial and error, the group has solidified. The women have chosen a butterfly theme (which is, for various reasons, Dominican). They sew, bead, and crochet. They recycle plastic bags and create beautiful clutches from them. In addition, they have been required to donate 10 percent of their profits to the Elizabeth Seton Nutrition Center, which provides a safe place for them to meet, and they are proud of the new plastic chairs their donations have purchased. The women have made a few thousand dollars as of this writing. They have paid for school uniforms and run down debt, and one woman, Carmen, was even able to save the $30 US it takes to open a bank account in the DR. The group is working on creating local sales opportunities. In a word, this messy, often frustrating long-distance project has brought a small amount of empowerment to a group of women willing to work for it. It has been a good lesson for both them and me.

James E. Saunders, MD, is associate professor of otology/neurotology at Dartmouth-Hitchcock Medical Center. He completed his MD at the University of Oklahoma and his residency and a research fellowship in otolaryngology–head and neck surgery at Duke University Medical Center. He then went on to a research and clinical fellowship at the House Ear Institute in Los Angeles, California, before returning to serve on the faculty of the University of Oklahoma Health Sciences Center for thirteen years. Jim obtained his board certification in neurotology in 2005. He has been involved in many projects in international medicine related to hearing loss. In 1998, he co-founded Mayflower Medical Outreach, a nonprofit organization that has been working to improve healthcare for hearing loss and ear disease in Nicaragua. MMO has led multiple teaching and surgical teams to Nicaragua, and has established a full-time otolaryngology and audiology clinic, as well as a residential home and educational center for children with hearing loss in Jinotega, Nicaragua.

Jim is currently coordinating a collaborative program with WHO and two other NGOs to develop a national program for hearing loss in Nicaragua. He has also been involved in multiple research projects to assess the root causes of hearing loss in Nicaragua and the developing world. Jim has served on several international expert advisory panels for hearing loss. He is the past chairman of the Humanitarian Efforts Committee of the American Academy of Otolaryngology–Head and Neck Surgery Foundation, is currently regional director for Africa, and has been selected to serve as the international coordinator for that organization.

Clyde Lanford Smith, MD, MPH, (Lanny) is a writer and a physician trained in primary care internal medicine and preventive medicine with an MPH from Harvard School of Public Health and a Diploma in Tropical Medicine and Hygiene from the London School of Hygiene and Tropical Medicine. From 1992 to 1998, he lived in El Salvador as country director of Médecins du Monde (Physicians of the World) France. Lanny is a fellow of the American College of Physicians and a member of the Alpha Omega Alpha Medical Honor Society. He has been the recipient of Davidson College's John Kuykendall Award for Community Service for "leadership in service to humankind" and of the Mid-Career Award in International Health of the American Public Health Association. He serves on the global steering committee of the People's Health Movement. Founder of Doctors for Global Health, he serves on its board as liberation medicine counsel. He is co-founder of the open-access online *Journal of Social Medicine* (www .socialmedicine.info) and serves on its editorial board. He is co-editor of the book *Women's Global Health and Human Rights*.

Lanny is associate professor of clinical medicine and clinical family and social medicine in the Residency Program in Primary Care and Social Internal Medicine, Montefiore Medical Center, Albert Einstein College of Medicine, and he serves as global health advisor at Einstein. He works in the Bronx Human Rights Clinic for Survivors of Torture, and cares for patients regularly as a primary care physician in the South Bronx Comprehensive Health Care Center. His research interests include social medicine, community-oriented primary care, art and health, tropical medicine, and health education. Lanny has lived in the Bronx since 2000 and works locally and globally to promote liberation medicine, "the conscious, conscientious use of health to promote social justice and human dignity." His book *Una Sola Vida: Lecciones hasta la Salud y la Justicia Social* (One life only: Lessons toward health and social justice) is available from Ediciones Corpus Libro, Rosario, Argentina.

Kim Wilson, MD, MPH, is assistant professor at Harvard Medical School and associate director for the Global Pediatric Program in the Department of Medicine at Boston

Children's Hospital. Her work has focused on improving healthcare for underserved populations domestically and internationally. In Boston, she has combined clinical care to underserved families with implementation of programs to improve health for children with chronic illness.

Kim's international work grew from her clinical pediatric practice in Boston working with transnational families from the Dominican Republic. Internationally, she leads a maternal and neonatal training and quality improvement program at hospital facilities in the DR. Her current research applies the technology of health to quality improvement, using cell-phone-based protocols as decision aids to improve newborn healthcare in Tanzania. Kim teaches at Harvard Medical School and Harvard School of Public Health, with a focus on global maternal child health and social determinants of disease. In addition, she developed and directs the Global Pediatric Fellows Program at Boston Children's Hospital, with pediatric fellows working in Haiti and Rwanda.

Index

Page numbers for tables and figures are italicized

207, 208–9, 210, 212; environmental issues, 189; geography, 206; global health work in, 225; and Haiti/Haitian immigrants, 188, 189, 207, 209, 211–14; healthcare system, 211–12, 214–20, 224; health inequities, 212–13, 216, 219–20; historical sketch, 206–8; identity as Hispanic, xvii; international aid collaborations, 214, 220–24; people, 206–7, 208–9, 213; politics, 207–8; US relationship with, 207–8, 209–10; violence in, xx, 208

Dominican Republic–Central America–United States Free Trade Agreement (CAFTA-DR), xxiii–xxiv, 48, 78

DOTS (directly observed therapy, short-course) protocol, 17, 35

downstream factors in socioeconomic inequality, 13

drug trafficking, xix–xx, 10, 33–34, 49, 158

Duvalier, François "Papa Doc," 187

Duvalier, Jean-Claude "Baby Doc," 187

earthquakes, xxii, 49, 76, 120, 191, 194–95, 197–99

Economic and Social Council, 77

economy: context for healthcare, xxii–xxiv; Dominican Republic, 207, 208–9, 210, 212; El Salvador, 77–79; free trade agreements, xix, xxiii–xxiv, 7, 11, 29–31, 48, 78; globalization's effect on health, xxv–xxvi; Guatemala, 42–43, 46, 48; Haiti, 189; Honduras, 100–101; Mexico, 4–5, 6–7, 11, 12, 28; Nicaragua, 118, 120, 122, 123, 124, 125–26, 128, 153. *See also* neoliberalism

education: El Salvador, 86, 88–91; Guatemala, 60, 63; Honduras, 99, 106–9, 110; Mexico, 9, 21; Nicaragua, 121, 124, 128–29, 139–40, 179

Ejército Zapatista de Liberación Nacional (EZLN), xix, 8, 31

Ejido system, Mexico, 6, 36

Elizabeth Seton Nutrition Center, 222–23

El Mozote massacre, 75

El Salvador: armed civil conflict, xix, 75–76, 78, 81, 83; economy, 77–79; environmental issues, 79, 86–88; healthcare system, 77, 80; health inequities, 74–75, 79–80; health outcomes, 79; historical sketch, 75–76; natural disasters, 76; NGOs in, 76, 81–88; politics, 76–77, 86; violence level in, xx, 75–76, 87

encomienda system, 45–46

environmental issues: Chiapas, Mexico, 11; El Salvador, 79, 86–88; Haiti, 189, 213; Nicaragua, 132–34, 153, 174, 175

epidemologic transition, 29, 80, 216

EZLN (Ejército Zapatista de Liberación Nacional), xix, 8, 31

faith-based organizations (FBOs): AMC, *xxix*, 152, 162, 165, 166–74, 175–76, 179–80; Catholic Action, 49; Catholic Church's social justice missions, 87; Daughters of Charity of St. Vincent de Paul, 32; Elizabeth Seton Nutrition Center, 222–23; HFSC, *xxix*, 106, 109–10

Farabundo Martí National Liberation Front (FMLN), 77

Farmer, Paul, xxviii–xxix, 35, 142, 192, 201

Flores Navarro, Hugo Ernesto, 18–22

folk medicine, 14, 24–26, 158–64, 168–69, 183n17, 188

food insecurity, xxii, 48, 59, 78, 169–70, 189, 192

Fox, Vicente, 9–10, 31

free trade agreements, xix, xxiii–xxiv, 7, 11, 29–31, 48, 78

Freire, Paolo, 89

French intervention in Mexico, 4–5

Frenk, Julio, 13

Frente Sandinista de Liberación Nacional (FSLN), 120

Funes, Mauricio, 77

The Fútbol Project, 109–10

HIV/AIDS: Dominican Republic, 194, 212, 213, 216; El Salvador, 84–86; Guatemala, 60; Haiti, 187, 192, 193–94, 196–97, 213; Honduras, 105; Nicaragua, 133, 166, 170, 172–73

Holy Family Surgery Center (HFSC), *xxix*, 106, 109–10

Honduras: coup by military, xxiv, 77, 101; culture, 103–4; economy, 100–101; geography, 96, 98; global health work in, 110–11; healthcare system, 101–3; health inequities, 102–3; historical sketch, 97–98; indigenous populations, 97; introduction, 96; natural disasters, 98, 99–100, 112; NGOs in, 100, 103, 104–10; people, 98–99, 114n8; politics, 77, 97–98, 100–101, 102; Río Lempa massacre, 76; violence level in, xx, 101; volunteer experience and impact, 96, 104–5, 110–13

horizontal public health program type, xxix

hot-cold dichotomy in traditional health beliefs, 24–26, 160

HSN (l'Hôpital de Saint Nicolas), 200

Hubbard, Brenda, 82

HUEH (l'Hôpital Université d'Etat d'Haïti), 191, 194, 198, 199

humanitarian medicine, potential pitfalls in, 143–45. *See also* global health work

human rights, xv, 74, 120

Hurricane Felix, 170

Hurricane Mitch, xxii, 76, 99–100, 112, 124, 170

Hurricane Stan, 35–36

ILEA (International Law Enforcement Academy), 77

illegal immigrants to US, 30

IMC (International Medical Corps), 199

immunization rates, 16, 79, 121, 133

import-substitution industrialization, 6–7

INCAP (Institute of Nutrition of Central America and Panama), 55–56

Incaparina, 56, 58

independence movements, xvii, 3, 46–47, 97, 117, 186, 207

indigenous populations: Dominican Republic, 206–7; El Salvador, 75; Guatemala, 42, 43, 49–50, *51*, 52–53, 64–65, 69n59; Haiti, 186; Honduras, 97; impact of European invasion on, xvi–xvii; Mexico, 2, 7–9, 12–13, 16, 32, 36; Nicaragua, 117, 122, 128, 152, 153–64, *154–55*, *157*, 168, 183n17; overview, xii, xviii

inequality, socioeconomic. *See* socioeconomic inequality

Infante Sano, 210, 220–22

infant mortality. *See* child mortality

infectious diseases: Dominican Republic, 194, 212, 213, 216; El Salvador, 80, 84–86; Guatemala, 60; Haiti, 187, 190, 192, 193–94, 196–97, 199–201, 213; Honduras, 102, 105; Mexico, 17–24, 35, 39n31; Nicaragua, 121, 132, 133, 134, 157, 166, 168, 170, 172–73

Institute of Nutrition of Central America and Panama (INCAP), 55–56

INTERFEROS, 100

international aid collaborations, xxvi–xxviii. *See also* NGOs (nongovernmental organizations)

International Law Enforcement Academy (ILEA), 77

International Medical Corps (IMC), 199

Iran-Contra Affair, 122–23

Ivers, Louise, 201

Juárez, Benito, 4

Juntas de Buen Gobierno (JBG), 9, 33

Kids to Kids, 223–24

Kim, Jim, xxviii–xxix, 142

Koehler, Reinhart, 104

LAC (Latin America and the Caribbean), xi–xii

Ladinos, 43, 46, 47

La Matanza, 75

land redistribution, 6, 47
languages: Chiapas, Mexico, 12, 32; Guatemala, 43, 49–50, 51, 52–53, 64–65, 69n59; Haiti, 188; importance of local knowledge, xiii–xvi, xv; Nicaragua, 128, 157–58, 159, 180
Latin America and the Caribbean (LAC), xi–xii
Leandre, Fernet, 201
Levitt, Peggy, 210
l'Hôpital de Saint Nicolas (HSN), 200
l'Hôpital Université d'Etat d'Haïti (HUEH), 191, 194, 198, 199
liberation medicine, 32–35, 81, 90
linguistic competency, xiii–xvi. *See also* languages
Lobo Sosa, Porfirio, 101

machismo (cult of virility), 114n5
Madero, Francisco, 5
malaria, 60, 121, 133, 157, 190
malnutrition: Dominican Republic, 212, 216, 222; El Salvador, 79; Guatemala, 55–60, 61; Haiti, 192; Mexico, 16, 29; Nicaragua, 133, 169–70; stunting, xxi–xxii, 16, 55, 59, 79, 212; wasting, xxi, 56
Managua, Nicaragua, 125–26
Managua earthquake, xxii, 120
maquilas, 78, 124
marginalization, 12–13, 211–13. *See also* indigenous populations; mestizo populations
Martelly, Michel, 187
Martín-Baró, Ignacio, 81
maternal health: Dominican Republic, 212, 217–22; El Salvador, 79, 82–83; Guatemala, 52, 59–60; Haiti, 192; Mexico, 16, 27, 28; Nicaragua, 127, 140, 157
Maxin, Guerre, 202
Maya calendar, 44, 66n16
Mayan language and indigenous people, xviii, 42, 45–46, 49–50, 51, 52–53, 64–65, 69n59

Maya religion, 43
Mayflower Medical outreach (MMO), *xxix,* 138–43
McGowan, Sister Catherine, 222–23
MDGs (Millennium Development Goals), xxiv–xxv, xxviii, xxix, 26, 80, 134, 224
Médecins Sans Frontières (MSF), 103, 200
medications, 15, 62, 63, 173, 196, 199
mental health services, 83–84, 157, 198
Mesoamerica, pre-Columbian, 44–45
mestizo populations, 3, 43, 46, 47, 98, 153, 209
Mexico: child health, 16, 23, 26–29; drug trafficking, xix, xx, 10; economy, 4–5, 6–7, 11, 12, 28, 29–31; fecundity, politics of, 16–17; healthcare system, 9, 13–15, 19–23, 27; health inequities, 15–16, 28; historical sketch, 1–10; inclusion in Latin America, xii; natural disasters, xxii, 4, 35–36; NGOs in, 19, 31–37; people, 2–3, 4–5, 11–12; politics, 5–6, 9–10; poverty and health status, 12–13, 15–24; traditional medicine, 24–26; violence level in, xix, xx, 10; Zapatista uprising, xix, 7–9. *See also* Chiapas, Mexico
middle class, growth of, 11, 46
Millennium Development Goals (MDGs), xxiv–xxv, xxviii, xxix, 26, 80, 134, 224
Ministry of Health (MINSA), 121, 129–32, 134, 138, 145, 156–57, 165–66, 177–78, 179
Mirabal sisters, 208
Miskito people, 122, 153, 157, 157–58, 159–64, 168, 183n17
Mojica Alvarez, Karen, 140–41
MSF (Médecins Sans Frontières), 103, 200
multidrug-resistant tuberculosis (MDR-TB), 17

NAFTA (North American Free Trade Agreement), xix, xxiii, 7, 11, 29–31

Nationalist Republican Alliance (ARENA), 76, 78

natural disasters: El Salvador, 76; Guatemala, xxii, 49; Haiti, xxii, 189, 191, 194–95, 197–99; Honduras, 98, 99–100, 112; impact on health, xxii; Mexico, xxii, 4, 35–36; Nicaragua, xxii, 120, 124, 157, 170, 174–76

NCDs. *See* noncommunicable diseases (NCDs)

neoliberalism, xxiii, 7, 29–31, 48, 76, 78, 88–90, 123

NGOs (nongovernmental organizations): Dominican Republic, 214, 220–24; El Salvador, 76, 81–88; Guatemala, 49, 54, 57, 58–59, 62–63, 64; Haiti, xxviii, 191, 192–93, 195–99; Honduras, 100, 103, 104–10; Mexico, 19, 31–37; Nicaragua, 131–32, 134–45, 164–74; overview, xxviii. *See also* global health work

Nicaragua: civil war, xviii, 118–21; dental health, 176–81; economy, 118, 120, 122, 123, 124, 125–26, 128; environmental issues, 132–34, 153, 174, 175; geography, 124–27, 152, 153, 155; global health work in, 116, 134–43, 145–46, 174; healthcare system, 127–28, 129–32, 155–57, 156–57, 177–78; health inequities, 157, 157–58; historical sketch, 116–24, 153; indigenous populations, 117, 122, 128, 152, 153–64, 154–55, 157; language and literacy, 128; natural disasters, xxii, 120, 124, 157, 170, 174–76; NGOs in, 131–32, 134–45, 164–74; people, 152; politics, 117–24; violence level in, xx, 127, 158

Nicaraguan National Guard, 118–21

NicaSalud, 134

noncommunicable diseases (NCDs): Dominican Republic, 216; El Salvador, 80, 82–83; Guatemala, 58, 60–64; Mexico, 28, 29, 31; Nicaragua, 132

North American Free Trade Agreement (NAFTA), xix, xxiii, 7, 11, 29–31

Northern Autonomous Atlantic Region (RAAN), 133, 152

NPH (Nuestros Pequeños Hermanos™) International, *xxix*, 104–9, 111–12

Nuss, Emily and Sarah, 223–24

nutrition. *See* malnutrition

Oportunidades (Progresa), 28

oral disease, Nicaragua, 176–81

orphanage, Honduras, 104–10

Ortega, Daniel, 121, 122, 124

Pacific Rim Mining Corp., 86–88

Palazuelos, Daniel, xiv

Panama, 118

Pan-American Health Organization (PAHO), xxvii, 178

Participatory Action Research (PAR), 168

Partido Acción Nacional (PAN), 9–10

Partido de la Revolución Democrática (PRD), 7, 10

Partido Revolucionario Institucional (PRI), 6, 9

Partners in Health (PIH), xiv, *xxix*, 19, 35–37, 192, 196–203

Pastora, Edén, 120

Paz, Octavio, 3

Peace Corps, xx, 103, 214, 224

Peña Nieto, Enrique, 10

Pérez Molina, Otto, 49, 57

pharmaceutical industry, 15, 173. *See also* medications

PIH (Partners in Health), xiv, *xxix*, 19, 35–37, 192, 196–203

point-of-care, 14, 201

politics: Dominican Republic, 207–8; El Salvador, 76–77, 86; Guatemala, 46–49; Haiti, 186, 187; history of dictatorship in LAC, xvii; Honduras, 77, 97–98, 100–101, 102; Mexico, 5–6, 9–10; Nicaraguan, 117–24

poverty and health: Dominican Republic, 212, 215; El Salvador, 78, 79; Guatemalan, 43, 52, 55, 59; Haiti, 191, 192–93, 212–13; Honduras, 97–98;